DEMENTIA CARE

Dementia Care

Patient, Family, and Community

edited by Nancy L. Mace

THE JOHNS HOPKINS UNIVERSITY PRESS
BALTIMORE AND LONDON

The Johns Hopkins University Press,
701 West 40th Street, Baltimore, Maryland 21211
The Johns Hopkins Press Ltd., London

The paper used in this publication meets the minimum
requirements of American National Standard for Information
Sciences—Permanence of Paper for Printed Library Materials,
ANSI Z39.48-1984.

LIBRARY OF CONGRESS CATALOGING-IN-PUBLICATION DATA

Dementia care: patient, family, and community / edited by Nancy L. Mace
    p. cm.—(The Johns Hopkins series in contemporary medicine and public
health)
Includes bibliographies and index.
ISBN 0-8018-3859-2 (alk. paper)
1. Dementia.   I. Mace, Nancy L.   II. Series.
[DNLM: 1. Community Health Services. 2. Dementia—therapy. 3. Family.
   WM 220 D37635]
RC521.D454 1990
362.1'968983—dc20
DNLM/DLC
for Library of Congress
                                         89-8106
                                           CIP

Note to the Reader: The science of medicine is constantly changing. Research and clinical experience keep broadening our knowledge, particularly regarding treatment. Where this book mentions dosages or specific applications, the authors, editors, and publishers strived to ensure that the information accurately reflects current knowledge. However, the reader is cautioned to examine all information accompanying the various drugs mentioned and to ascertain whether currently recommended dosages or considerations regarding contraindications agree or disagree with those presented in this book. This is especially important when rarely used or recently introduced drugs are involved or in the case of restricted-use drugs.

Contents

Foreword

In 1980 Ebbinghaus said of psychology that it had
a long past but a short history. This remark is even more apt as a
description of the systematic study of the dementias, for when Ebbinghaus spoke the history of that work was exactly one year old. We
mark the beginning of the systematic and scientific study of the dementias with the publication of Alzheimer's paper in 1907. There, for
the first time, a clear differentiation of dementia from the general
infirmities of aging was connected to a specific neuropathological
condition identifiable by both gross and microscopic changes in the
brain. We are a little more than eighty years into the history of this
subject and can reflect on that history to advantage.

It has not been a history of steady progress since Alzheimer. I
suppose no emerging discipline demonstrates a stability of direction
and purpose in its infancy. Rather, as here, we find the hesitation and
contradictions of individuals working somewhat at cross purposes
and vacillating in their vision. Within general medicine and even
among some neurologists, the specificities identified by Alzheimer
were submerged within the concepts of some natural process of aging
such as "hardening of the arteries." Psychiatrists, on the other hand,
blurred all distinctions between dementia and other brain-based disorders by lumping them under the ugly rubric of "organicity." Much
of the first sixty years or so of the history of this subject was a prolonged period of stumbling around in the dark with an occasional
happy reemphasis of Alzheimer's achievements. This was the result
of the different roles assumed by neurologists and psychiatrists in the
management of dementia during this time: neurologists diagnosing
the conditions and psychiatrists caring for the patient with little or

no cross-referencing or mutual interest in each other's experiences. As a result, a treasure trove of information and a set of opportunities for comprehending important distinctions in prognosis and treatment were deferred. Doctors and patients alike remained bewildered.

From out of this period of vacillation and cross purposes, however, there has emerged in the last twenty years a stability of direction that marks the maturation of this discipline. The linkages that brought this about are not difficult to identify but are hard to date. They are, however, all recent. There was the emergence in neurology, for example, of the interest in neuropsychology that began with a particular interest in the specific conditions of amnesia and aphasia. Raymond Adams and Maurice Victor beginning in the 1950s and Norman Geschwind in the 1960s were the charismatic leaders of this research at its start. On the other hand, the acceptance by psychiatrists of the crucial importance of diagnostic criteria and as well the concept that we should separate the psychological symptoms from their pathological underpinnings as did Alzheimer were other important themes that became general in the early 1980s. These were crucial because they permitted psychiatrists to see that the diagnosis of dementia should not be identified by aspects of prognosis and treatment such as "relentlessly progressive" or "incurable." They came to know what neuropathologists had long known, that these aspects of a dementia syndrome depended upon the particular pathological mechanism at work in the patient and not upon the clinical appearance alone.

This book is a contemporary culmination of that convergence of interest and understanding between neurologists and psychiatrists. It displays the confidence that comes from an understanding of basic principles and it lays out the intriguing new findings that can be turned to practical account for our study in the future. It is thus a vital interest to all.

But where is it leading? Clinically this book demonstrates that this systematic study of dementia is leading to a progressive sophistication and assessment of the various brain disorders that produce dementia and to a greater capacity to take reciprocating advantage of the advances of contemporary technology, particularly brain imaging, in their study. At the same time this book combines solid clinical descriptions of mental disorders with up-to-date descriptions of the neural systems under pathological attack, and thus it opens up our comprehension of the basis of human cognitive capacity. Disease as the experiment of nature has its most obvious psychological example here in the neuropsychiatric domain.

What we have before us is the edited and compiled foundations for the future of this clinical discipline that began in 1907. None of us can speak for others in our enthusiasm for this work but I am sure that every reader can see within the details of these chapters and their careful empirical studies issues crucial to the comprehension and care of patients with dementia. We can note as well, the elements that are here subject to disorder and that in health are coordinated into human cognitive skill. The emergent properties of human mental capacities that physicians are committed to preserve and that disease attacks represent the central drama of this text and the source of its greatest excitement. If Alzheimer was the beginning paragraph in this history, here are the opening chapters in the volume of the future.

Paul R. McHugh, M.D.
Henry Phipps Professor of Psychiatry
The Johns Hopkins University School of Medicine

Preface and Acknowledgments

Alzheimer's disease and the other currently irreversible dementing illnesses have an impact that extends far beyond the individual victim. They place heavy burdens on families and on the community. They threaten to overwhelm the long-term care system. The family, aptly called the second victim, provides about 80 percent of all care. Yet the cost to the nation of institutional care alone is estimated in billions of dollars. Treatment means change not just in the person with the dementing illness but in the family and the greater community as well. It also means change in professional practice. Interdisciplinary care is necessary, and the patient's environment—the immediate physical environment and the psychosocial environment—should be used as a preferred treatment tool.

Treatment of the environment and the family often benefits the patient. For example, in the absence of a treatment for the person with dementia, many of our intervention efforts have focused on the family. Respite care and support groups were begun to relieve the caregiver; they are now observed to benefit the patient as well. There is reciprocal interaction among patient, family, and community; thus, this book addresses all three.

This book begins with the heart of the problem, the patient, and the second victim, the family. The degree to which the patient suffers and the amount of damage resulting from the family's burden are determined not only by clinical skills but also by knowledge of and ability to manipulate long-term care resources. Thus, this book must discuss not only clinical care, but also the environment, law, finance, and the reasons that resources are often fragmented, inappropriate, or nonexistent.

What treatment goals are possible? Dementia care has long been considered as palliative and *un*rewarding. There is nothing in the arsenal of medications or surgery that will halt or reverse the course of the most common dementing illnesses and, because they destroy the mind, their courses are especially horrible to watch. However, when I visited the Helping Hand Day Care Center in Lexington, Kentucky, I asked the volunteers why they worked in the program there. They replied, "Because it's so rewarding." The contributors to this volume and people around the world who work with people who have dementing illnesses are reporting exciting changes in their clients and rewards in their work. Has the tragedy of these diseases driven them to take refuge in fantasy? Repeated observation and research are confirming these positive observations. With good care, cognitive function is maximized. Evidence of fear, anxiety, hopelessness, and despair in these patients is reduced, and their problem behaviors (which in part reflect the ill person's anguish) are diminished. Some patients resume sleeping through the night, their wandering behavior and agitation decline, and they participate in personal care tasks. Even more impressive, some people begin to smile, to laugh, and sometimes to joke.

The two dementia units at Eastern State Hospital in Virginia accept residents who were unmanageable in nursing homes. At Eastern State, there have been reductions of many disturbed behaviors without an increase in the use of behavior-controlling drugs or restraints. Patients appear happier, calmer, and more relaxed than they had in their previous placements. Staff members told me—and a survey confirmed—that they like their jobs and find working with these people fulfilling.

There are no changes in symptoms such as the underlying aphasia, memory impairments, and apraxia, but the changes that are observed, in psychosocial function and behavior, indicate significant gains in the quality of life. As we have with other chronic illnesses, we are learning how to help people with dementia live more comfortably and fully with their disease. Better quality of life for the patient means a better quality of life for the family—and other caregivers. These are legitimate treatment goals in chronic illness.

Several years ago I asked a group of day care directors about their philosophies of dementia care. One wrote, "We love them and we try to understand them." This is where good dementia care began, but as we enter the last decade of this century we can go far beyond this affective approach. Although more clinical research is needed, we now have a coherent body of knowledge based on good clinical experience and research. We have the tools to provide treatment—not mere maintenance—even while we cannot arrest the chronic disease itself.

It is with great pleasure that I bring together in one volume the expertise of these clinicians and researchers. They are aware of the realities of dementia. They will not assert that care of people with dementia and their families is easy; it is not. They write soberly and practically, without hyperbole, but they also write, between the lines, of the benefits to be gained for people with dementia and for their families and of the professional rewards of the work.

A critical part of care is the recognition that each person with dementia is an individual who will need a unique plan of care. Dementia afflicts both men and women. Therefore we have chosen to use the singular pronouns "he, him" and "she, her" randomly through the text because we are writing about individuals of both sexes. We have avoided using *demented* as an adjective; the term refers to a condition, not to a person.

Many people have contributed to the development of this book: people with dementia, their families, and care providers have taught us much. Each of these chapters was read and critiqued by colleagues whose help and encouragement are gratefully acknowledged. I also appreciate the work of Wendy Harris, my editor; Linda Forlifer, copy editor; and others at the Johns Hopkins University Press.

Contributors

Virginia Bell, M.S.W., Family Counselor, Sanders Brown Center on Aging, University of Kentucky

David F. Chavkin, public interest lawyer specializing in health and disability issues, Silver Spring, MD

Robert Mullan Cook-Deegan, M.D., Acting Executive Director, Biomedical Ethical Advisory Committee, U.S. Congress, and Senior Research Fellow, Kennedy Institute of Ethics, Georgetown University

Dorothy H. Coons, Project Director, Alzheimer's Disease Projects on Environmental Intervention, Institute of Gerontology, University of Michigan

Lisa P. Gwyther, M.S.W., Director, Center for Aging Family Support Programs, and Assistant Professor, Department of Psychiatry, Duke University

Lorraine G. Hiatt, Ph.D., consultant in environmental psychology and aging

Nancy L. Mace, M.A., Consultant, Office of Technology Assessment, U.S. Congress and Alzheimer's Association; formerly Assistant in Psychiatry, Johns Hopkins University School of Medicine; Coordinator, Sir James McCuster Training Programme, Perth, Australia

Jane L. Marks, R.N., M.S., Coordinator, Continence Program, Beacham Ambulatory Care Center, Francis Scott Key Medical Center

Richard J. Martin, N.D., R.N., Advanced Clinical Nurse, Alzheimer Center, University Hospitals of Cleveland

Katie Maslow, M.S.W., Policy Analyst and Project Director, Office of Technology Assessment, U.S. Congress

Joseph G. Ouslander, M.D., Medical Director, Jewish Homes for the Aging of Greater Los Angeles

Marian B. Patterson, Ph.D., Associate Professor, Department of Neurology, Case Western Reserve University School of Medicine

Diana M. Petty, Executive Director, Family Survival Project for Brain-Damaged Adults, Inc., San Francisco

Shelly E. Weaverdyck, Ph.D., Instructor, Department of Psychology, University of Michigan

Peter J. Whitehouse, M.D., Ph.D., Associate Professor of Neurology and Director, Division of Behavioral Neurology, Case Western Reserve University School of Medicine, and Director, Alzheimer Center, University Hospitals of Cleveland

Jitka M. Zgola, Psychogeriatric Clinic, Ottawa General Hospital

I   THE PATIENT

1

The Diagnostic Assessment of Patients with Dementia

MARIAN B. PATTERSON, PH.D.,
AND PETER J. WHITEHOUSE,
M.D., PH.D.

The diagnostic assessment of a patient with dementia includes both medical and psychosocial aspects. A medical diagnosis is necessary to establish, to the extent possible, the disease causing the dementia, as well as any concurrent illnesses contributing to the cognitive impairment. A process of history taking, physical examination, laboratory testing, and brain imaging is necessary to establish a diagnosis. Equally important, however, is the psychosocial assessment of the patient and the family, which leads to an understanding of the impact of the disease on the patient and on the functioning of the individual and the family. The psychosocial assessment also requires an understanding and evaluation of available community resources. Medical and psychosocial assessments frequently involve an interdisciplinary team including physicians, nurses, social workers, psychologists, occupational and physical therapists, nutritionists, and speech therapists.

The medical diagnostic process and psychosocial assessment are not independent processes. Information obtained during the medical diagnostic process is helpful to the psychosocial assessment. A close collaboration among different health care professionals is necessary when gathering information and communicating it to the patient and caregivers. The physician working independently, without benefit of a team, will need to take special care to explore all relevant areas of the interdisciplinary evaluation. In such a situation, it is especially useful to develop a set of available and reliable resource persons to whom the patient can be referred for consultation and for support in the community. The primary purpose of this assessment process is to identify problems that are remediable. A program of management

tailored to the individual patient and caregiver is developed and presented to the family for their consideration. During the assessment
period, the team members learn how this particular family has reacted
to the disease and can best judge how to present the new information
obtained as a result of the assessment process. Considerable individual
variations exist in the patient's and family's expectations concerning
the assessment process, their sophistication concerning the disease,
and their psychological strengths, which allow them to adjust to information presented during the assessment process. In our clinic, we
usually assess the patient and family on a single day, discuss the
assessment among the team members, and present our evaluation to
the family at a second meeting—the summary conference. During this
summary session, time is spent communicating the results of our
assessment and assuring that the information is transmitted as accurately as possible.

This process of medical and psychosocial assessment is ongoing
because many of the diseases that cause dementia are progressive.
Every six months to one year, the patient, caregivers, and support
systems should be reevaluated and the care plan adjusted based on
any changes that may have occurred during the interim.

Differential Diagnosis

Dementia is a term used to describe the loss of cognitive abilities
in someone who was previously intellectually intact. It is usually
defined as a disturbance of memory and other cognitive functions
that is severe enough to interfere with work or other social activities
(American Psychiatric Association 1987). Mental retardation is not
considered dementia because the intellectual impairment was present
at birth (McKhann et al. 1984); however, it is possible for mentally
retarded individuals to develop a superimposed dementia in which
there is a generalized deterioration from previous levels of functioning. Many dementias are progressive, but some are not (e.g., those
resulting from head trauma). Dementias frequently occur in older
individuals, although some forms of dementia occur in children and
younger adults. Dementias should also be differentiated from psychiatric conditions in which there are alterations in thought process
and content, frequently associated with affective symptoms. In some
psychiatric syndromes, such as schizophrenia and depression, cognitive impairment can occur. Although as a rule the cognitive im-

pairment is not as major as in the dementias, differentiation can be difficult during the earliest stages of dementia. Delirium or acute confusional states can also sometimes be confused with dementia, especially in older persons, who may not show other acute symptoms. Delirium often develops more rapidly than dementia and is associated with changes in level of arousal. Deliria are often caused by medical illnesses that disrupt the metabolic support of the brain and are frequently reversible by appropriate treatment of the underlying medical condition.

The evaluation of an older person with progressive cognitive impairment requires knowledge of the normal age-related changes in intellectual functions. As we all age, certain cognitive abilities change, including recent memory and the speed of thought processes. Vocabulary and general comprehension are less affected by the aging process. Very early dementia is often difficult to discriminate from normal age-related changes on the initial evaluation and requires follow-up to establish the rate of progression of the impairment to make the diagnosis.

The process of differential diagnosis in dementia is one of exclusion. One starts with a long list of potential medical conditions that can cause dementia and, by appropriate history taking, physical examination, and laboratory testing, rules out as many conditions as possible. The primary purpose of the evaluation is to determine whether any treatable conditions are contributing to cognitive impairment. The most common causes of dementia are Alzheimer's disease (AD) and related degenerative diseases of the nervous system, and multi-infarct dementia caused by multiple strokes. These disorders, occurring either separately or together in the same individual, probably account for 80 percent of all dementias. Alzheimer's disease accounts for over 50 percent of dementia cases and is diagnosed clinically by excluding other forms of dementia (Consensus Conference 1987; Katzman and Terry 1983; U.S. Congress 1987; Civil and Whitehouse 1988). The confirmation of the diagnosis of AD requires examination of brain tissue at autopsy or upon brain biopsy. Characteristic pathological features of AD include loss of nerve cells, senile plaques, and neurofibrillary tangles out of proportion to what one would see in a normal aged individual. Multi-infarct dementia is diagnosed in the setting of a history of stepwise deterioration, often with abrupt onset, associated with a history and physical examination suggestive of previous vascular disease and strokes. The Hachinski

TABLE 1.1 Ischemic Score

	Weight
Abrupt onset	2
Stepwise deterioration	1
Fluctuating course	2
Nocturnal confusion	1
Relative preservation of personality	1
Depression	1
Somatic complaints	1
Emotional incontinence	1
History of hypertension	1
History of strokes	2
Evidence of associated atherosclerosis	1
Focal neurological symptoms	2
Focal neurological signs	2

Note: Scores of ≥7 suggest that vascular disease plays a role in the dementia, whereas scores of ≤4 are more likely in AD.

Scale (Table 1.1) can be used to differentiate AD and multi-infarct dementia in many cases (Hachinski 1983; Hachinski et al. 1975). A score of ≤4 is suggestive of AD; a score of ≥7, multi-infarct dementia. A score of 5 or 6 suggests that possibly both diseases may be affecting an individual.

Several medical conditions can present as progressive cognitive impairment, including thyroid and other endocrine diseases, vitamin B_{12} deficiency, and a variety of other body system malfunctions. Table 1.2 lists some of the conditions that present as dementia. Many of these conditions are at least partially treatable and, therefore, require careful evaluation. Several neurodegenerative diseases besides AD are associated with dementia. Parkinson's disease, which is characterized by motor slowness, tremor, and rigidity, is associated with dementia in approximately 30 percent of the cases. Huntington's disease is a rare form of dementia occurring in younger individuals, which is characterized by abnormal movements called chorea. Several psychiatric conditions can also present with progressive cognitive impairments as part of their picture. Depression is common in older people and can present with slowed thinking and memory impairment. Depression should be considered in every patient, but particularly when there is a past history of depression, sudden onset of

TABLE 1.2 Causes of Dementia

Alzheimer's disease	Encephalitis
Huntington's disease	Meningitis
Parkinson's disease	Drug toxicity (iatrogenic)
Wilson's disease	Chemical substance abuse,
Progressive supranuclear palsy	including alcohol
Spinocerebellar degeneration	Heavy metal intoxications
Multiple sclerosis	Industrial exposures
Multi-infarct dementia	Postanoxic encephalopathy
AIDS	Carbon monoxide
Head injury	Cardiopulmonary disorders
Subdural hematoma	Metabolic disturbances
Dementia pugilistica	Endocrine disorders
Tumors	Vitamin deficiency
Hydrocephalus	Connective tissue disease
Syphilitic general paresis	Chronic schizophrenia
Jakob-Creutzfeldt disease	Depression

symptoms, stressful environmental events, and changes in appetite and sleep pattern. Chronic schizophrenia and, in older individuals, paraphrenia, can include cognitive impairment, although the psychiatric manifestations are usually predominant. Alzheimer's disease and other dementias can have associated secondary psychiatric symptoms including hallucinations, illusions, paranoia, delusions, and affective signs. It is sometimes difficult to establish whether one is dealing with a primary psychiatric syndrome such as depression with secondary cognitive symptoms or primary cognitive impairment with secondary psychiatric symptoms.

One major treatable form of cognitive impairment in older patients that must be specifically ruled out is drug misuse or abuse. Aged people frequently see several physicians, who may prescribe several different drugs, which interact to produce cognitive impairment. A careful history of drug usage from both patient and caregivers is essential to the evaluation process. A drug without clear-cut medical indications can often be stopped to assess its role in adding to confusion.

Methods of Evaluation

History

The history of the development of the cognitive impairment is the most important aspect of the medical diagnostic process and includes a careful definition of the onset and progression of the cognitive problems. The initial symptoms are characterized, followed by any additional symptoms that developed later in the course. Factors that make the cognitive problems worse or better are explored. This information must be obtained from both the patient and a caregiver to assure as much accuracy as possible. The results of any previous medical tests should be reviewed. The past medical history is explored to determine whether any other medical illnesses, such as strokes or heart attacks, may have contributed to the current problems. The process of history taking allows the examiners to develop a personal relationship with the family and caregivers, which is necessary to facilitate understanding and cooperation during the remaining parts of the assessment.

Neurological Examination

The purpose of the neurological examination is to disclose signs of illnesses that may be contributing to the cognitive impairment. Neurological examination begins with mental status testing. Every nurse and physician involved in assessing patients with progressive cognitive impairment should examine different aspects of cognitive performance, including arousal, attention, memory, language, judgment, praxis, perception, and psychiatric symptoms. The use of a screening mental status instrument, such as the Mini-Mental State examination (Folstein et al. 1975; Anthony et al. 1982), is recommended because this objective test allows one to compare a patient's performance to those of other patients and to follow the course of the illness in a particular individual. As with any cognitive screening test, however, the test score can serve only as a rough guideline and should never form the sole basis for making a clinical judgment.

Mental status examination is followed by examination of cranial nerve function, including eyes, ears, and sensation and motor control above the neck. Assessment of the patient's ability to use muscles, looking for signs of weakness or abnormal movements, is followed by a sensory exam. Assessment of coordination, gait, and reflexes completes the neurological examination.

TABLE 1.3 Screening Tests for Dementia

Blood Determinations
  Hematological
    Hematocrit
    White blood count
    Platelets
    Differential
    Indices
    Sedimentation rate
  Chemical
    Electrolytes (Na, K, carbonate, chloride, Ca, Mg)
    Liver function tests (transaminases)
    Renal function
    Urea creatinine
    Vitamin B_{12}
    Thyroid function tests
    Serology for syphilis
Brain Imaging
  Computed tomography, or
  Magnetic resonance imaging
Optional Tests Depending on Clinical Indications
  Chest x-ray
  Electrocardiogram
  Vascular work-up
  Cerebrospinal fluid exam

Medical Examination

Every patient who presents with symptoms of dementia requires a general physical examination searching for evidence of vascular disease, heart disease, pulmonary disease, joint disease, or liver or kidney failure, which could relate to the patient's symptoms. Patients with dementia may also suffer from other illnesses commonly found in older people, which may contribute to "excess disability" (see Chapter 2).

Laboratory Testing

Examination of blood specimens of every patient is also required to determine whether there are any metabolic or endocrine abnormalities. Table 1.3 is a listing of the routine screening tests to detect treatable causes of dementia. A computed tomographic (CT) or magnetic resonance imaging (MRI) scan is used to examine the brain structurally for evidence of brain lesions such as previous strokes or tumors that could contribute to the symptoms. In addition, a CT scan allows evaluation of the possibility of normal pressure hydrocephalus. Normal pressure hydrocephalus is characterized clinically by progressive dementia, gait abnormalities, and incontinence in association with ventricular enlargement out of proportion to the degree of atrophy on CT scan.

Psychological Testing

All patients should receive mental status assessment, but some patients will require more comprehensive neuropsychological testing. This process is described in Chapter 3. Reasons for considering full neuropsychological assessment include early dementia, in which the distinction from normal, age-related cognitive impairment is difficult, assessment of the interaction between psychiatric and neurological diseases, and the development of a better profile of the patient's abilities and impairments to advise patients and families concerning management. A detailed neuropsychological evaluation can be extremely useful in providing specific recommendations for management that capitalize on the patient's remaining capabilities to compensate for his deficits.

The processes of medical diagnosis and psychosocial assessment cannot be separated. Moreover, the diagnostic process cannot be separated from the formulation of a treatment program. It is during the diagnostic process that the clinician gains the greatest amount of information concerning the patient and the family/caregiver. The manner in which the diagnostic process is accomplished allows the family to learn about the caregiving team and to trust them. With trust, the information obtained during the assessment process can be successfully communicated to the family to help them deal better with the disease.

Psychosocial Formulation

Psychosocial Strengths and Deficits

The term *diagnosis,* when applied to the psychosocial formulation, means making a considered determination or judgment on the basis of critical scrutiny of a psychosocial problem. Because Alzheimer's disease touches the whole fabric of the patient's life, the accuracy of diagnosis and the success of treatment hinge on making an accurate diagnostic assessment of the psychosocial situation. It is not enough simply to identify problem areas or symptoms; if the diagnosis is to lead to a useful and individually meaningful plan of treatment, the psychological, intellectual, and functional resources of the patient must be discovered and their strength determined.

When one attempts to reach an understanding of the patient's psychological strengths and deficits, it is useful to look at both personal style and coping mechanisms, as they were in the past and as they are at present. A clinical approach to incorporating this current and historical information is described by Pfeiffer (1980) in his discussion of the psychosocial evaluation of the elderly patient. Past personal style refers to those attributes that characterize this person's life and make the person unique. A picture of a person's style may be filled in with information provided by the patient and by family members or friends who are questioned about the patient's affective, interpersonal, and intrapersonal qualities. Although information about each of these spheres should be obtained, what is needed is not an exhaustive accounting but a highlighting of those features that the patient and those close to the patient think are most salient.

Affective facets of personal style include temperament, mood, and reactivity. For example, was the person short-tempered or patient, ebullient or pessimistic, impulsive or cautious? Did the personal overreact to even minor stresses or seem to take everything in stride? Did people see the patient as alert and energetic or placid and dull? Even if there was no psychiatric history, was the patient's life marked by mood swings from low to high or by periodic spells of depressed mood? If so, it is particularly useful to characterize the nature and duration of such affective features because they are important in evaluating the presence of an ongoing depressive disorder.

It is especially helpful to find out how the patient has coped with past stresses. Life events such as a death or major illness in the family, a natural disaster, or an economic reversal are major stresses that can elicit a variety of coping responses. Did the patient become depressed or anxious and unable to function normally for a period? Did he throw himself into activities, and were they productive or random and ineffectual? Was she the sort of person who never allowed feelings to surface or to be discussed, or did she grieve openly? Knowing how a patient has coped with major stresses in the past will help the clinician both in assessing what personality changes have taken place and in finding ways of managing present stresses.

Interpersonal aspects of personal style include the patient's relationships with family members and those outside the family, such as friends, lovers and associates, those in authority, or even strangers. Of particular interest are the number, quality, intensity, and persistence of interpersonal relationships. For example, does the patient seek out others or become involved only with family and a few friends? Is the patient independent of others or dependent and needing of support, assertive or timid, rebellious or compliant? Have relationships been maintained over long periods, or have relationships been interrupted in some way? Because interpersonal relationships are one of the biggest sources of conflicts in a person's life and at the same time are one of the major sources of satisfaction, this area can often be a highly useful source of information in diagnostic formulation and treatment planning.

The intrapersonal aspects of the patient refer to those qualities that reflect activities, aspirations, and self-concept. Two pieces of such information routinely obtained are education and occupation. It is often very instructive to elaborate on these. In addition to knowing how far someone has gone in school, one may want to know what kind of student the patient was. Was school enjoyed? Was there frequent trouble? What were the patient's best and worst subjects? This information serves at least two important purposes in the diagnostic formulation. First, it helps to determine a baseline estimation of intellectual functioning from which evaluation may be made of present decline. Second, it may reveal individual interests and skills that can be supported in structuring the patient's activities. Similarly, one's past vocational and avocational pursuits can provide information both on the premorbid intellectual level and on likely interests in the present.

An individual's aspirations and self-concept are more subtle personal qualities that must be inferred from the patient's conversation and others' descriptions. Sometimes it is the loss of or change in these qualities that is especially painful for the family to observe, and their reactions to such changes will affect their handling of the patient's management. For example, a formerly ambitious and perfectionistic person who seems to have become sloppy and lazy may provoke hurt and anger in caretakers. Understanding not only the present behavior but also the extent of the changes that have taken place will help the clinician to find an appropriate intervention to relieve the psychosocial stress created by the caretaker's reactions.

Also, having a conception of the patient's self-image will often be of great assistance in interpreting behavior that might seem peculiar or inappropriate. Thus, a patient who poses a problem because of inappropriate sexual remarks to the staff may really be trying to restore a self-concept of physical attractiveness in the past. If in the past, physical attractiveness had been used as a way of coping, for example, to gain support or make new friends, it would not be surprising if the patient were to fall back on old and tried methods when faced with a confusing interpersonal situation.

Such formulations as those described are really founded on a commonsensical assessment based on fairly obvious information. Our goal is not to make an in-depth psychodynamic interpretation but to obtain practical information that can be used in practical ways to resolve some current problem. This information can be easily obtained during the course of conversations with the patient and family if one gives them the opportunity to talk a little about their personal history, while keeping in mind the essential elements of the psychosocial picture that are likely to be relevant. These include *affect* (temperament, mood, and reactivity), *interpersonal qualities* (relationships with family, friends, and authorities), and *intrapersonal qualities* (activities, aspirations, and self-concept).

Information about the patient's past pattern of psychological functioning is needed if one is making a diagnosis in the *Diagnostic and Statistical Manual* of the American Psychiatric Association (American Psychiatric Association 1987). Particularly in Axis II, in which personality disorders are diagnosed, it is necessary to have a sense of long-standing adaptive and maladaptive behaviors that characterize the patient's adjustment. Although such Axis II diagnoses are often not considered in patients with dementia, it can be argued that a good deal of present behavior can be made more understandable if the persistent patterns of the past are revealed.

A second practical use of past psychosocial information lies in its ability to convey a sense of uniqueness about each patient. Especially helpful are facts that emphasize the more positive aspects of the patient's life and convey a sense of the person's achievements and special interests, for example, that the patient was a skilled dancer, a world traveler, or an avid gardener. This information enables non-family caregivers to regard the person as special and unique.

Having come to some understanding of a patient's lifelong affective, interpersonal, and intrapersonal patterns, one can assess the patient's present behavior. A problem-oriented approach will properly orient the clinician to diagnostic scrutiny of the most relevant areas. At the same time, however, the development of an effective treatment strategy requires a broader conception of the patient's remaining psychological assets.

In assessing problems identified in the patient's present psychological functioning, one will need to examine emotional state, interpersonal relationships, and intrapersonal qualities and to view them in relation to previous patterns of functioning. For example, a family might give as a presenting complaint that they are having difficulty dealing with their relative's anxiety. Although one might decide merely to treat the target symptom of anxiety, a more comprehensive approach seeks to diagnose its source, rather than simply to add a medication or intervention of questionable value. In this example, one could start by asking questions regarding the nature of the anxiety. Is it pervasive or intermittent, diffuse or specific to some particular stimulus or situation? Is this patient's anxiety part of a lifelong pattern? What provoked it in the past, and what eased it? What are the present stressors? Are the resources for coping with stress that the patient used in the past still available? Can substitutes be found for lost resources?

It is occasionally observed that long-standing personality traits have become exaggerated to the point that they present problematic behaviors in a patient with dementia. A formerly cautious and thrifty individual may begin to hoard all sorts of items, no longer able to discriminate those that are potentially valuable from those that are not or to inhibit the desire to save even things that are known to be valueless. A formerly dependent and self-centered person may begin refusing to do any self-care. A formerly critical and hypersensitive individual may have come to believe that people are actively hostile and may develop paranoid fears of being harmed. Where such pre-existing personality features can be identified, the endpoint of treatment may be defined differently, as some degree of amelioration of symptoms, because long-standing underlying traits are likely to be unaffected by treatment. Clearly, when frank psychopathology is present, appropriate interventions should be devised.

Finally, personality changes may reflect the losses of intellectual capacity and self-regulation associated with the disease, but they may also be reflections of increased stress or counterproductive interactions with caretakers and, as such, may be potentially treatable. Thus, it is important to know what is producing stress and maintaining it and how the caregivers respond to the patient's maladaptive behavior in ways to encourage or discourage it.

Intellectual Assets and Liabilities

A discussion of issues that must be considered in assessing the intellectual status of a demented patient is presented in Chapter 3, and it will not be repeated here. The aim of this section is to illustrate the role of intellectual factors in the diagnostic formulation. Clearly, the intellectual state of the patient cannot be viewed in isolation because it has a profound impact on all aspects of the patient's psychosocial functioning. This influence is reciprocal, in that psychosocial factors such as anxiety, depression, or a high degree of stress may exacerbate the extent of the intellectual disability. This point cannot be overemphasized, as the excess cognitive disability caused by anxiety or stress can usually be reduced through appropriate interventions and may have a significant impact on the patient's (and family's) quality of life. Furthermore, information about the precise nature and extent of a patient's memory and cognitive problems may be critical in making a differential diagnosis and is essential in formulating treatment plans. Finally, repeated assessment of intellectual functioning is often necessary to track the progression of disease and to reformulate plans as changes in intellectual capacity occur.

As was the case with the psychological factors in the psychosocial formulation, understanding the intellectual status will entail first obtaining a good cognitive history (Albert and Moss 1988). The patient's baseline functioning and premorbid intellectual capacity and sophistication will have to be inferred from previous accomplishments, such as education, occupation, hobbies, and past problem-solving efforts. Second, the history of the intellectual problems should be determined as precisely as possible and related to other life events. For example, did past experiences of impaired attention and memory occur during episodes of depression, or did a cognitive decline follow a closed head injury or a lengthy period of substance abuse? Also important are the patient's past attempts to compensate for or cope with cognitive changes and their success.

The implications of impaired intellectual functioning for the patient's psychological and functional adjustment are in many respects

rather obvious. For example, poor memory interferes with social relationships in that it limits the patient's ability to participate in meaningful conversation and to meet responsibilities. Impaired judgment
and problem-solving ability may necessitate constant supervision, and
visual-spatial deficits may make it unsafe for the patient to drive. The
combination of concreteness, misperceptions, and faulty memory may
lead the patient to erroneous conclusions that reinforce suspiciousness
and delusions. As intellectual resources become more constricted, the
patient's psychological adaptiveness becomes concomitantly more restricted, and rigidity and seemingly irrational behaviors may result.

Although the identification of such problems is clearly necessary,
it is equally important to assess the spared and preserved abilities at
each stage of the illness. Thus, even patients with serious memory
problems may be able to learn under some circumstances. For example, a patient may be able, with sufficient repetition, to pick up a
sequence of motor behaviors although not being able to remember
how or where it was learned (Schachter 1987). Also, in many patients,
particularly during the early stages of the disease, cognitive functions
are affected unevenly. Thus, a patient who has some verbal difficulties
may still be able to derive satisfaction from activities in a nonverbal
sphere. A comprehensive care plan will aim at helping the patient to
utilize spared functions to compensate for deficits.

Finally, it is often important to note the circumstances under
which the deficits appear. Thus, attentional problems may be markedly exacerbated by environmental distractions; sensory deficits interfere with information processing, especially in noisy and poorly
illuminated settings; and emotional factors, such as anxiety, may be
present under some circumstances. The validity and usefulness of a
neuropsychological assessment, in particular, will depend upon how
successfully these factors can be controlled or at least factored into
the interpretation.

Functional Abilities

The third aspect of the psychological assessment is determining
the patient's functional abilities, what the patient can and cannot do,
and why. This means examining the patient's practical, everyday
activities and integrating this information with the medical and diagnostic information. For example, a patient unable to dress alone
may no longer be able to remember or keep straight the correct sequence of actions, may not see well enough, may have limited move-

ment due to arthritis, or may be affected by many other deficits. The solution to the problem will depend on the particular combination of causes.

Once again, it is worth remembering that a history of the patient's past patterns of functioning is also relevant. As an obvious example, a man who had never cooked until his wife died a couple of years previously might be expected to deteriorate in that skill earlier than someone who has cooked for a lifetime. One commonly observes a patient who presents as demented for the first time after the death of a spouse. Although sometimes the impairment reflects the onset of depression, it is often found that the deceased spouse had for some time been quietly caring for and protecting the patient.

Family and Support Systems

Just as formulating a diagnosis and a care plan requires an assessment of the patient's resources and shortcomings, both lifelong patterns and present changes, so too is the success of a treatment plan dependent upon an accurate assessment of the patient's support systems. The elements of the support systems can be regarded as parallel to those of the individual patient, with the nature of the system determining which features are particularly relevant.

For example, for a patient living within a family, one can ask about the present psychological and practical resources of the family and how the patient's illness has necessitated changes. How do members of this family react emotionally to problems? Are they ordinarily anxious, impatient, tolerant, flexible? What are their preferred methods of coping? Are they stoic or expressive; do they avoid problems or actively seek solutions? What is the interpersonal style within the family? Are they cooperative or argumentative, inclined to take on too much responsibility or to shift responsibility and blame others? An understanding of both the psychological and the practical resources and problems within the family will help the clinician to avoid making a care plan that is beyond the capacity of the family to carry out. Obvious examples are the family that has neither the money nor the transportation to get the patient to a recommended day care program, or the family that is psychologically unable to move their patient to a nursing home even though it is clearly needed.

Different facets of the psychosocial formulation may be more relevant if the support system is different, for example, a nursing home. In examining the resources available and the problems that pertain to the patient's care, one must adapt the care plan to the features of that particular setting. For example, the clinician may have determined that a patient's hoarding behavior represents an expression of lifelong tendencies exacerbated by boredom, anxiety about losses, and defects of memory and inhibition. A care plan is formulated that permits the hoarding of a limited amount of material and attempts to reduce hoarding through the gentle application of behavior modification techniques. Unless the nursing home has sufficient practical resources—a large staff and flexible policies about keeping objects in the room—and the individual staff members assigned to the patient are sufficiently flexible and have the time, training, and sensitivity to give consistent positive and negative reinforcements, the plan will have little chance of succeeding.

Using Diagnostic Information in a Problem-Solving Approach

The information that has been obtained through the process of differential diagnosis and psychosocial formulation will quite readily be adapted to a problem-solving approach to treatment planning. Problems that have been identified are targeted for intervention if they are treatable or remediable on any level (medical, intellectual, functional, psychosocial). The planned intervention is likely to be successful only if the targeted problem has been adequately characterized on all relevant levels as well. As an example, a patient's presenting symptom of confusion may be identified as arising from a toxic state resulting from overmedication. Two associated problems may be uncovered: the patient is taking too much medication because he cannot remember that he has just taken his pills, and the family cannot stand up to demands of the patient to control the medication alone. Clearly, the treatment plan must be individually tailored to account for all of these relevant levels of the problem if it is to be successful.

One aspect of the diagnostic and planning process that is often not given enough attention is how to present the diagnosis to the patient and the family. Hearing the diagnosis of Alzheimer's disease can be a devastating experience for the patient and family, and giving it is difficult for the clinician, especially in early cases when the diagnosis may be only probable. It is wise to plan ahead how the diagnosis is to be presented. Important considerations are knowing how much the patient and/or family can understand, are ready to hear, and can absorb at one sitting. Often the clinician finds that recommendations go unfollowed simply because the family has been so preoccupied with assimilating the diagnosis of AD that they have not processed the rest of what was said during the session.

Usually a follow-up visit is needed to reiterate the recommended treatment plan, to see how well the initial recommendations have been followed and to deal with any problems that the plan has created, and to answer the many questions that may have arisen since the previous visit. At this time, as well as during the initial diagnostic summary, the clinician can explore fears and expectations of the family and patient and help them work through their emotional reactions. If other consultants have been involved in the case, it is important to know what the family has been told and what they expect the consultant's role to be. The clinicians most directly involved with the patient's ongoing care must be responsible for coordinating the inputs of consultants. Finally, through regular contacts with the family, the primary physician or case manager will usually have the major role in helping the patient and family work through and cope with the implications of living with a dementing disease.

One source of anxiety that is often overlooked by clinicians is the family's fear of the financial burden of caring for a demented relative. Some families may be unrealistically worried, whereas others may not have adequately considered the financial situation. Furthermore, legal questions may have to be resolved, such as who should handle the patient's finances or to what extent the patient is competent to participate in making such decisions (see Chapter 11). The family's decisions may be colored by emotional reactions, such as the difficulty of taking over control from a parent, particularly one who does not understand why this is happening and may disagree strenuously. It is often the clinician's role to help the family work through such difficulties.

A second major task as the diagnosis and care plan are presented is enlisting the family's participation. The clinician must assess their understanding of the plan and its purpose and their willingness and ability to comply. Even the most elegant and well-thought-out plan can be unsuccessful if it is beyond the capacity of the support system to effect, and it may be necessary to be flexible and devise a more practical if less adequate plan.

Continuing Diagnosis

The diagnostic process should not end with the initial diagnosis of AD but should include regular reevaluation of the patient, the caregivers and the support systems. It is important to monitor the progression of dementia, any concurrent illness and the general medical condition, the effectiveness of and continued necessity for medications, and the potential side effects of medications. It is also important to keep abreast of the family situation and the level of stress experienced by caregivers. For the patient in a nursing home, one needs to keep abreast of any changes in staff, physical environment, or policies that may have affected the patient's health or behavior.

In conjunction with the reevaluation of the medical and psychosocial diagnostic picture, the care plan must be reconsidered. It is necessary to know what has worked and what hasn't—and why. If there have been changes in the patient or in the situation (e.g., a progression of dementia or an increase in caregiver stress), the plan may no longer be appropriate and may have to be modified. On the other hand, problems previously present may have been resolved, and the specific intervention may be terminated. This is particularly notable in the case of medications given to patients in nursing homes. It is sometimes found that a patient is continuing to be given a medication, often a neuroleptic, when indications for it no longer exist.

A part of the continuing diagnosis is a reevaluation of the family's long-term expectations about the patient and their fears about their own vulnerability. A challenging aspect of working with AD families is maintaining a delicate balance between clinically assessing family members' personal needs, anxieties, weaknesses, and stress and maintaining a relationship with them as colleagues and equal partners in the care plan.

Conclusion

In this chapter, we reviewed the medical and psychosocial aspects of the assessment of patients with dementia. We discussed a multidisciplinary approach to assessment that is designed to identify the diseases contributing to the patient's cognitive impairment—to determine the patient's particular problems and strengths, and to assess the adequacy of the family and support system to carry out the care plan. There is no abrupt transition between diagnosis and treatment, and the building of rapport during diagnosis is essential to successful management after the diagnostic process is completed. The process of evolution is ongoing as changes in the patient's and the caregiver's status must be monitored through the course of the illness.

References

Albert, M. S., and M. B. Moss. 1988. *Geriatric neuropsychology*. New York: Guilford Press.

American Psychiatric Association. 1987. *Diagnostic and statistical manual of mental disorders (DSM III-R)*. 3d ed. – revised. Washington, DC: American Psychiatric Association.

Anthony, J. C., L. LeResche, U. Niaz, M. R. Van Korff, and M. F. Folstein. 1982. Limits of the Mini-Mental State as a screening test for dementia and delirium among hospital patients. *Psychological Medicine* 12:397–408.

Civil R., and P. Whitehouse. 1988. Alzheimer's disease. In *Current Neurology*, ed. S. Appel, 227–50. Philadelphia: Yearbook Publisher.

Consensus Conference, Office of Medical Applications of Research, National Institutes of Health. 1987. Differential diagnosis of dementing diseases, 1987. *Journal of the American Medical Association* 256:3411–16.

Folstein, M. F., S. E. Folstein, and P. R. McHugh. 1975. Mini-Mental State: A practical method for grading the cognitive state of patients for the clinician. *Journal of Psychiatric Research* 12:189–98.

Hachinski, V. C. 1983. Differential diagnosis of Alzheimer's dementia: Multi-infarct dementia. In *Alzheimer's disease: The standard reference*, ed. B. Reisberg, 188–92. New York: Free Press.

Hachinski, V. C., L. E. Iliff, E. Zilhka, G. H. Du Boulay, V. L. McAllister, J. Marshall, R. W. R. Russell, and L. Symon. 1975. Cerebral blood flow in dementia. *Archives of Neurology* 32:632–37.

Katzman, R., and R. D. Terry. 1983. *The neurology of aging*. Philadelphia: F. A. Davis.

McKhann, G., D. Drachman, M. Folstein, R. Katzman, D. Price, and E. M. Stadlan. 1984. Clinical diagnosis of Alzheimer's disease: Report of the NINCDS-ADRDA work group under the auspices of Department of Health and Human Services Task Force on Alzheimer's Disease. *Neurology* 34:939–44.

Pfeiffer, E. 1980. The psychosocial evaluation of the elderly patient. In *Handbook of geriatric psychiatry*, ed. E. W. Busse and D. G. Blazer, 275–84. New York: Van Nostrand Reinhold.

Schachter, D. L. 1987. Implicit memory: History and current status. *Journal of Experimental Psychology: Learning, Memory and Cognition* 13:501–18.

U.S. Congress. Office of Technology Assessment. 1987. *Losing a million minds: Confronting the tragedy of Alzheimer's disease and other dementias*. OTA-BA-323. Washington, DC: U.S. Government Printing Office. April.

2

The Clinical Care of Patients with Dementia

RICHARD J. MARTIN, N.D., R.N.,
AND PETER J. WHITEHOUSE,
M.D., PH.D.

The interdisciplinary assessment process described in Chapter 1 results in a care plan to address the identified medical, behavioral, and psychosocial problems. In this chapter, we will consider the medical management of dementia patients. Knowledge of the disease causing the cognitive impairment, concern for the presence of other medical problems, and careful attention to the prevention of future health problems are essential to the health of patient and family. We will not discuss the specific medical or surgical treatment of potentially reversible dementias due to metabolic or endocrine malfunction or structural brain lesions as the management of these illnesses can be found in standard medical textbooks. Rather, we will consider general principles to guide the medical practitioner in the management of the patient with cognitive impairment.

First, we will consider what biological therapies are available for the cognitive impairment itself. Second, we will outline the use of drugs to treat the secondary psychiatric and behavioral symptoms often found in patients with dementia. Then we will discuss some principles of preventive medicine important for the care of the person with dementia to prevent what is called "excess disability." Patients with dementia are often elderly and therefore at risk for other medical illnesses that are common to the aged and that can compound cognitive functioning. It is essential to remember that the medical management should be part of a care plan that includes attention to psychosocial problems as well. Through regular reassessments of patient and family, the care plan should be modified as necessary as the disease progresses.

The Biological Treatment of Cognitive Impairment

Pharmacological approaches to the treatment of the cognitive impairment in irreversible dementias are limited. Ideally, the development of effective drug therapy should be based on an understanding of the biological mechanisms underlying the dementia. Although our current understanding of dementing illnesses such as Alzheimer's disease (AD) and related disorders remains incomplete, a growing knowledge of the neurochemistry in these diseases combined with new computer-guided methods of drug design allow hope for the development of therapeutic agents. At present, no consistently effective clinical pharmacological treatments are available for the cognitive symptoms of Alzheimer's disease. Various drugs, including cerebral vasodilators, cerebral metabolic enhancers, nootropics ("mind growth"), psychostimulants, and agents that act on specific chemical messenger systems (neurotransmitters) have been tried. Some of these agents have demonstrated positive effects on psychological tests in small numbers of subjects but have failed to have consistent beneficial effects in more carefully done larger studies. Hydergine (Sandoz, Inc., East Hanover, N.J.) is the only compound approved for use in treating cognitive impairment in the elderly by the Food and Drug Administration. It may have minimal benefit in some patients, perhaps by its effect on mood and arousal. Cholinergic agents such as physostigmine and tetrahydroaminoacridine (THA) may also have some effects in some patients. Acetylcholine is a neurotransmitter important for memory that is reduced in concentration in the brains of patients with AD. Large, multicenter trials of these compounds are now under way to define better their efficacy in AD. Different methods of delivering drugs to the brain, such as injecting directly into the fluid spaces in the brain (ventricles) through an implanted pump, have been tried experimentally but are not recommended because results have been disappointing and the procedure is invasive. For patients and family who need to feel that no therapeutic avenue has been left unexplored or who want to contribute to finding new answers, referral to a research center is appropriate.

As noted in Chapter 1, the second most common cause of dementia is the cumulative damage of small strokes called multi-infarct dementia. The strokes may be quite small, sometimes not visible upon computed tomographic scan examination. Although no current therapy can remediate the effects of multi-infarct dementia, a program of

stroke prevention can minimize the continued occurrence of the in-
farcts. Stroke prevention includes control of illnesses that increase the
likelihood of strokes such as hypertension and high blood cholesterol.
Often, the blood-thinning properties of low doses of aspirin taken
daily can inhibit continued strokes. There are some patients for whom
an anticoagulant such as Coumadin (warfarin; Endo Laboratories,
Inc., Garden City, N.Y.) may be indicated. The dangers of bleeding
episodes related to injury or hemorrhagic (bleeding) strokes must be
considered when using anticoagulant therapy.

The Biological Treatment of Behavioral Symptoms

Although dementia is defined by the impairment of memory,
language, and reasoning, the most troubling aspects of dementia are
often problems of behavior. Reasonably well defined psychiatric terms
can be used to label some of the behavior disturbances, including
depression, paranoia, and anxiety. Other behaviors, such as wandering and agitation, are less easy to fit into standard psychiatric
categories and are often particularly difficult to manage. Such problems range in severity from incessant repetition of questions to impairment in driving and cooking skills, which leads to major concerns
about safety. The behavioral manifestations of dementia occupy a great
deal of the caregiving energy of family members, nursing staff, and
primary care physicians and contribute frequently to the need for
respite services and institutionalization.

Behavioral disturbance and psychiatric symptoms occur as a result
of damage to the brain and unsuccessful attempts to adjust psychologically to the dementing illness. As is well stated in the recent report
from the Office of Technology Assessment:

> The division between behavioral and cognitive symptoms is arbi-
> trary. A person suffering from damage to nerve cells or changes in
> brain chemistry can be expected to exhibit behavior that results
> from neurological illness. It can also be reasoned that persons who
> cannot communicate their needs or thoughts, who cannot get
> dressed or who do not know where they are or who is caring for
> them might experience depression, fear, anxiety, or anger. Thus
> these symptoms are not so much "psychiatric" as they are the clear
> result of the neurological illness. They may be due both to brain
> damage and to an understandable reaction to the loss of mental
> abilities caused by that damage. (U.S. Congress, OTA, 1987, p. 73)

Behavioral interventions (i.e., making modifications in the environment) are generally preferable to medications for the treatment of most behavioral problems. These techniques are discussed throughout this book. There are a number of common behavioral problems in dementia for which the use of medications is appropriate, however. Depression, psychosis (hallucinations, delusions, paranoia), anxiety, and sleep disturbances can be treated with antidepressants, major tranquilizers, anxiolytics, and soporifics, respectively.

Although cautious use of psychoactive drugs can contribute to optimal functioning for the cognitively impaired patient, few studies have systematically examined the use of these medications in Alzheimer's disease and related disorders. The use of medications should be guided, however, by a few basic principles. First, purposeful treatment demands that the target symptoms be well defined. The behavioral assessment should focus treatment specifically on depression, anxiety, agitation, psychotic behavior, or insomnia, as appropriate. Before the initiation of therapy, the magnitude of the problem must be assessed so that the positive or even negative effects of therapy can be judged. The use of agents for their nonspecific, sedative effects to produce a more "cooperative" patient is to be avoided.

The second principle relates to drug usage. Employ as few drugs as possible, start with low doses, increase dosages slowly, and monitor carefully for side effects. Delayed side effects and adverse reactions to medications occur with greater frequency and severity in the aged than in younger individuals because of the slowed hepatic and renal function of the aged. Polypharmacy (the use of multiple medications whose effects may interact) often clouds the differentiation of desirable effects and side effects and puts the patient at risk for adverse reactions. Not infrequently, the discontinuation of all psychotropic medication to evaluate the patient's drug-free baseline is beneficial diagnostically and therapeutically. In general, medications with short half-lives should be favored to avoid buildup of cumulative toxicity. Many of these psychoactive agents produce substantial side effects including paradoxical agitation, somnolence, hypotension, and movement disorders such as Parkinsonism, as well as increased confusion. Small incremental changes in medication and subsequent effects on behavior must be closely monitored. Family and nursing staff members must be educated about the symptoms of medication overdose. Finally, the use of medications should always occur with appropriate psychological counseling with patient and family or with adequate training of paid caregivers.

Antidepressant therapy (tricyclic antidepressants and mono-amine oxidase (MAO) inhibitors) in the elderly person with dementia is less predictable than in younger patients. Depression can itself cause cognitive impairment and may respond dramatically to medication. Many patients suffer from both a degenerative dementia and depression and may not respond as readily. As it is often difficult to know how great a role the depression is playing in producing the cognitive symptoms, a therapeutic trial may be indicated. The cardiovascular and sedative effects may limit the usefulness of some tricyclic drugs. The long period (2 to 4 weeks) before the onset of action of some tricyclics may further complicate therapy. Agents with lower anticholinergic effects are generally best. The role of MAO inhibitors is somewhat controversial in the aged. If successful, antidepressant therapy should be stopped after several months to evaluate the need for continuing therapy. Electroconvulsive therapy (ECT) offers an option for some severely depressed patients. The deleterious effects of ECT on memory, as well as contraindications for patients with cardiovascular or pulmonary illness, limit its use in elderly people with dementia.

Anxiolytics are indicated for reducing anxiety and associated somatic symptoms. Most antianxiety agents have substantial sedative properties and are sometimes used to induce sleep. Patients differ greatly in their susceptibility to sedative effects. Disturbed sleep patterns, often accompanied by nighttime wandering, are a common problem. Barbiturates or benzodiazepams can impair daytime alertness, thus further impairing the next night's sleep. Continued use can lead to accumulation and potential toxicity. Mild sedatives, such as the antihistamine diphenhydramine (Benadryl; Parke, Davis & Co., Detroit, Mich.) or chloral hydrate, are often the best drugs to try first.

Severe behavior disturbances such as profound suspiciousness, agitation, or violence often require the use of antipsychotic (neuroleptic) agents. Although these medications can be useful, many toxic effects can occur, including confusion, sedation, hypotension, and changes in blood chemistries. Monitoring for extrapyramidal symptoms is necessary. Acutely dystonic reactions with uncontrollable twitching of muscles can occur. Increased muscle rigidity and stiffness with slowing of motor activity (Parkinsonism) occurs as doses are increased. Finally, irreversible abnormal movements, particularly of the face (tardive dyskinesia), are a risk with long-term therapy. Patients will sometimes experience paradoxical effects such as worsening of agitation or akathisia (restlessness). These effects should be considered before increasing the dose of an agent in response to increased behavioral symptoms.

The Prevention of Excess Disability

The focus of the clinician should be directed not only to the treatment of current problems but also to the prevention of future difficulties. The patient with dementia is at risk for suffering "excess disability." Excess disability is a reversible deficit that increases the degree of functional impairment beyond what would be expected based solely on the underlying cause of dementia (Kahn 1965; Brody et al. 1971). Physical illness, psychological stress, sensory difficulties (hearing or vision loss), and social problems can all exacerbate cognitive impairments. As other areas are addressed in subsequent chapters, we will limit our discussion to excess disability secondary to concurrent physical illness (and side effects of treatment) and sensory deficits.

Concurrent Physical Illness

Elderly patients with dementia are susceptible to the many acute and chronic medical conditions that affect other aged persons. A recent study demonstrated an average of 3.4 additional medical problems per patient with dementia, predominantly gastrointestinal, cardiac, and vascular disease (Fisk and Pannill 1987). Cognitive dysfunction, which affects self-care, hygiene, and mobility, often places an individual at higher risk for physical illness. Successful management of multiple medical problems in a person with dementia requires a good working relationship both with the family and with other professional caregivers.

Communication difficulties stemming from the dementia complicate taking a history about concurrent medical illnesses. Often, the primary presenting symptom of physical illness or intoxication is delirium (see Chapter 1). Delirium is characterized by acute clouding of consciousness, disorientation, and perceptual aberrations often including hallucinations. In the person with dementia, clinicians and caregivers should be alert to a sudden decline in cognitive or functional level or the abrupt onset of behavioral disturbance ranging from sullenness to agitation. As Winograd and Jarvik pointed out: "the dull confusion, bewilderment, urinary incontinence, and apathy interrupted by noisy restlessness overlap with the dementia syndrome and may be misinterpreted by both family and physicians as a worsening of the dementing process" (Winograd and Jarvik 1986; Lipowski 1983). Rather than accepting an abrupt change as a "normal" progression, one should recognize it as a symptom that requires examination. Almost any medical condition can trigger delirium, including cardiac disease, infection (urinary tract infection, pneumonia), and any metabolic problem that would interfere with support of brain function including dehydration, hypo/hyperglycemia, and hypotension. Taking a medical history, performing a physical examination, and checking appropriate laboratory studies should be part of the assessment. The prescription of psychoactive medications for agitation without examination of the acutely confused patient is obviously inappropriate.

Untoward effects of treatment for physical illness, including medications, hospitalization, and surgery, can also cause delirium (iatrogenic causes). Elderly people with multiple physical illnesses are often cared for by multiple physicians and are particularly susceptible to polypharmacy. Table 2.1 lists common drugs that can cause delirium.

Delirium is not uncommon when patients with dementia are hospitalized. Acute confusion may be caused by a strange environment and hospital procedures, as well as the effects of illness and physical discomfort. Physical pain, in particular, can cause delirium. Often this occurs in patients who are unable to communicate their discomfort because of their cognitive deficits in language and reasoning. The family and nursing staff should be forewarned of the potential for confusion while the patient is in the hospital and of the possible need for physical restraint and/or sedating medications. Restraint is to be used only for the maintenance of safety and the support of medical treatment, such as intravenous therapy. Patients should be provided with familiar items from home and should have frequent contact with caregivers and family. Comfort measures should be undertaken by family and nursing staff. Attempts should be made to minimize the hustle and bustle common to acute care units. Frequent mental status monitoring throughout acute care treatment is obviously essential.

The delirium may not resolve completely before discharge, making discharge planning and aftercare essential. Effective discharge

TABLE 2.1 Drugs That Can Cause or Contribute to Delirium and Dementia

Analgesics	*Cardiovascular*
Narcotic	Atropine
Codeine	Digitalis
Meperidine	Diuretics
Morphine	Lidocaine
Pentazocine	*Hypoglycemics*
Propoxyphene	Insulin
Nonnarcotic	Sulfonylureas
Indomethacin	*Psychotropic drugs*
Antihistamines	Antianxiety drugs
Diphenhydramine	Benzodiazepines
Hydroxyzine	Antidepressant drugs
Antihypertensives	Lithium
Clonidine	Tricyclics
Hydralazine	Antipsychotics
Methyldopa	Haloperidol
Propranolol	Thiothixene
Reserpine	Thioridazine
Antimicrobials	Chlorpromazine
Gentamicin	Hypnotics
Isoniazid	Barbiturates
Antiparkinsonism drugs	Benzodiazepines
Amantadine	Chloral hydrate
Bromocriptine	Others
Carbidopa	Cimetidine
L-Dopa	Steroids
Trihexyphenidyl and other	
anticholinergics	

Source: R. L. Kane, J. G. Ouslander, and I. B. Abrass. *Essentials of clinical geriatrics.* New York: McGraw-Hill, 1984, p. 66.

planning will include systematic monitoring for resolution of the delirium state and return to baseline cognition. Unfortunately, some patients never return to their previous level of cognitive ability after an acute confusional episode.

Behavioral interventions directed toward health maintenance and compensation for self-care deficits can minimize excess disability. Education for patients and caregivers should include discussion of nutrition and hydration, exercise and mobility, aids for stable elimination (including bowel and bladder routines for the management of incon-

tinence), personal hygiene, and home safety. Areas frequently neglected include dental and foot care. Often, referral to a gerontological
nurse knowledgeable in the management of dementia is helpful in
dealing with these practical and preventive measures.

Sensory Deficits

Sensory deficits, particularly in vision and hearing, frequently
contribute to increased functional disability in the patient with dementia. Visual-spatial impairment, comprehension difficulties, and
problems of attention frequently limit the dementia patient's ability
to perceive sensory messages (and our ability to test sensory abilities).
Patients with dementia will need reminders to use eyeglasses and
hearing aids. New adaptive devices such as a "first time" hearing aid
may not be acceptable to the patient with dementia. If such devices
are likely to be necessary, it is best to introduce them early in the
course of the disease when the patient is best able to learn to use
them.

Continuing Care

As stated previously, clinical care of the patient with dementia
and of the caregivers is based on a care plan developed during diagnosis. The patient and caregivers should be seen on a regular basis
(generally every 6 months in the absence of acute problems) for reevaluation and reappraisal of the care plan. Episodic, problem-oriented
treatment alone does not adequately provide for the ongoing care of
a patient with progressive dementia.

The complexity of these patients and the current limitations of
medical treatment often prompt compromises with regard to care.
Problems cannot always be solved to complete satisfaction. Side effects
of medications are often accepted because of safety risks without the
medications. The risks of ambulation and the potential for falls must
be weighed against the risks of restraint. Later in the course of the
illness, the physician or nurse will often be the first professional
consulted about institutionalization. Decisions regarding life support
(i.e., treating acute illnesses or even, in later stages, the maintenance
of nourishment) should be addressed within a supportive clinical
relationship.

The primary care physician is the professional most capable of
teaching the family about the importance of autopsy. The family

should make early preparations with the mortician, hospital, nursing home, coroner's office, etc., to expedite this process and minimize stress for the family. Examination of brain tissue currently provides the only definitive way of making the diagnosis of AD. As knowledge of the familial occurrence of AD spreads, more families will want the certainty of an autopsy diagnosis. Although our understanding of the genetic risks in AD and related disorders is limited, the clinician has the responsibility of ensuring that genetic counseling is available for families who request it.

Conclusion

The clinical care of the patient with dementia starts with a care plan based on medical diagnosis and psychosocial assessment. The rapport established during the diagnostic process is essential to ongoing care. Medical management includes the treatment of remediable cognitive and behavioral symptoms as well as the prevention of excess disability due to physical illness, drug intoxication, and sensory deficits. Periodic reassessment of the patient and family should lead to appropriate modifications in the care plan as the disease progresses.

References

Brody, E. M., M. H. Kleban, M. P. Lawton, and H. Silverman. 1971. Excess disabilities of mentally impaired aged: Impact of individualized treatment. *Gerontologist* 11:124–33.

Fisk, A. A., and Pannill, F. C. 1987. Assessment and care of the community-dwelling Alzheimer's disease patient. *Journal of the American Geriatrics Society* 35 (4): 307–11.

Kahn, R. L. 1965. Comments. In *Mental impairment in the aged,* ed. M. P. Lawton and F. G. Lawton, 109–14. Philadelphia: Philadelphia Geriatric Centre.

Lipowski, Z. J. 1983. Transient cognitive disorders (delirium, acute confusional states) in the elderly. *American Journal of Psychiatry* 140:1426–36.

U.S. Congress. Office of Technology Assessment. 1987. *Losing a million minds: Confronting the tragedy of Alzheimer's disease and other dementias.* OTA-BA-323. Washington, D.C.: U.S. Government Printing Office. April.

Winograd, C. H., and Jarvik, L. F. 1986. Physician management of the demented patient. *Journal of the American Geriatrics Society* 34 (4): 295–308.

3

Intervention-Based Neuropsychological Assessment

SHELLY E. WEAVERDYCK, PH.D.

Premises Underlying and Explored in This Chapter

I. There are *many* possible explanations for behaviors or impairments in dementia (in response to the assumption that it's simply the dementia or brain damage that's "making them act that way"). These include:
    A. "nonperson" explanations, such as environment, task, caregiver;
    B. noncognitive explanations, such as motivation, affect, physical disorder (e.g., impaction or flu);
    C. cognitive explanations, such as problems with sensory, perceptual, executive, expressive, or motoric functions;
    D. competencies usually masked by impairments or by an appearance of overwhelming impairment resulting in assumptions of helplessness.
II. Four targets must be assessed: environment, task, caregiver, person.
III. A model of task complexity can be useful for assessment and intervention (for task modification) purposes.
IV. The following analyses are required in responsible assessment and intervention:
    A. task analysis—breaking tasks down into component steps;
    B. analysis of the cognitive functions underlying each task step;
    C. analysis of the cognitive functions underlying the execution of ADLs;

   D. analysis of the cognitive functions underlying undesirable behaviors.

V. Impairments and competencies can be localized along a theoretical cognitive path by which information is processed, including sensory, perceptual, executive, expressive, and motoric functions.

VI. An ecological approach to assessment and intervention is necessary.

VII. Caregivers and assessors must work hard to discern and respect the goals of the person with dementia.

VIII. Competencies, not primarily impairments, must be emphasized. Identification and description of competencies will:

   A. help the caregiver respect and appreciate the person with dementia;

   B. provide a basis for intervention that relies on and reinforces remaining skills;

   C. contribute to the general research and knowledge regarding dementia;

   D. alert the caregivers. Competencies are usually not obvious or recognized by caregivers in the face of the overwhelming impairments.

"Sir, do you know how to get back to this country?" Bea[1] asked as she emerged from the bathroom. Bea lived in a residential dementia unit and, upon emerging from the bathroom, she was seeking directions from the first person she encountered. The person from whom she sought help was a woman who was also a resident of the unit. The woman replied that she was going "home" and moved on.

Bea was the subject of some concern among the staff of the dementia unit. Two major changes had been evident in Bea's functioning level over the past few months: increasing difficulty in finding the bathroom and other rooms and increasing difficulty in dressing herself independently. The staff wondered whether these changes reflected

1. Bea was the subject of an intense neuropsychological case study of Alzheimer's disease presented in a Ph.D. dissertation by the author (Weaverdyck 1987). ("Bea" was referred to as "B" in the dissertation.) Some of the incidents, comments, and examples regarding Bea in this chapter are fictitious, but are based on fact as described by the author in the dissertation. Both names (Bea and B) are fictitious.

further brain degeneration or whether some other cause, perhaps more susceptible to intervention, was precipitating the changes. The apparent disorientation upon *emerging from* the bathroom seemed to be a recent development.

The staff noted that, although Bea had great difficulty finding the bathroom when she needed it, she did not usually seem to have as much trouble finding the kitchen, diningroom, livingroom, or her bedroom. A red awning hung over the bathroom door as a visual cue, but such cuing did not seem to enable Bea to find the bathroom without asking for directions. Staff members were concerned about the potential for incontinence resulting from this "disorientation" and were sometimes impatient with Bea's repeated requests for directions and occasional inability to respond to directions when given. They requested an assessment of Bea to develop an appropriate intervention for her apparent disorientation.

Staff members also were concerned about Bea's difficulty in getting dressed. Within a period of approximately six months, she had deteriorated from being able to dress herself with only occasional assistance in choosing clothes or fastening awkwardly placed hooks and eyes to an apparent need for extensive assistance throughout the entire dressing task. Some staff members claimed that she could do much more of the dressing task independently if allowed. It was unclear whether the deterioration in Bea's functioning resulted directly from her brain disease or from excessive staff assistance, which gradually encouraged Bea to "forget" how to dress out of disuse of her skills.

The staff wondered how useful an intervention, such as skill retraining, would be. They also wondered how cost effective any intervention, particularly one that involved retraining, would be. Much staff time would likely be devoted to the retraining and monitoring process because Bea was so slow. Would the resulting savings in staff time when Bea was more independent be worth the initial cost in staff time? If the deterioration were a direct manifestation of the increasing severity or spread of brain pathology, wouldn't the independence resulting from retraining be short-lived? Would the amount of staff time and attention available to other residents on the dementia unit be reduced while the potentially lengthy retraining was in process? In an attempt to answer some of the many questions of the staff, an assessment of Bea's current and potential levels of functioning was requested. From such an assessment, staff members hoped to develop with Bea reasonable goals and intervention strategies.

With their requests for an assessment of Bea, the staff had even more questions to consider. Who should conduct the assessment? What information would be gained, and how would it be useful? How extensive could the assessment be before the assessment, itself, became cost ineffective?

These, along with other questions that frequently confront caregivers of people with dementia, will be addressed in this chapter. The value and potential role of neuropsychological assessment (the assessment of cognition and of the relationship between behavior and the brain) in the development of interventions in dementia will be emphasized. There will be particular emphasis on the relevance of the assessment of cognition and of the general context in which cognition occurs to the understanding of a person's behavior (including "management problem behaviors") and performance on tasks of everyday living.

The conceptual outline of a suggested protocol for assessment is presented in this chapter, which is intended to enable a caregiver to explore the larger question, Why does Bea act this way? The assumption is that, once a caregiver has asked such "why" questions and attempted to discover the context and the roles of various factors contributing to the behavior or functioning level of an individual, ideas of what to do about the behavior or functioning level (i.e., ideas regarding intervention) will come more easily.

This chapter is not intended to be a review of the literature or of neuropsychological assessment protocols already in existence, nor is it an instructional text on how to administer successfully or interpret neuropsychological assessments of dementia victims, although both a review and a "how to" text are certainly needed (Brink 1986; Cohen 1982; Gilleard 1984; Hamsher 1983; Poon 1986; Zarit 1980). Instead, this chapter outlines some issues particularly relevant or unique to dementia and identifies the various types of questions and targets that should be focused upon when assessing an individual for the purpose of determining appropriate adaptations or interventions. [For specific methods or protocols for developing an intervention program based on systematic assessment of situations and individuals, see Weaverdyck (1987) and Weaverdyck (in preparation).]

The ultimate potential of success of a given intervention is dependent upon the patient's functional and behavioral status. Only a trained neuropsychologist can draw conclusions regarding the possible effects of brain pathology on that status, as evident in the cognitive functioning explored by the types of questions raised in this chapter. When the types of questions that allow such exploration of cognitive functioning and of noncognitive factors that affect cognitive functioning are identified, however, non-neuropsychologists can also see their value. Such questions can be used to understand and attempt intervention in the skill and behavior changes that frequently occur with dementia (Goldenberg and Chiverton 1984).

Whether or not the services of a neuropsychologist or a cognition specialist are available, the protocol conceptually presented here can be used by nonneuropsychologists. One advantage of the protocol outlined here is that a caregiver of nearly any level of sophistication can produce optional interventions after gaining a better understanding of "why the person seems to be doing that." The protocol enables any caregiver to ask questions that could enhance the understanding of causes of behaviors.

In this chapter, the issues pertinent to the assessment of someone with dementia will be discussed through the identification of the types of questions that must be asked by the caregivers (and by the person with dementia if able) and/or by the person conducting the assessment. Bea's difficulties in dressing and finding the bathroom will be used as examples throughout the chapter. By asking the types of questions raised here, the fundamental question of "Why does Bea act this way?" can perhaps be addressed.

The primary issues to be discussed are the objectives, targets, and methods of assessment. The targets of assessment are identified as the environment (including the physical, social, emotional, and intellectual environments), the tasks, the caregivers, and the person with dementia (see Table 3.1). The person as a target is discussed in sections that address the person's medical and physical status, history, stage of dementia, behavior, affect, social functioning, performance on activities of daily living, response to previously attempted interventions, and cognition.

The cognitive functioning of the individual is explored in detail in sections devoted to the various functions or skills involved in cognition. The specific skills are generally organized along a theoretical path through which information can be seen to be processed, including the ability to receive physically through the senses information

TABLE 3.1 Targets for the Assessment of Dementia

Environment
  Physical
  Social
  Emotional
  Cognitive
Task
Caregiver
Person
  Medical/physical status
  Premorbid history
  Stage of disorder
  Behavior
  Affect
  Social Functioning
  ADL performance as a measure of cognitive functioning
  Interventions attempted
  Cognition
    Sensory functions
    Perception and comprehension
    Attention
    Executive functions
      Memory
      Logic
      Abstraction
      Quantity appreciation
      Sequencing
      Choosing among options
      Planning
      Shifting mental set
      Initiation
    Expressive functions
    Motoric functions

from the environment, the ability to understand the information received, the ability to organize and manipulate the information, the ability of the brain to tell the body what to do (praxis), and the ability of the body to act motorically on the instructions of the brain. A section of general issues and difficulties in assessment concludes the chapter.

The Objectives of Assessment

Assessment generally serves two purposes, diagnosis and description. The diagnostic role of assessment includes the use of assessment to identify the disorder causing the assessed signs and symptoms. It might also suggest prognosis or the potential for reversal or retardation of disease progression. It sometimes defines a specific problem or objective.

The description role of assessment has as its objective the identification and description of the signs and symptoms of a disorder. It usually focuses on more detail and subtleties than does the routine diagnostic assessment. Descriptive assessment is used to monitor change over time, to classify (e.g., for "placement" purposes), to document (e.g., for reimbursement or for the purpose of demonstrating the effectiveness of a particular intervention), and to formulate a more detailed basis for intervention development. Descriptive assessment can inform decisions regarding the appropriate type and amount of intervention and the advisability of intervention. The questions raised in this chapter are important to both the diagnostic and the descriptive roles of assessment.

Before meeting the person to be assessed, it is important to identify the basic objectives of the assessment itself. Initially, one must answer the following questions: Why is the assessment to be conducted? Is it primarily for research, theory, or clinical purposes? Who is asking for the assessment (caregiver, professional specialist, the patient)? Who will use the information resulting from the assessment (the same person who asked for the assessment, a specialist who will simply file the information, a caregiver)? How will the information be used (to "place" someone in an appropriate intervention program or care setting, to build an individualized intervention program, to compare this individual with a described population with dementia)? What are the ultimate goals of the user (improvement of quality of life for the patient and the caregiver, reduction of certain undesirable behaviors, improvement of performance on activities of daily living tasks)?

In this chapter, we will assume that assessment is primarily for the purpose of intervention development and for the environmental adaptation to the person's functioning and/or behavior. For such general purposes, a variety of objectives usually exist:

1. identification of the individual's competencies and deficits with regard to specific tasks;
2. evaluation of the individual's cognitive functioning (i.e., the extent to which various cognitive skills remain intact or are impaired);
3. establishment of a baseline of behaviors and functioning levels and ongoing monitoring of change;
4. determination of the extent to which functioning and/or behaviors may be attributed to each of the following common sources: environment, affective factors (such as motivation and psychopathology), excessive caregiver assistance, physical/medical disability, and brain dysfunction; and
5. determination of the conditions under which the individual is competent or incompetent and under which specific behaviors occur.

There may be more objectives, particularly as the fundamental objectives of the anticipated intervention become clear (Weaverdyck 1987). The five objectives outlined are described and elaborated upon throughout the chapter.

In the case of Bea, the questions asked by the staff reflect a concern both with a disruptive behavior (repetitive requests for directions which, according to staff members, are distracting and annoying) that they would like to reduce and with an increasing impairment of functioning on a task of daily living (dressing), which may reflect increasing cognitive impairment. The staff seemed to want information that would allow them to reduce the impairments and to enhance successful independent dressing skills without unduly increasing demands on staff time. In Bea's case, both undesirable (to the caregiver) behavior and cognitive functioning were of concern. The primary objective of the staff seemed to be enhancement of self-esteem and satisfaction on the part of Bea, herself.

Although Bea's own objectives may be difficult for the staff to discern, it is very important to discover and articulate them as clearly and accurately as possible. The accurate identification of Bea's goals is necessary to the success of the resulting intervention and to the enhancement of Bea's own self-esteem. The objectives of Bea and those of the staff may at some points conflict. Such conflicts, including those among any other interested parties, require resolution before an assessment satisfactory to all can be conducted.

Targets of Assessment

Assessments may be situational or general. In situational assessments, specifically targeted behaviors or tasks are observed and the conditions under which they occur are documented. Some of these documented conditions include the cognitive demands of the tasks or situation, affective factors such as the expectations of the person and of others in the environment for the person's behavior or for that of others in the environment, physical environmental factors (including other people present), stress levels and demands (Hall and Buckwalter 1987), antecedent events (Hussian and Davis 1985), and the time and duration of the event or behavior. General assessments attempt to document an individual's general level of functioning or the general pattern of factors affecting the manifestation of particular behaviors. The protocol conceptually outlined here applies to both situational and general assessment; both are necessary to the development of effective intervention.

There are four targets of an assessment in dementia: the environment, the task, the caregiver, and the person with the dementia (see Table 3.1). One objective of an assessment is to determine the actual and potential role and degree of impact of each of these targets on the individual's behaviors and functioning levels. This teasing out of the various contributing factors is a major step in the identification of possible sources of impairment and of conditions under which competent functioning could potentially be enhanced.

Environment

In this context, environment includes the physical, emotional, social, and cognitive or intellectual environments. Environment is usually considered to be the personal, immediate environment of the individual, such as the dementia unit for Bea. It also includes the immediate context of observed behaviors and cognitive functioning, both temporally and spatially. For example, the situations in which Bea asks for help in getting to the bathroom would be assessed. Where is she usually when she asks? What time of day is it when she asks? What occurs before and immediately after her requests for help? Sometimes the larger environment, such as society in general, is considered. The role of society's perception of Bea in her social environment, for example, may have a significant impact on her behavior (Wolfensberger 1972). Chapter 9 discusses in more detail the role and potential of the environment. (Also see Weaverdyck, in preparation.)

The fundamental question asked when assessing the environment is, How does this person's environment affect (i.e., help or hinder) this person's functioning? In examining Bea's physical environment, the assessor may consider the extent to which the environment cues and orients Bea. Are there directional signs? Is the lighting helpful or distracting (e.g., glaring for older people)? Is the bathroom door clearly visible from all vantage points (e.g., is the visual cue three-dimensional, so that it can be seen down the hall)? When Bea asks for help, is she near the bathroom door or in another room? What are the relative distances between the bathroom, bedroom, kitchen, and livingroom? The last two questions may suggest the possibility that Bea remembers how to get to the bathroom for a particular duration but then forgets before she actually gets there. It may be, too, that she has more difficulty remembering locations that are more distant (and therefore less frequently seen and rehearsed, perhaps) from her usual hub of activity. On Bea's dementia unit, in fact, the bathroom was approximately thirty feet in one direction and the diningroom approximately twenty feet in the opposite direction from her bedroom. The livingroom and kitchen were immediately next to the diningroom, so the frequency with which Bea saw or inhabited the diningroom, livingroom, or kitchen was probably greater than the frequency with which she saw or inhabited the bathroom. Furthermore, the bathroom was behind a closed door and therefore less visible, whereas the other rooms had open doors and were inhabited more visibly (Weaverdyck 1987).

The social environment includes the general social milieu and its demands, as well as the frequency and nature of Bea's social interactions. Bea's emotional attachment to or investment in her various social interactions would also be assessed. What are the social expectations of Bea? Do staff members expect her to be able to dress herself, or is passivity subtly encouraged? Are there specific individuals with whom Bea seems to have personality clashes? Whom does she usually ask for help? Does she dress more independently with some caregivers than with others? Does Bea find visiting with peers rewarding?

The emotional climate may be a major factor contributing to Bea's functional and cognitive performance. Is the ambience of the unit envigorating, stimulating, and light-hearted, or is it oppressively dull or depressing? Is there an air of urgency or anxiety promoted by rushing or impersonal caregivers? Bea frequently exhibited anxiety, through behaviors such as restless pacing or withdrawal, when there was an unexpected change in routine or when staff members were particularly rushed.

The extent to which an environment is intellectually stimulating may affect a person's arousal or energy level (Kendrick 1972; Miller 1977a, 1977b). Does the environment in terms of its expectations, opportunities, level of general activity, sensory stimulation, and cognitive demands appropriately stimulate the individual to think creatively, problem solve, and take responsibility? Does the environment provide motivation to maintain or improve cognitive functioning?

Of particular concern in dementia assessment is the consistency in and congruency among the physical, social, emotional, and intellectual environments. Are cues, for example, consistent? Are the same cues used each time a task is attempted, or do the cues change unpredictably? When staff members give Bea directions to the bathroom, does each staff person give Bea identical or at least similar directions? Are the identification signs on the bathroom door permanent, or do they change depending on the staff working that day?

Environmental congruency is particularly important, although perhaps more difficult to maintain (Weaverdyck and Coons 1988; Weaverdyck, in preparation). Is there environmental congruency among cues, for example, as well as within the various environments? Is there congruency with the person's past? Do the cues in the person's environment match the caregiver's or others' expectations of the individual? Is the social environment (i.e., the caregiving staff), for example, encouraging Bea to dress independently in a physical environment with no cues to tell her where her clothes are? Do family members implicitly tell Bea that she is an independent resident of an apartment or hotel room, while the physical and social environments implicitly tell Bea that she is a patient in a hospital-like setting?

One illustration of the effects of incongruency among environmental cues and expectations occurred when the author was conducting some cognitive assessments of persons with dementia in a long-term care facility. A group was sitting around a table appropriately performing tasks with small assessment blocks. When a staff person entered and put bibs on each of the group members in preparation for lunch, several of the members suddenly began putting the blocks into their mouths as though to eat them! Clearly, the bibs introduced conflicting environmental cues and expectations.

The nature of environmental cues and the extent to which the cues accommodate the individual's preferences and skills are also assessed. Are cues emotionally and aesthetically appealing? If the person cannot read, or cannot remember the existence or location of rooms that are not visible from where he is standing, or is unable to articulate or even recognize his own desires at the moment, are the available cues effective with him? Are there cues that attract at an emotional level rather than simply at an intellectual level? For example, instead of signs with arrows pointing to a quiet, cozy den area, is there a path created by a series of strategically placed attractive, luxurious plants? Each of these plants could be seen (and therefore, could attract or lure a person at an emotional level) around each corner until the person reaches the den. When he sees each plant and the den, he is, perhaps unconsciously, drawn to it when he is in the mood for a quiet, cozy den.

Interventions currently in use, such as environmental interventions [e.g., milieu therapy (Coons 1983)], behavioral therapy (Hussian 1986), or individualized intervention programs (Beck et al. 1985; Weaverdyck 1987) would also be examined in an environmental assessment. The examination would include the nature, frequency, duration, and effectiveness of the attempted interventions.

Task

The task or activity in which the individual with dementia is engaged or is expected to be engaged must be assessed to evaluate or predict the individual's performance and to assess the extent to which the task is appropriate to that individual. Such an assessment could also aid in the selection of the type of help (e.g., prompting versus encouragement versus demonstration) that would most closely match the task demands with the individual's cognitive functioning (Weaverdyck 1987; Weaverdyck, in preparation).

The task must be assessed in terms of its cognitive, emotional, social, physical, and sensory demands (Weaverdyck, in preparation). The nature of the materials or objects manipulated in the task must also be examined. Are the stimuli or task objects concrete or abstract, visual or auditory? Are they conducive to left-handed or right-handed use (such as in a pair of scissors)? In an assessment of a task, the task is usually broken down into its component steps or skill requirements. Each step of the task is analyzed for its demands and properties. The individual's ability to perform each step is also analyzed after as-

TABLE 3.2 Model of Task Complexity

Feature	Task Steps	Content Elements	Body Parts
		Task Component	
Number			
Variety			
Abstractness			
Novelty			

Source: Adapted from Weaverdyck 1987.

sessment through direct observation (Coons 1983; Diller and Gordon 1981; Gold 1980; Hodge 1984; Kennedy and Kennedy 1982; Robinson et al. 1987; Weaverdyck 1987).

Frequently, the most appropriate intervention is one in which the task is modified to suit an individual's particular competencies and impairments. There may be specific dimensions to a task that determine its general level of complexity for someone with dementia and, hence, the ease with which an individual with dementia can successfully accomplish it. Table 3.2 identifies some possible dimensions.

As shown in Table 3.2, increased complexity can be defined as an increase in number, variety, abstractness, or novelty (positioned along the vertical axis) in one or more of three components (positioned along the horizontal axis): task steps, content elements, and personal body parts to operate (Weaverdyck 1987). Content elements refer to the objects or materials manipulated in the task, such as clothing in the dressing task.

Presumably, by reducing any one or more of the task features identified in Table 3.2 in terms of one or more of the task components, the task can be simplified to allow successful and independent execution by the person with dementia. An example of this would be the dressing task. With its many varied content elements (garments) and its involvement of nearly all parts of the body in many task steps, the number and variety of task components are very high. The abstract and novel qualities of the task components are, however, generally much lower. It is perhaps the latter two features, the concreteness and familiarity of the task, that allow people with dementia to continue to dress themselves as long as they do.

As the person's functioning becomes increasingly impaired, reducing the number of task steps by having the caregiver do the first steps or reducing the number of content elements by having the caregiver put on the dress and shoes may be all that is needed to allow the person to perform the rest of the task independently. (For one possible delineation of the steps involved in the dressing task and for possible modifications of a task's complexity, see Weaverdyck 1987.)

To some extent, a neuropsychologist could also identify the cognitive functions underlying each of the steps of a task and ascertain the level of intactness of the various brain structures that mediate each cognitive function. Such an analysis would depend, of course, upon the results of the assessments of each of the other assessment targets, including the environment, the caregiver, and the person with dementia.

Caregiver

Zarit and colleagues (1985) and Cohen and Eisdorfer (1986) noted the integral role of the health of the caregiver in the care of a victim of dementia. Zarit et al. (1985) referred to the family members of the affected individual as the hidden victims of the disorder. No intervention program and hence no assessment protocol can succeed without the willingness and ability of the caregiver (whether family member or staff member of a care facility) to implement the intervention. In fact, to a great extent, as we saw in the vignette introducing this chapter, the intervention plan must in some way also benefit the caregiver for it to be beneficial in the long term to the individual with dementia.

The care of someone afflicted with dementia is exceedingly stressful and fatiguing, both physically and emotionally. This overwhelming fatigue is evident in the deteriorating social and mental health of family caregivers (Chenoweth and Spencer 1986; Cohen and Eisdorfer 1986; Zarit et al. 1985) and in the high rate of staff burnout in long-term care facilities (Hoffman et al. 1987; Kane and Kane 1982).

The quality of care and resulting level of functioning depends to a great extent upon the skill, tolerance, patience, flexibility, and endurance of the primary caregiver. Assessment of the caregiver, then, would include evaluation of the caregiver's mental health, physical health, and social support systems. It would also include assessment of the family's financial status and the legal relationship between the caregiver and the individual with dementia because aspects of finances and legal guardianship and power affect directly the emotional relationships in the care of people with dementia (Mace and Rabins 1981; Cohen and Eisdorfer 1986).

Particularly important in the cognitive functioning of the individual with dementia are the specific nonverbal and verbal interactions between the caregiver and the individual (Bartol 1979; Burnside 1981). Are the interactions generally supportive, encouraging, appropriately challenging, affectionate, and sensitive to specific cognitive changes? Is the caregiver alert to and trained to attend to the particular cognitive competencies and deficits experienced by the dementia victim? Are the caregiver's expectations of the individual appropriate? Does the caregiver know when to wait, when to assist, and when to do something for the individual?

Alertness and sensitivity on the part of the caregiver can make the difference between apparent competence and incompetence on the part of the person with dementia. Frequently, when a caregiver subtly organizes information for a person or subtly gives reminders of pertinent information, the person is able to participate meaningfully in a conversation or interaction.

Is the caregiver trained and invested in the implementation of intervention in general? Is the caregiver ready and willing to engage in a particular intervention plan? Such assessment of the caregiver is critical to the health of both the caregiver and the dementia victim, as well as to the success of the intervention (see Weaverdyck, in preparation).

Person

The most complex and the most recognized target of dementia assessment, of course, is the person with dementia. This is the primary target of assessment in diagnostic evaluations. In descriptive assessments, it is also the most enigmatic.

There are nine basic aspects upon which to focus when assessing the individual for the purposes of intervention development:

medical/physical status;
premorbid history;
stage or position in the progression of the disease state;
behavior;
affect;

social functioning;
performance in activities of daily living (ADL);
interventions attempted; and
cognitive functioning.

Medical/Physical Status

Because individual and combinations of medications in the older person can frequently cause unpredictable side effects, such as confusion or "exaggerated" impaired functioning, it is important to examine a person's medications early in the assessment process (see Chapter 1). A diuretic may be the primary source of Bea's problems.

A physical or medical abnormality or change, including fecal impaction, dehydration, or fever, can also cause cognitive impairment (see Chapter 1). Therefore, the individual's medical status must also be constantly monitored.

It is important to assess the individual's physical status. How is this person's range of motion, for example? Can she reach her arms up high enough to put her arms into the dress sleeves? Sometimes, such a relatively minor difficulty can be enough to cause the individual to abandon a task completely. Are there any other major or minor disabilities in any of the person's extremities? Does she use a walker? Is the pace at which Bea walks slow enough that she cannot retain a memory long enough to find the bathroom? Obviously, Bea would be checked thoroughly for urinary tract infection, etc. Along with the physical status, the chronological age of the person is noted, as are any other physical conditions common to that particular age group.

Premorbid History

As noted in Chapters 1 and 2, history is an essential component of the diagnostic evaluation, and it is just as essential in a descriptive assessment. Although information should be confirmed by a reliable source, the dementia victim's ability to recall events, places, and people from the past when contemporary events and people are forgotten has been mentioned frequently by clinicians and researchers (Kral 1970; Miller 1977a; Moscovitch 1982). Such past events and people may play a much more significant part in the person's own world or reality than do the people or events in the contemporary (i.e., objectively real) situation.

Clearly, the more a caregiver knows about the person's social, emotional, occupational, educational, geographic, family, and medical history, the more effective will be the care giving. The caregiver may be more able to decipher a person's needs, desires, and abilities or to engage in meaningful conversations about events or people important to the individual. Changes in the person's level of functioning or in life-style can also be identified. In the face of such overwhelming deficits, it is frequently difficult to imagine, much less recall, the sophistication and integrity of the person that once was. A detailed history makes it much easier for paid caregivers, in particular, to treat the individual with respect and with a genuine interest.

With regard to cognition, the history is extremely important in identifying lasting habits and preferences. If Bea has always put her socks and shoes on before her dress, it would likely enhance her independent functioning if she were encouraged to continue that order of dressing. In dementia, there may be an increasing reliance on routines (particularly overlearned routines in which the person has engaged throughout her life) that allow the individual to avoid consciously attending to the task (Moscovitch 1982; Weaverdyck 1987). In this regard, habits are crucial to independence.

Similarly, habits and preferences for particular sleep patterns and periods of alertness are important. Someone who has always been a "night person" may continue to function better in the evening than in the morning.

Of particular importance are the individual's past experiences with coping strategies and "cognitive style" (Kogan 1982). It is frequently useful to be familiar with the individual's past successes and mistakes and with past strategies for coping with stress or traumatic life events. Such familiarity can also help in identifying the coping strategies that the individual may be adopting currently in response to the dementing disorder. An individual's cognitive style, the manner in which an individual perceives and uses information (Kogan 1982), can also be examined by analyzing evidence of the individual's premorbid cognitive behavior. A neuropsychologist is particularly interested in discerning the individual's premorbid intelligence so that changes in specific cognitive skills can be identified.

Perhaps most importantly, the person's own values and life goals may become more apparent through an examination of the premorbid history. In developing intervention strategies, adoption of the person's own goals are of crucial importance to both the integrity and the effectiveness of the intervention. It is, at times, extremely difficult to detect such goals in the person's current behaviors, particularly when the person is unable to articulate reactions or desires verbally. Frequently, the person states apparent goals that may not be true goals or unconsciously acts on goals that are obscure to the caregiver or contradictory to the individual's stated intentions or desires. An examination of the premorbid history may lend some perspective to the discernment of the person's genuine lifelong and short-term goals.

The Stage of the Disorder

There is some controversy regarding the necessity and validity of identifying stages of a disease such as Alzheimer's disease (Miller and Cohen 1981, 55; Reisberg et al. 1982). For the purposes of this chapter, we will simply note that the manifest signs and symptoms of the particular diagnosed disorder in this individual are important to identify and monitor. Which symptoms appear to be "typical"? Which are unusual? How long has the disorder been evident (i.e., time since onset)? What is the genetic history of the disorder in this person's family? What were the behaviors and symptoms of similar disorders among family members? What changes in cognitive functions might be anticipated? Such an assessment may suggest to caregivers those symptoms that might be amenable to interventions and those that might be more resistant.

Behavior

Some behaviors, such as wandering, pacing, combativeness, incontinence, sexual inappropriateness, repetitive actions or questioning, and hoarding are frequently found among people with dementia (Burnside 1980; Gwyther 1985) (see Chapter 4). To what extent are these behaviors evident in the person to be assessed? Usually, the frequency, duration, and context (temporal, spatial, and social) of the behaviors are assessed.

As was noted in the section on environments, the context in which a specific behavior occurs is usually important. The impetus for the behavior may be environmental or internal. The assessor observes a series of occurrences of the identified behavior to note commonalities among the contexts and the emotional or cognitive status of the individual. Such commonalities may be a clue to the locus of the impetus, thereby suggesting a possible target for intervention.

Very frequently, a behavior identified as undesirable by the caregiver precipitates an assessment. In such an assessment, it is important to identify the reasons that the caregiver perceives the behavior as undesirable, as well as to discover how the person with dementia experiences the behavior. Hussian and Davis (1985) described from a behavioral point of view various motives for excessive behaviors (behaviors that are unusually or undesirably frequent) and deficient behaviors (behaviors or abilities that are manifest too infrequently). They also described behavioral assessment and intervention techniques to address those behaviors.

A neuropsychologist would analyze behaviors (both excessive and deficient) from a cognitive point of view. To what extent are the excessive behaviors, such as pacing and repetitively buttoning and unbuttoning a sweater, self-stimulatory (possibly resulting from stimulation deprivation within the environment), and to what extent are they perseverative (resulting from, for example, frontal lobe dysfunction)? Bea, who frequently paced, seemed to pace primarily when she was restless, bored, or anxious. This was determined by, among other methods, observing when she paced, the commonalities among her facial and verbal expressions as she paced, and the behaviors and events that usually preceded her pacing. Although the actual cause of her pacing was not clear, caregiver familiarity with the conditions surrounding her pacing could help accommodate, avert, or reduce the pacing considerably.

Affect

The emotional status of the individual plays a major role in that patient's response to interventions and to the symptoms of the disorder. Depression, which frequently accompanies dementia and which is a major cause of confusion among older people, may be related to the individual's capacity for insight into her or his own cognitive and mental health status, to an affective disorder, or to the disease process itself. Assessment and intervention in the depression may alleviate the identified behavior or cognitive dysfunction. (See Chapters 1 and 2.)

The assessment is an attempt to identify the role of affective factors (such as anxiety, motivation, paranoia, psychosis, emotional lability, anger, and catastrophic reaction) in the behavioral and cognitive performance of the individual. An evaluation of incidences of combativeness, for example, may suggest that the individual is unusually sensitive to controlling behaviors by the caregiver and responds by striking "back." On the other hand, the evaluation may suggest that the person is too anxious and frightened to comprehend objectively the benign intentions of the caregiver. In many cases, affective and cognitive factors interact to create undesirable behavioral excesses or impairments in the activities of daily living. It may be discovered through the assessment that an affective factor such as paranoia has been long-standing, in which case the probability of alleviating it is reduced.

Bea's frequent apparent inability to find the bathroom may have a variety of affective explanations. Among them could be the following three. Bea experiences a psychopathological avoidance of the responsibility of acknowledging or using the bathroom. Bea relieves her loneliness or boredom by using requests for directions as an opportunity to establish contact with staff. A generalized or specific anxiety prompts Bea to seek reassurance by receiving assistance from staff. There are more possible factors. The roles of as many such factors as possible are investigated during a proper assessment.

Social Functioning

It is not uncommon for people with Alzheimer's disease to retain their ability to, at least superficially, interact socially with appropriate verbal and behavioral clichés. They know how to make "small talk," for example, so that frequently an observer does not recognize the disorder until several minutes into the conversation when the person either begins to repeat statements or begins to state obviously erroneous "facts."

The extent to which a person seems to care about and is able to monitor her or his social image may be indicative of intact cognitive functioning. Such an ability to self-monitor, however limited, may be helpful in planning the specific contexts, consequences (e.g., reinforcement in behavioral interventions), and inducements in intervention development.

An awareness of the quality and quantity of the individual's social contacts may be useful in intervention planning. How does this individual interact with peers, caregivers, family members, or friends? Assessment of Bea's social interactions, for example, could have implications in a search for someone to assist her to the bathroom.

ADL Performance as a Measure of Cognitive Functioning

A detailed assessment of the individual's performance on each step of a variety of activities of daily living (ADL), such as dressing, toileting, bathing, and eating, is important for classification (e.g.,

determination of appropriate placement within a long-term care facility) and documentation purposes. It is also useful for monitoring
change, as in evaluation of the efficacy of a given intervention (when
performance on ADL is assessed before and after an intervention is
introduced), and for evaluating the individual's cognitive functioning.

An evaluation of cognitive functioning through assessment of
ADL performance involves breaking the particular ADL task down
into component steps and identifying the cognitive functions mini-
mally required for the successful and independent execution of each
step. (See under "Task" in this chapter.) Such cognitive functions may
include, for example, a particular type of memory, object recognition,
attention, sequencing, or various aspects of spatial organization. The
specific roles of factors such as the environment, caregiver, task demands, and affective elements in the performance of each step must
be accounted for. An examination of the role of the individual's cognitive functioning includes the discovery of patterns of impairment
and competency in the individual's cognitive functioning by noting
the frequency with which the various cognitive functions identified
as underlying the task steps seem to be implicated in those steps
successfully and unsuccessfully executed. [See Weaverdyck (1987) for
further elaboration and examples.]

The implications of such a "cognitive skill-task analysis" for intervention purposes were briefly noted in the section on the task as
a target for assessment. Not only can the task be analyzed and then
modified to increase independent functioning, but the cognitive functions themselves can be addressed in an intervention. By targeting
the underlying cognitive functions rather than simply the manifest
behavior or skill, one may encourage gains from the intervention that
may generalize more readily to other tasks and contexts. For example,
if through assessment and analysis it is determined that the inability
to recognize an object's orientation in space relative to other objects
is the problem underlying some of Bea's dressing difficulties, then
environmental adaptations to compensate for or to remediate the
disability by, for example, highlighting salient orienting features of
important objects may result in improved functioning in general. To
help her dress, a staff person may position her dress sleeve near her
arm; to help her find the bathroom, staff may verbally inform Bea of
the location of the bathroom relative to the other doorways.

In dementia, it is important to assess actual performance on the
ADL task itself, in addition to performance on tasks manipulated and

structured by the examiner (as in conventional neuropsychological tests and most dementia screening instruments) (Albert 1981). Observation of the actual ADL performance can increase the ecological validity (i.e., the ability of the measure to reflect actual functioning in the individual's own environment) of the assessment. In dementia, ecological validity is particularly important for many reasons.

First, people with dementia seem to perform optimally on tasks and in contexts that are familiar to them. In fact, the functioning level clinically seems to increase with increasing familiarity; on overlearned tasks, performance may often appear to be entirely intact (Mace and Rabins 1981; Cohen and Eisdorfer 1986; Fuld 1983). (Systematic investigation of the cognitive and behavioral aspects of dementia is relatively recent. As a result, very few clinical observations of cognitive functioning in dementia have been corroborated by empirical research.) The introduction of an esoteric, standardized laboratory test or pencil and paper test may reduce the subject's performance by virtue of its unfamiliar and anxiety-producing content, procedures, and assumptions. Most dementia victims have not taken such tests at all recently or perhaps ever. An accurate assessment of the person's optimal or even prevalent level of cognitive or behavioral functioning, therefore, is very difficult with conventional assessment measures and procedures.

Second, for intervention purposes, caregivers generally prefer information that can be directly translated into practical applications. By assessing Bea's performance on the dressing task directly, the examiner may be able to suggest more specific modifications in the task, environment, or caregiver-person interaction. The examiner would also probably be able to offer more applicable impressions regarding the potential for functioning by the individual and perhaps possible reasons for impaired performance. Understanding of the specific cognitive functions involved and the implications of cognitive impairments with respect to everyday functioning and intervention may also be enhanced. For behavioral modification interventions, it is of course important to know which steps of the task need attention by the caregiver and which can be performed by the individual with no intervention (McEvoy and Patterson 1986). The limitations of relating neuropsychological assessment, both in clinical settings and in the laboratories of experimental research, to everyday functioning and intervention for the general population (Diller and Gordon 1981; Heaton and Pendleton 1981) and, in particular, for older impaired adults (Baddeley et al. 1982; Vitaliano et al. 1984; Weintraub et al. 1982) have been the subject of much discussion and concern.

ADL tasks to be assessed could include bathing, dressing, toileting, brushing teeth, eating, grooming, setting the table, clearing dishes from the table or counter, washing/drying dishes, vacuuming the carpet, and watering plants. Even simple tasks such as donning a hat could be usefully assessed.

Interventions Attempted

It may be obvious that an evaluation of past and current caregiver-initiated interventions could be useful in identifying successes to emulate and mistakes to avoid in subsequent intervention planning and implementation. Assessment of past and current interventions could also include those initiated and conducted by the individual. It is particularly instructive to note which strategies an individual has adopted in response to the disorder. These strategies may reflect preferences or retained abilities on the part of the individual.

One important strategy to be assessed is the individual's own help-seeking behaviors. Is help sought when needed/not needed? From whom is help usually sought? How frequently is it sought? Is help generally effective when it is received? What type of help seems to be most effective?

Cognition

The final aspect of the person to be assessed, and in this chapter of central concern, is the individual's cognitive functioning. As was noted in the section on ADL, cognitive functioning can be assessed through conventional cognitive assessment instruments and techniques or through skilled observation of performance on ADL.

Cognition is, of course, the primary focus of neuropsychological assessment. The primary goal of the neuropsychological assessment is the identification of intact and impaired cognitive functioning, which may reflect the function/dysfunction of various brain structures. Neuropsychological assessment also lays the foundation for responsible and efficacious cognitive intervention. Cognitive intervention is an attempt to address the cognitive functions that underlie the performances seen on tasks such as those of ADL and others. By focusing on the cognitive functions, rather than simply on the task performance, a more precise intervention focus can be defined, which may therefore lead to increased generalization of the intervention results. (See the previous sections on tasks and ADL.)

A neuropsychological understanding of the disease progression may aid in prognosis or in a tentative identification of cognitive skills that may be retained for a longer period. These "longer-lasting" skills could possibly be relied upon and trained to compensate for the cognitive skills that are lost earlier in the disease process.

The procedures by which neuropsychologists conventionally assess cognitive functioning rely primarily on inferences drawn from directly observed performance on psychological tasks presented and controlled by the examiner. These tasks are usually pencil and paper tasks, verbal tasks, or tasks that involve small motor manipulation of objects (Lezak 1983).

Neuropsychologists have been encouraged to adopt a more ecological approach to the assessment of dementia. This approach involves either directly observing subjects in spontaneous performance of tasks typically executed by them throughout their daily lives and in their own familiar environment or observing subjects in typical (for the subjects) daily tasks that are elicited and manipulated by the examiner.

Through cognitive (i.e., neuropsychological) assessment, the assessor attempts to identify the individual's premorbid level of intelligence to allow a comparison with the current level of cognitive functioning. A second major task of the assessor is to differentiate the lower (sensory and motoric) cognitive functions from the higher (e.g., thinking, problem solving, memory, and creativity) cognitive functions (Smith 1975). There is some evidence that, in dementia, the lower cognitive functions are generally more intact than the higher cognitive functions (Fuld 1983; Lezak 1983; Woods and Britton 1985). This has major implications for intervention in, for example, the selection of task steps that an individual is encouraged to perform. The person with dementia will more likely need help with those steps that require memory than with those that require primarily seeing or hearing.

In this chapter, the assessed cognitive functions are discussed in the order in which information can be seen to be processed (see Table 3.1). First, the sensory functions (physical reception of a stimulus), then perception and comprehension (recognition of the stimulus), the executive functions (the ability to organize and manipulate the received information), the expressive functions (the ability of the brain to tell the body what to do), and, finally, the motoric functions (the physical response to the brain's commands) are discussed. By analyzing each aspect of functioning, one may be able to determine the extent to which cognitive processing breaks down at each point in a given individual's case.

Sensory

Assessment of the individual's ability to see, hear, feel, taste, and smell is important in the cognitive assessment. Many times, particularly among older dementia victims, one or more of these senses are impaired. The effectiveness of environmental cues depends upon the integrity of the sensory system.

Identification of apparently preferred sensory modalities is also necessary. In Bea's case, assessment suggested that she had a preference for auditory over visual stimuli. If the red awning over the bathroom door had been replaced or augmented by an auditory cue, such as running water, it might have been more effective.

Perception and Comprehension

The person's ability to understand instructions and conversations and to recognize an object is included in comprehension and perception. Also assessed, for example, is the person's ability to judge distance and the relative orientation of objects in space. When Bea sees the red awning or the bathroom door, does she recognize where she is in relation to it? Does she recognize how far she must go to get to it? Does Bea know where her arm is relative to the armhole of the dress? If she moves her arm, does she recognize the actual change in distance and spatial orientation of her arm relative to the armhole? Does she recognize the distance between two landmarks in her environment?

Does Bea recognize size and the relative size of objects? Does she recognize some colors or shapes better than others? Does she recognize her own body parts and her right from her left side?

Sometimes a person sees an object but does not recognize it and does not associate the object with its typical use. Does Bea recognize what a dress is and that it is typically worn on the body? Perhaps Bea simply does not recognize objects in part of her visual field. Does Bea recognize only the rooms on the wall to her left? If she were to approach the bathroom from the other end of the hall, would she recognize it more often? Does Bea sometimes seem to "forget" to dress on one side or part of her body? Does she tend to wear only one shoe or comb only one side of her hair? (See Wolanin and Phillips 1981.) Does Bea seem unable to distinguish the individual parts of a whole object or, conversely, is she able to see only the parts of an object but not the whole object (Lezak 1983)? Does Bea recognize faces, particularly those that are familiar to her?

Frequently, music is a valuable source of stimulation or soothing influence. Does the person recognize the pitch and rhythm of music? Is this person able to recognize individual letters and the combination of letters into words? Can Bea understand the directional signs posted on the wall and on the door of the bathroom? Does she have more difficulty understanding oral instructions or written instructions?

Orientation can also be considered to be perceptual in some respects. When Bea is in the hall, does she recognize where she is? Does the bathroom look and feel familiar to her? Orientation for time and for person is also assessed.

Attention

The ability of the person to concentrate or to attend is important to note. Does Bea listen to the staff give directions to the bathroom? Does she hear the first part and then get distracted by another stimulus? Does the time required to deliver the directions simply exceed the length of time that Bea is capable of focusing on one item?

What role does an inability to attend possibly play in Bea's difficulties with dressing? Does she get distracted part way through the task or even part way through each task step?

Is Bea able to recognize and react selectively to the various stimuli that bombard her simultaneously, or does she seem to react only to the most powerful stimulus at any given time? Would the use of very powerful stimuli at a multiple sensory level or the reduction of powerful distracting environmental stimuli focus her attention more effectively in interventions? What role are internal stimuli (such as fatigue and stomach pains) playing in her distraction from possibly weaker environmental stimuli?

Is Bea sometimes better able to accomplish a task, such as buttoning up her sleeve cuffs, when she is not attending to it and is, instead, thinking about something else (Weaverdyck 1987)?

Executive Functions

There are many cognitive functions involving organization and manipulation of information, which could be classified as "executive" (Lezak 1982, 1983). In this chapter, memory, logic, abstraction, appreciation of quantity, sequencing, choosing among options, planning (including the generation of options), shifting mental set, and initiation are identified (see Table 3.1). There are, of course, other executive functions.

Memory

Memory, as defined here, includes both new learning (the ability to acquire and retain unfamiliar information) and the retrieval of stored information that was acquired in the past. The increasing reliance, in dementia, on familiarity and overlearned task performance has been noted (Fuld 1983; Weaverdyck 1987; Weaverdyck and Coons 1988). Also common in dementia is impairment of the ability to acquire new information.

In a cognitive assessment, the individual's ability to learn is examined. When a person has difficulty learning new information, the effectiveness of intervention that involves retraining and the acquisition of new skills or information is jeopardized.

Several aspects of memory are examined in an assessment, including the registration, storage, and retrieval of various types of content. These types of content may include information (such as names of siblings), motor skills (Moscovitch 1982), and events (Kral 1970). (See also Poon 1986.) For example, does Bea remember what a bathroom or door is? Has she learned that the red awning means women's bathroom? Does she remember skills such as tying shoes or buttoning sleeve cuffs? Many times a person is able to perform a skill such as donning a dress but is unaware of having the ability (Martin 1987; Moscovitch 1982; Schacter et al. 1983). Does the individual require reassurance or feedback to perform a task? Of events such as a birthday party, is the whole or parts remembered? Are only the emotional aspects of the event remembered?

When learning new information, such as the changed location of a chest of drawers or the face of a new assistant, is the information recorded? Is the information stored, or is it lost immediately? When the information is actually recorded and retained, can it be retrieved by the individual when wanted? Does retrieval (or any stage of new learning) of both recently and previously learned content depend upon conscious or unconscious attempts by the individual? For example, can Bea put a sweater on when she concentrates on the task? Can she don a sweater when she is focused on another event or concern, such as "going home"?

Particularly for intervention purposes, it is important to identify the conditions under which learning or memory is enhanced. How is Bea's memory affected by the situation (e.g., the number of people in the room), by the complexity of the task or the content to learn or remember (see under "Task" in this chapter for a model of task complexity), by the modality involved (e.g., visual versus auditory), and by the type of content involved (e.g., concrete versus abstract or verbal versus nonverbal). Does the memory task or new learning require Bea, for example, to create in her mind or recall an image or standard? When she looks in a mirror, does she remember how a person who is dressed and groomed should look, so that she can compare what she sees with an appropriate standard? Does she have difficulty recalling something but then recognize it when she sees or hears it?

A final aspect of memory and learning to be assessed is the degree to which an individual processes single behaviors or details versus whole events and contexts. This includes an assessment of the size of the "chunks" in which the individual processes information (Birren 1969; Labouvie-Vief 1979; Miller 1956; Tulving 1962). Is a task such as dressing or tying a shoe a ritualized habit for Bea (i.e., overlearned), enabling her more easily to perform the task in its entirety (or in large chunks that include many task steps) rather than as isolated individual task steps? A chunk of task steps may be successfully executed by Bea only when the chunk (sequence of task steps) itself remains intact. If Bea is distracted or the sequence is in some way disrupted, can Bea still complete the task? For example, Bea may have always put her slacks on in a certain order (sit on bed, lean over, put left foot in, pull leg sleeve up, insert right foot, pull leg sleeve up, stand up, pull slacks up to waist). When her nose itches, or when a caregiver enters just after Bea pulls her left leg sleeve up, can Bea recover the sequence after such a distraction and continue, or is the chunk "lost"?

Bea's ability to engage in polite social "small talk" or clichés may also reflect the size of the chunks in which she retains skills and information. When politely refusing more crackers, for example, does she use an explanation that accomplishes her goal (refusal of crackers) but is not quite appropriate to the particular situation (e.g., "No, thank you, I have some at home" while she sits in her home). To what extent does this reflect Bea's reliance on her memory of a context (serving food socially) that includes appropriate phrases to say and her inability to generate or recall phrases that are specifically appropriate to the immediate context (Weaverdyck 1987)?

Similarly, does Bea recall the entire context of the dressing task (including the environmental features) but not the individual events (the task steps)? Is Bea's dressing performance enhanced when she consistently dresses in the same place in her bedroom or with the same introductory comments by the caregiver? Is it enhanced when she consistently dresses in one place but undresses in another spot?

Logic

Both induction and deduction are usually assessed in dementia (Mattis 1976). This includes an individual's ability to draw conclusions from observations and to recognize the relative importance of elements in a situation. It also includes the ability to recognize similarities among objects or events and to categorize them. When Bea sees a cue (such as a picture of a watering can by her actual plant) or an unfinished task (such as a piece of toast lying next to a plate of butter, jelly, and a knife), does it occur to her to water the plant or to butter the toast? When she is cold, does it occur to her to close the window, pull up another blanket, or put on a sweater? When she selects clothing to wear, does she choose an article of clothing rather than something else, and is the clothing article appropriate?

Abstraction

Can Bea create or use an image in her mind to facilitate the dressing task (e.g., an image of how her dress should look on her)? Does Bea recognize the significance of a cue such as a red awning over a door, which has no inherent meaning relevant to a bathroom door? Would a picture of a toilet be more effective? Bea may need progressively more concrete stimuli to cue or orient her as her dementia progresses. For example, cues to her bedroom door may progress from a particular color on her door, to a name plate, to a photograph of her, to a picture of a bed, to the door standing open so that she can see her bed in the bedroom. When Bea was assessed, it was noted that she could recognize herself in a mirror but not in a photograph.

Quantity Appreciation

Most of the executive functions identified here are interrelated and overlapping. Quantity appreciation is similar to abstraction. Does Bea recognize and can she create or manipulate quantitative aspects of tasks? For example, does she recognize the error of three socks for two feet? Does she recognize a one-to-one relationship? Distance appreciation could be included here. Does she recognize relative distances from the bathroom door?

Sequencing

Most neuropsychologists are particularly interested in a person's ability to sequence because of implications regarding brain functioning. Can the person order objects or events spatially and temporally? Bea may remember the task steps involved in dressing, but can she order them effectively? Bea may know where the bathroom is, but does she recognize that it comes before or after certain doorways or other landmarks?

Sequencing as a basic skill is a primary requisite to learning new tasks or landmarks in a new setting. Even a slight impairment in sequencing can have important consequences for the method in which new skills are taught or earlier skills are retrained effectively.

Choosing among Options

Decision making is often impaired in dementia (Holden and Woods 1982; Reisberg 1981). When Bea is confronted with two doors, one of which has a blue awning and one of which has a red awning, can she determine which door to choose? (On Bea's residential unit, a blue awning hung over the men's restroom and a red awning hung over the women's restroom.) Decision making requires judgment and generation of or memory for criteria upon which to base a decision. Even when the options are before her and her goal seems to be clear to her, can she choose? Is Bea able to recognize the need for strategy and then to generate strategy when faced with a decision to make or a problem to solve?

Planning

Related to decision making are planning and problem solving. Planning represents an attempt to change a situation to achieve one or more goals. It implies the development and application of a strategy or strategies toward the resolution of a dysfunctional situation or toward the creation of an unrelated desired situation (such as a picnic). Planning requires the organization and coordination of multiple steps and goals. It obviously depends heavily upon the individual's ability to understand a situation and the relationships within it. It is highly complex and abstract.

The person assessed may be able to anticipate only one step at a time. Bea did seem to recognize the need for the bathroom and to recognize and use the strategy of seeking help. An analysis of the role of planning in the dressing task and of Bea's competence with such planning might be helpful.

Shifting Mental Set

In patients with dementia, a neuropsychologist is particularly alert to evidence of perseveration, the repetition of behaviors or thoughts that seems unintentional and uncontrolled (Fuld 1978; Goldberg 1986; Sandson and Albert 1987). A person with dementia may be unable to shift easily into another thought pattern or behavior. How easily can Bea shift from focusing on eating breakfast to the goal of getting dressed? How easily can she shift from putting on a dress to putting on shoes or from walking down the hall to turning in through a door, such as the one to the bathroom?

During assessment, one may ask a related question about the type or intensity of stimulus that is most conducive to facilitating a person's ability to change direction, focus, or goal. If Bea is getting dressed, how powerful must a stimulus be to "pull" her away from the dressing task? Once she is "pulled away" momentarily, how easily does she return to the dressing task? How intentional is her typical change in mental set? When she stops dressing and begins to crawl into bed, is it because of a conscious decision to rest, because of an internal stimulus indicating fatigue, or because of simple distraction by the sight of the bed? A person may shift mental set very easily (highly distractible) or with great difficulty (perseveration). A related question is therefore, What conditions facilitate the continued concentration and focus on a task and then a recognition of completion and the ability to "release" a task? Perhaps powerful stimuli that are well timed and placed will allow Bea to shift from one task to another or keep her returning to the necessary task at hand.

Initiation

Related to shifting mental set is the ability to get started on one's own. Bea may know that she needs the bathroom and may even know what she must do next to get there, but how easily can she actually initiate the movements and the decision making required to address her need? If she takes too long to initiate her intended set of behaviors, the need to urinate may become powerful enough to generate anxiety, which could in turn preclude her ability to think or behave efficiently.

Expressive Functions

Expressive functions, as described in this chapter, reflect the ability of the brain to dictate to the body what to do. Two major types of expressive dysfunctions are aphasia (disorders of language expression) (Bayles et al. 1986; Nicholas et al. 1985; Woods and Britton 1985) and apraxia (disorders of intentional coordination of actions or movements into meaningful tasks) (Hecaen 1981; Holden and Woods 1982; Lezak 1983). Apraxia in dementia was referred to in the previous sections on attention and memory. In apraxia, the inability to perform a task occurs when an individual attempts to focus on or intentionally execute the task. The person is able to perform the task when not thinking about it.

It is important to identify evidence of aphasia with respect to both comprehension and expression (see Perception and Comprehension, above). A common problem in dementia is the inability to find the exact word that one wants to use (Kirshner et al. 1984; Miller 1981). This is sometimes called amnestic aphasia or anomia (Mattis 1976). When this person speaks, does she or he say what is intended? How fluent is the speech? Does the person require time to organize thoughts and words? Does the person understand, or does it take longer to understand instructions? How easily does the person write? Does the person write what he or she intends to write? How often does this person use profanity? Is the use of profanity a direct reflection of brain impairment (as it sometimes is), or does it arise from anger and frustration alone?

What type of language seems to be intact—novel phrases, clichés, verses? What is the quality of grammar and syntax? For what purposes is language usually used by this person (to obtain information, to socialize, to express emotions)? Clear identification of precise disorders in language may facilitate language intervention, which could, in turn, allow the person to participate more easily in the identification of how help could be most useful in, for example, the dressing task. Clear identification of language disorders may also indicate to the caregiver the optimal length and level of complexity of sentences that most effectively communicate to the person.

To what extent can impairments be attributed to higher cognitive dysfunction versus the inability to do what the person wants to do? It may be that Bea knows quite clearly the steps required to get dressed, but her body simply won't do the motions in the way that she wants it to. Apraxia may be evident in a variety of ways, including an inability to organize and place objects in space, to construct three- and two-dimensional objects in space, to pretend to execute tasks and actually to execute tasks, and to move oneself appropriately in space. A person may be able to perform a task but unable to do it upon command. It is also very useful to assess the ability of the person to respond to and to create music, including rhythm, pitch, and tonal progressions.

Motoric Functions

Finally, the individual's ability to respond physically to appropriate messages from the brain is assessed. How much physical control does Bea have over her arms and legs? Strength, coordination, and range of motion are measured. There may be differences between left and right sides. Because most inferences regarding brain function and cognitive functioning are drawn from observation of behaviors that depend upon intact motor skills, accurate measurement of motor skills is essential to any assessment.

Issues in Cognitive Assessment of Dementia

In conclusion, some of the general issues pertaining to the assessment of individuals with dementia are briefly summarized. Assessment is essentially the systematic observation of a person's behaviors. Assessment is usually conducted with specific goals in mind. Dementia is a disorder, sometimes progressive, in which a person's cognition or ability to think is impaired. The affected person is usually much less impaired physically than cognitively (Lishman 1978). The assessment focuses to a large extent, therefore, upon the specific cognitive disorders in evidence.

When the dementia is progressive, the content and procedures of the assessment may vary considerably across the duration of the disorder. Early in the course, a person may be able to perform some tasks or comprehend some instructions that later are simply impossible. Because of the progressive nature of the disorder, interval assessments are important. At present, the ability to maintain consistency in test procedures and test items (which helps to ensure validity) is compromised (Teri and Lewinsohn 1986). Few currently standardized assessment measures are adequate in their ability to measure the small decremental or incremental changes occurring over time, or to handle the range of abilities exhibited across the course of the disease. Many do not measure mild (ceiling effect) or severe (floor effect) disability (Kane and Kane 1981; Mattis 1976; Miller 1981).

Furthermore, most of the assessment measures currently available do not accommodate the particular needs, habits, and preferences of a dementia population or of the older population from which many dementia patients are drawn (Labouvie-Vief 1977). The use of measures and procedures that are more ecologically or naturalistically based (i.e., based on more direct observation of performance on tasks that are spontaneous and familiar to the individual and are conducted in the individual's familiar living environment) will probably be required throughout the course of the dementia.

The specific content and procedures of an assessment will also vary according to the goal of the assessment. Assessments may be conducted to establish baselines, to measure the effectiveness of interventions, or simply to document competencies and deficits for classification purposes (Burnside et al. 1984). Possible objectives of assessment have been discussed in detail. In this chapter, the ultimate goal of the assessment was appropriate intervention development. Of particular importance is discernment of and respect for the goals held by the individual with dementia. These goals of the individual may conflict with those of the caregivers or the assessor.

It is important to avoid stressing primarily the impairments over the competencies. A careful identification and description of the individual's competencies is essential to incisive intervention development.

The need for flexibility in timing has been noted. The duration of an assessment session will vary according to the fluctuations in the individual's preferences, energy level, and abilities. The quality of a person's performance may depend upon the time of day, the day itself, the particular antecedent events, or any of a variety of environmental factors. Both the time of initiation and the duration of the assessment session will depend upon whether the assessor is at-

tempting to evaluate optimal or typical functioning. Optimal functioning can best be assessed through naturalistic observation during
which spontaneous behaviors can be captured. This type of assessment, however, is very time-consuming and costly. Perhaps by training caregivers (including nurse assistants and other direct service staff
of long-term care facilities) in some forms of cognitive assessment,
such drawbacks can be accommodated (Parachek 1986).

The interpretation of the assessment data must account for the
impact of the environmental context of the assessment session itself.
More than most populations, people with dementia are unusually
susceptible to environmental conditions and are therefore more difficult to assess (and interpret) with accuracy and validity.

A major difficulty in the assessment of dementia is the definition
of norms. With whom is this person to be compared: young healthy
adults (the population used for most studies in which norms and
standardized procedures were established) (Baltes and Labouvie
1973), healthy adults of comparable age and/or gender, or with other
people with dementia? Is the frequency or quality of performance
measured? Does a rare occurrence constitute competency? Is the norm
for that individual the current baseline data or the historical baseline
data (how the person always used to do that task)? Answers to these
questions depend, of course, upon the objectives of the assessment,
the availability of norms, and the feasibility of various assessment
procedures.

It is important to distinguish the role of dementia and the role
of aging in the interpretation of assessment data. Frequently, impairments resulting from dementia are exacerbated by environmental
insensitivity to normal age-related changes, such as sensory changes
(Lawton 1986).

Particularly for intervention purposes, it is important to assess
the timing requirements of each individual. A task that takes more
time than it used to for an individual may indicate a type of cognitive
impairment. In some cases, simply allowing more time for the person
to process, react to, or execute a particular aspect or step of a task
may allow that person to accomplish the task successfully and independently. Reaction time and the time required to perform each
cognitive function are therefore noted in an assessment.

An assessment must also identify the individual's threshold for
stimulation. What level (how powerful) and type of stimulation fa-

cilitate optimal performance? Such a threshold may, of course, vary with circumstances, which also must be identified.

An interpretation of assessment data should yield some recommendations regarding the preferred type (e.g., abstract or concrete) and amount of content, modality demands (visual, hearing, tactile), and contextual properties (type of cueing, people involved, time of day, etc.) of tasks that an individual is expected to undertake. In addition, the extent to which a person is conscious of or able to discern her or his own level of abilities or desires should be identified.

As research and documented experience yield more insight into cognitive functioning in dementia, we may develop a protocol for assessment that would predict with some precision the nature of impairments to come and methods that might appropriately forestall or prepare for the changes. To make such predictions, we must assess any given individual at regular intervals and consistently.

A dementia assessment examines carefully the environment, the task, the caregiver, and the person with dementia in an effort to identify contributions each makes to the type and level of impairment, to the competency of the individual with dementia, and to the occurrence of "management problem" behaviors. This chapter presented a conceptual outline for the assessment of each of these four targets. It also introduced a model for the analysis of task complexity in dementia.

It is important to note the extent to which impairments result from brain damage or from other factors, such as the environment or excessive caregiver assistance (Kahn 1977). It is also important to identify how each of these targets (the environment, task, caregiver, and person with dementia) could be modified to foster optimal functioning and satisfaction on the part of the individual (Brody et al. 1971; Weaverdyck 1987).

There are many possible explanations, some treatable, for the behaviors and disabilities or deficits encountered in a person with dementia. These explanations are frequently complex, interactive, and idiosyncratic. They include factors such as environmental conditions, inappropriate task requirements, caregiver misperceptions and interactions, and factors arising directly from the dementia victim. These latter factors arising from the person can include cognitive and noncognitive aspects.

Contributing factors that are noncognitive include motivation, habits, affect, and physical or medical conditions. When the explanatory factor is primarily cognitive, the type of cognitive skills involved could be sensory, perceptual, executive, expressive, or motoric, as described in this chapter.

It can be very difficult, yet rewarding and important, to differentiate among the various explanatory factors and to identify the extent to which each plays a role. Specific factors can then be selected to be addressed in the resulting intervention program. Sometimes only a slight adjustment can reverse an apparent impairment.

The cognitive functioning of any individual is very complex. Most cognitive functions, including those identified in this chapter, are interdependent and overlap. Those identified here were discussed simplistically and superficially and constitute only a small portion of the types and aspects of cognitive functions or skills affected in a dementing disorder. Rarely is there an impairment in only one discrete function in any disorder.

Despite the complexity and magnitude of the undertaking, cognitive or neuropsychological assessment is of utmost importance to the intelligent development of effective intervention (Miller 1984). To the extent that assessment can identify, in detail, the competencies of an individual and not simply the impairments, it will also enhance respect for and appreciation of the person with the dementia on the part of the caregiver. To both the individual and the caregiver, such an appreciation renders immeasurable emotional support.

Although neuropsychological assessment is valuable for the development of any intervention program (Holden and Woods 1982; Zgola 1987), it is particularly useful in the design of cognitive interventions (Coons and Weaverdyck 1986; Weaverdyck 1987). By identifying the cognitive competencies and impairments underlying the execution of tasks and behaviors, the assessment aids caregivers in the selection of intervention goals (e.g., compensation, remediation, maintenance at present level, avoidance), strategies (e.g., practice, reinforcement, demonstration, training, feedback), and contexts (e.g., recreational programming, activities of daily living, structured therapy or retraining, caregiver-person interactions, environment) (Weaverdyck 1987).

Our current state of knowledge regarding dementia is, at best, limited and likely erroneous in many respects (U.S. Congress, Office of Technology Assessment 1987). Assessment that is valid, reliable, and comprehensive in its focus will make a valuable contribution not only to immediate intervention planning but also to the long-term study of dementia.

References

Albert, M. 1981. Geriatric neuropsychology. *Journal of Consulting and Clinical Psychology* 49:835–50.

Baddeley, A., A. Sunderland, and J. Harris. 1982. How well do laboratory-based psychological tests predict patients' performance outside the laboratory? In *Alzheimer's disease: A report of progress in research*, ed. S. Corkin, K. Davis, J. Growden, E. Usdin, and R. Wurtman. New York: Raven Press.

Baltes, P., and G. Labouvie. 1973. Adult development of intellectual performance: Description, explanation, and modification. In *Psychology of adult development and aging*, ed. C. Eisdorder and M. Lawton. Washington, DC: American Psychological Association.

Bartol, M. 1979. Nonverbal communication in patients with Alzheimer's disease. *Journal of Gerontological Nursing* 5:21–31.

Bayles, K., A. Kaszniak, and C. Tomoeda. 1986. *Communication and cognition in normal aging and dementia*. New York: Little, Brown.

Beck, C., P. Heacock, R. Thatcher, S. Mercer, C. Sparkman, and M. Roberts. 1985. *Cognitive skills remediation with Alzheimer's patients*. Presented at the meeting of the International Congress of Gerontology, New York, July.

Birren, J. 1969. Age and decision strategies. In *Interdisciplinary topics in gerontology*, ed. A. Welford and J. Birren. Basel: Karger.

Brink, T., ed. 1986. *Clinical gerontology: A guide to assessment and intervention*. New York: Haworth Press.

Brody, E., M. Kleban, M. Lawton, and H. Silverman. 1971. Excess disabilities of mentally impaired aged: Impact of individualized treatment. *Gerontologist* 11:124–32.

Burnside, I. 1980. Symptomatic behaviors in the elderly. In *Handbook of mental health and aging*, ed. J. Birren and R. Sloane. Englewood Cliffs, NJ: Prentice Hall.

Burnside, I. 1981. *Nursing and the aged*. New York: McGraw-Hill.

Burnside, I., J. Baumler and S. Weaverdyck. 1984. Group work in a day care center. In *Working with the elderly: Group processes and techniques*. 2d ed., ed. I. Burnside. Belmont, CA: Wadsworth.

Chenoweth, B., and B. Spencer. 1986. Dementia: The experience of family caregivers. *Gerontologist* 26:267–72.

Cohen, D. 1982. Issues in psychological diagnosis and management of the cognitively impaired aged. In *Treatment of psychopathology in the aging*, ed. C. Eisdorder and W. Fann. New York: Springer.

Cohen, D., and C. Eisdorder. 1986. *The loss of self: A family resource for the care of Alzheimer's disease and related disorders*. New York: W. W. Norton.

Coons, D. 1983. The therapeutic milieu. In *Clinical aspects of aging.* 2d ed., ed. W. Reichel. Baltimore: Williams & Wilkins.

Coons, D., and S. Weaverdyck. 1986. Wesley Hall: A residential unit for persons with Alzheimer's disease and related disorders. In *Therapeutic interventions for the person with dementia,* ed. E. Taira. New York: Haworth Press.

Diller, L., and W. Gordon. 1981. Rehabilitation and clinical neuropsychology. In *Handbook of clinical neuropsychology,* ed. S. Filskov and T. Boll. New York: Wiley.

Fuld, P. 1978. Psychological testing in the differential diagnosis of the dementias. In *Alzheimer's disease: Senile dementia and related disorders,* ed. R. Katzman, R. Terry, and K. Bick. New York: Raven Press.

Fuld, P. 1983. Psychometric differentiation of the dementias: An overview. In *Alzheimer's disease: The standard reference,* ed. B. Reisberg. New York: Free Press.

Gilleard, C. 1984. Assessment of cognitive impairment in the elderly: A review. In *Psychological approaches to the care of the elderly,* ed. I. Hanley and J. Hodge, 1–21. London: Croom-Helm.

Gold, M. 1980. *Try another way.* Champaign, IL: Research Press.

Goldberg, E. 1986. Varieties of perseveration: A comparison of two taxonomies. *Journal of Clinical and Experimental Neuropsychology* 8:710–26.

Goldenberg, B., and P. Chiverton. 1984. Assessing behavior: The nurse's mental status exam. *Geriatric Nursing* 2:94–98.

Gwyther, L. 1985. *Care of Alzheimer's patients: A manual for nursing home staff.* Chicago: Alzheimer's Disease and Related Disorders Association.

Hall, G., and K. Buckwalter. 1987. Progressively lowered stress threshold: A conceptual model for care of adults with Alzheimer's disease. *Archives of Psychiatric Nursing* 1:399–406.

Hamsher, K. 1983. Mental status examination in Alzheimer's disease: A neuropsychologist's role. *Postgraduate Medicine* 73:225–28.

Heaton, R., and M. Pendleton. 1981. Use of neuropsychological tests to predict adult patient's everyday functioning. *Journal of Consulting and Clinical Psychology* 49:807–21.

Hecaen, H. 1981. Apraxia. In *Handbook of clinical neuropsychology,* ed. S. Filskov and T. Boll. New York: Wiley-Interscience.

Hodge, J. 1984. Towards a behavioural analysis of dementia. In *Psychological approaches to the care of the elderly,* ed. I. Hanley and J. Hodge, 61–87. London: Croom-Helm.

Hoffman, S., C. Platt, and K. Barry. 1987. Managing the difficult dementia patient: The impact on untrained nursing home staff. *American Journal of Alzheimer's Care and Research* 2:26–31.

Holden, U., and R. Woods. 1982. *Reality orientation: Psychological approaches to the confused elderly.* New York: Churchill Livingstone.

Hussian, R. 1986. Severe behavioral problems. In *Geropsychological assessment and treatment,* ed. L. Teri and P. Lewinsohn, 121–43. New York: Springer.

Hussian, R., and R. Davis. 1985. *Responsive care: Behavioral interventions with elderly persons.* Champaign, IL: Research Press.

Kahn, R. 1977. Excess disabilities. In *Readings in aging and death: Contemporary perspectives,* ed. S. Zarit. New York: Harper & Row.

Kane, R., and R. Kane. 1981. *Assessing the elderly: A practical guide to measurement.* Lexington, MA: Lexington Books.

Kane, R., and R. Kane. 1982. *Values and long-term care.* Lexington, MA: Lexington Books.

Kendrick, D. 1972. The Kendrick battery of tests: Theoretical assumptions and clinical uses. *British Journal of Social and Clinical Psychology* 11:373–86.

Kennedy, R., and A. Kennedy. 1982. Absence of purposeful behavior: Issues in training the profoundly impaired elderly. In *Mental health interventions for the aging,* ed. A. Horton. New York: Praeger.

Kirshner, H., W. Webb, and M. Kelly. 1984. The naming disorder of dementia. *Neuropsychologia* 22:23–30.

Kogan, N. 1982. Cognitive styles in older adults. In *Review of human development,* ed. T. Field, A. Huston, H. Quay, L. Troll, and G. Finley. New York: Wiley-Interscience.

Kral, V. 1970. Clinical contribution towards an understanding of memory function. *Diseases of the Nervous System* 31:23–29.

Labouvie-Vief, G. 1977. Adult cognitive development: In search of alternative interpretations. *Merrill-Palmer Quarterly* 23:227–63.

Labouvie-Vief, G. 1979. Adaptive dimensions of adult cognition. In *Transitions of aging,* ed. N. Datan and N. Lohmann. New York: Academic Press.

Lawton, M. 1986. *Environment and aging.* Monterey: Brooks/Cole.

Lezak, M. 1982. The problems of assessing executive functions. *International Journal of Psychology* 17:281–97.

Lezak, M. 1983. *Neuropsychological assessment.* 2d ed. New York: Oxford University Press.

Lishman, W. 1978. *Organic psychiatry.* London: Blackwell Scientific Publications.

Mace, N. L., and P. V. Rabins. 1981. *The 36 hour day.* Baltimore: Johns Hopkins University Press.

Martin, A. 1987. Representation of semantic and spatial knowledge in Alzheimer's patients: Implications for models of preserved learning in amnesia. *Journal of Clinical and Experimental Neuropsychology* 9:191–224.

Mattis, S. 1976. Mental status examination for organic mental syndrome in the elderly patient. In *Geriatric Psychiatry,* ed. R. Bellak and T. Karasu. New York: Grune & Stratton.

McEvoy, C., and R. Patterson. 1986. Behavioral treatment of deficit skills in dementia patients. *Gerontologist* 26:475–78.

Miller, E. 1977a. *Abnormal aging: The psychology of senile and presenile dementia.* New York: Wiley.

Miller, E. 1977b. The management of dementia: A review of some possibilities. *British Journal of Social and Clinical Psychology* 16:77–85.

Miller, E. 1981. The nature of the cognitive deficit in dementia. In *Clinical aspects of Alzheimer's disease and senile dementia*, ed. N. Miller and G. Cohen. New York: Raven Press.

Miller, E. 1984. *Recovery and management of neuropsychological impairments*. New York: Wiley.

Miller, G. 1956. The magical number seven plus or minus two: Some limits on our capacity for processing information. *Psychological Review* 63:81–97.

Miller, N., and G. Cohen. 1981. *Clinical aspects of Alzheimer's disease and senile dementia*. New York: Raven Press.

Moscovitch, M. 1982. A neuropsychological approach to perception and memory in normal and pathological aging. In *Aging and cognitive processes*, ed. F. Craik and S. Trehub. New York: Plenum.

Nicholas, M., L. Obler, M. Albert, and N. Helm-Estabrooks. 1985. Empty speech in Alzheimer's disease and fluent aphasia. *Journal of Speech and Hearing Research* 28:405–410.

Parachek, J. 1986. *Parachek geriatric rating scale*. 3d ed. Phoenix: Center for Neurodevelopmental Studies.

Poon, L. ed. 1986. *Handbook for clinical memory assessment of older adults*. Washington, DC: American Psychological Association.

Reisberg, B. 1981. *Brain failure: An introduction to current concepts of senility*. New York: Free Press.

Reisberg, B., S. Ferris, and T. Crook. 1982. Signs, symptoms, and course of age associated cognitive decline. In *Alzheimer's disease: A report of progress in research*, ed. S. Corkin, K. Davis, J. Growdon, E. Usdin, and R. Wurtman. New York: Raven Press.

Robinson, A., B. Spencer, S. Weaverdyck, and S. Gardner. 1987. *Helping people with dementia in activities of daily living*. Ann Arbor, MI: PhotoMotion. Video and slide-tape production.

Sandson, J., and M. Albert. 1987. Perseveration in behavioral neurology. *Neurology* 37:1736–41.

Schacter, D., J. Harbluk, and R. Kirshbaum. 1983. *Laboratory simulation of memory disorders: Source amnesia*. Presented at the meeting of the International Neuropsychological Society, Mexico City, February.

Smith, A. 1975. Neuropsychological testing in neurological disorders. In *Current reviews of higher nervous system dysfunction*, ed. W. Friedlander. New York: Raven Press.

Teri, L., and P. Lewinsohn, eds. 1986. *Geropsychological assessment and treatment: Selected topics*. New York: Springer.

Tulving, E. 1962. Subjective organization in free recall of "unrelated" words. *Psychological Review* 69:344–54.

U.S. Congress. Office of Technology Assessment. 1987. *Losing a million minds: Confronting the tragedy of Alzheimer's disease and other dementias*. OTA-BA-323. Washington, DC: U.S. Government Printing Office. April.

Vitaliano, P., A. Breen, M. Albert, J. Russo, and P. Prinz. 1984. Memory, attention, and functional status in community residing Alzheimer type dementia patients and optimally healthy aged individuals. *Journal of Gerontology* 39:58–64.

Weaverdyck, S. 1987. A cognitive intervention protocol: Its derivation from and application to a neuropsychological case study of Alzheimer's disease. Ph.D. diss., University of Michigan. *Dissertation Abstracts International.* September 1987. Available from University Microfilms International, 300 N. Zeeb Road, Ann Arbor, MI 48106. Publication #8712237.

Weaverdyck, S. In preparation. Assessment for intervention planning. *Living environments for persons with Alzheimer's disease or related dementias*, ed. D. Coons. Baltimore: Johns Hopkins University Press.

Weaverdyck, S., and D. Coons. 1988. Designing a dementia residential care unit: Addressing cognitive changes with the Wesley Hall model. In *Housing the very old*, ed. G. Gutman and N. Blackie. Burnaby, British Columbia: Simon Fraser University.

Weintraub, S., R. Baratz, and M. Mesulam. 1982. Daily living activities in the assessment of dementia. In *Alzheimer's disease: A report of progress in research*, ed. S. Corkin, K. Davis, J. Growdon, E. Usdin, and R. Wurtman. New York: Raven Press.

Wolanin, M., and L. Phillips. 1981. *Confusion: Prevention and care.* St. Louis: C. V. Mosby.

Wolfensberger, W. 1972. *The principle of normalization in human services.* Toronto: National Institute on Mental Retardation.

Woods, R., and P. Britton. 1985. *Clinical psychology with the elderly.* Rockville, MD: Aspen.

Zarit, S. 1980. *Aging and mental disorders: Psychological approaches to assessment and treatment.* Riverside, NJ: Macmillan.

Zarit, S., N. Orr, and J. Zarit. 1985. *The hidden victims of Alzheimer's disease: Families under stress.* New York: New York University Press.

Zgola, J. 1987. *Doing things: A guide to programming activities for persons with Alzheimer's disease and related disorders.* Baltimore: Johns Hopkins University Press.

4

The Management of
Problem Behaviors
NANCY L. MACE

People suffering from dementing illnesses often exhibit behaviors that endanger themselves or others; that stress, frighten, or exhaust their caregivers; or that are socially unacceptable. These behaviors have been identified as precipitants of institutionalization (Smallegan 1985; Knopman et al. 1988). Nursing homes report that managing behaviorally disturbed patients is difficult and costly. Behavior problems increase the physical demands of caregiving (searching for a wanderer, dealing with resistance to the bath). Watching a loved one whose actions are so changed (making accusations, cursing, propositioning a daughter) is painful for caregivers. Yet these behaviors have not been clearly defined or studied, and until the beginning of this decade they were almost completely overlooked. A review (Cohen-Mansfeld and Billig 1986) found that the existing literature is largely on pharmacological topics. Cornbleth (1977) and Hiatt (1980) studied wandering. Ryan et al. (1988) defined and described noisemaking in institutions. Rubin et al. (1988, 1987a, 1987b) grouped symptoms and examined the frequency with which these groups appear. Clinicians disagree over these observations, however, indicating that much more study is needed.

The presence of behavior problems is not a defining characteristic of dementia. Similar behaviors can occur in persons suffering from mental disorders, personality disorders, or physical illnesses and in normal but angry or upset individuals. Yet few articles distinguish between underlying causes.

Whether a behavior is a problem may depend on the setting and on the judgment of the carer. The attitude of the carer can change a behavior from problematic to acceptable. The setting may determine whether a behavior places someone at risk. Some settings are much more accepting of deviant behavior than others, yet some behaviors are generally agreed to be serious problems.

Behaviors are often described with general terms such as "wandering," "accusatory," "agitated," "combative," or "incontinent." These terms are rarely defined and can include a range of different behaviors, further confusing our understanding of the problem. Although instruments describing the degree of behavior problem have been difficult to develop and good studies have been challenging to design, clinical experience has shown that the difficulty that behaviors create can be reduced by training carers—family members, volunteers, and paid staff.

This chapter will use the term *problem behaviors* to refer to those behaviors that endanger the person with dementia or others; that stress, frighten, or exhaust the caregivers; or that are perceived as socially unacceptable. Passive behavior (when the person does not participate in personal care or social activities although able to do so) is also included. The patients targeted are those who have dementing illnesses and are exhibiting problem behaviors. Behaviors are probably related to the degree of cognitive impairment and also to the stage of the illness (Teri et al. 1988). They may not necessarily conform to particular models of aging, however. Clinicians report that those patients who present behavior problems have also lost skills, insight, and self-control but have language skills or motor skills sufficient to carry out the behaviors. Those in the late stages may be too impaired to wander, argue, or be combative.

Although families and providers report that even simple interventions are helpful, behavior management alone probably will not completely relieve the burden on carers. Implementing the changes that reduce problem behaviors is itself demanding, and these interventions do not change the need for constant vigilance and care. Behavior is difficult to predict; interventions may prevent the behavior in some situations but not in others. Providers in congregate settings often report remarkable changes in client behavior, but the most skilled providers in the best settings cannot eliminate all behaviors. Finally, behaviors depend on the intervention; when the intervention is withdrawn, the behavior may resume. The following changes in behavior are often reported by the staff of successful congregate settings for ambulatory individuals who are moderately to severely impaired:

decrease in wandering;

decrease in episodes of agitation;

no screaming or decrease in screaming;

few or no drugs needed to control behavior;

improved orientation (e.g., person knows that he or she belongs here);

decrease in socially unacceptable behaviors (masturbation, rummaging in other patients' rooms, etc.);

weight gains or improved eating;

decrease in depression;

greater ability to sleep through the night;

a sense of humor;

a happy, relaxed appearance;

the formation of friendships;

reduction or elimination of incontinence;

the initiation of interpersonal exchanges; and

decrease in hallucinations (U.S. Congress 1987).

Cleary et al. (1988) reported similar gains in a low-stimulus unit.

An important argument in favor of treating behavior problems is the observable change in the individual's affect. Problem behaviors often communicate painful feelings (anger, fear, being lost), whereas treated patients indicate satisfaction, affection, and security more often. In this chapter, the prevalence of behavior problems in dementia, theories of the causes of behavior problems, possible goals of behavior management, and strategies for management are discussed.

Prevalence

Problem behaviors are quite common among individuals with dementia, although their true prevalence is not known. Not all patients exhibit disturbed behaviors, and the behaviors that do occur vary from person to person. Little is known about the distribution of behavior problems within the population of people who have dementing illnesses. Little is known about the impact of the underlying disease process or the premorbid personality (Shomaker 1987). Reisberg (1983), Teri et al. (1988), and Rubin et al. (1987a, 1987b) reported an association between certain behaviors and the stage of the illness, but others found little association beyond the patient's declining physical ability to continue behaviors such as wandering or making accusations (Cohen et al. 1984).

TABLE 4.1 Patients' Behavior Problems Cited by Families

Behavior	Number of Families Reporting	Families Reporting the Behavior		Families Reporting the Behavior and Citing It as a Problem	
		No.	(%)	No.	(%)
Memory disturbance	55	55	(100)	51	(93)
Catastrophic reactions	52	45	(87)	40	(89)
Demanding/critical behavior	52	37	(71)	27	(73)
Night waking	54	37	(69)	22	(59)
Hiding things	51	35	(69)	25	(71)
Communication difficulties	50	34	(68)	25	(74)
Suspiciousness	52	33	(63)	26	(79)
Making accusations	53	32	(60)	26	(81)
Needing help at mealtimes	55	33	(60)	18	(55)
Daytime wandering	51	30	(59)	21	(70)
Bathing	51	27	(53)	20	(74)
Delusions	49	23	(47)	19	(83)
Physical violence	51	24	(47)	22	(92)
Incontinence	53	21	(40)	18	(86)
Cooking	54	18	(33)	8	(44)
Hitting	50	16	(32)	13	(81)
Driving	55	11	(20)	8	(73)
Smoking	53	6	(11)	4	(67)
Inappropriate sexual behavior	51	1	(2)	0	(0)

Source: Adapted from P. V. Rabins, N. L. Mace, and J. T. Rabins, "The Impact of Dementia on the Family," *Journal of the American Medical Association* 248:334, 1982.

Rabins et al. (1982) reported a high prevalence of problem behaviors in a population of patients whose caregivers were seeking help for the patient (Table 4.1). A survey by the Office of Technology Assessment (OTA) of a group of individuals at all stages of their illnesses and not necessarily seeking help revealed lower but still significant rates of behavior problems (Table 4.2). A survey of day care programs serving people with dementia also reported frequent problem behaviors (Mace and Rabins 1984). Zimmer et al. (1984) reported that behavior problems are common among nursing home residents. Thus, although it seems that behavior problems are com-

TABLE 4.2 Frequency of Dementia Patients' Engagement in Certain Behaviors

	Percentage of Total Respondents			
	Very Frequently	Occasionally	Rarely/ Never	Don't Know/No Answer[a]
How frequently does patient:				
Have periods of restlessness and agitation?	39	33	10	18
Become listless and apathetic?	32	29	14	26
Get in a depressed mood?	27	32	12	29
Wander away from home unless watched?	29	24	36	
Have inappropriate angry outbursts?	19	32	30	19
Engage in crying episodes?	13	26	38	23
Engage in actions (hit, pinch, throw things) that physically hurt people?	9	17	53	22

[a]Respondents who are not the primary caregiver may not know the frequency of behavior problems.
Note: This table is percentaged horizontally. Also totals may not add because of rounding.
Source: U.S. Congress. Office of Technology Assessment. 1987. *Losing a million minds: Confronting the tragedy of Alzheimer's disease and other dementias.* OTA-BA-323. Washington, DC: U.S. Government Printing Office. April.

mon in all caregiving settings, in no study did caregivers report that all patients presented serious behavior problems. Further studies of the relationship of the disease process to behavior problems, of those patients who do not present major problems, and of the distribution of disruptive behaviors by setting will yield valuable information on the care of these patients.

Theories of the Cause of Behavior Problems

The cause of behavior problems in dementia is not well understood. It is probably the sum of (1) the brain damage itself, (2) the patient's premorbid coping style, (3) affect, (4) concurrent conditions that cause excess disability, and (5) the physical, interpersonal, and internal environments. The weight of each of these factors in influencing behavior is not known.

The Role of Brain Damage in Behavior

Dementing illnesses cause extensive changes in brain chemistry and structure. The nature and location of the damage vary with the specific disease.

Although the damage to the brain is organic, the symptoms of the disease are behavioral, placing problem behavior squarely between neurology and psychiatry. Families, the patient, and professional providers must deal with strange behaviors, but these behaviors do not have a familiar explanation—personality, mental illness, drug intoxication, etc. The cause of the observed behaviors is, to a great extent, damage to a highly complex and poorly understood organ— the brain (U.S. Congress 1987).

The damage to the brain is usually not uniform. Until the late stages of the disease, some abilities will remain fairly intact while others are significantly impaired. This uneven decline explains many seemingly paradoxical behaviors. (For a description of the course of the illnesses and the behavioral symptoms, see Chapter 2 of the OTA report.) Behavior problems are probably related to the severity of cognitive impairment (Teri et al. 1988).

The behavioral symptoms can be loosely grouped into three categories: cognitive or neurological symptoms, impairments in the ability to do normal tasks, and behavioral or "psychiatric" symptoms. The terminology used to describe symptoms varies; this chapter will follow that used in the 1987 OTA report. Categorization is rather arbitrary; many symptoms can easily fit into more than one category.

An understanding of which cognitive functions have been spared or impaired in an individual can enable the clinician to explain seemingly bizarre behaviors and to devise interventions to circumvent the problem, reduce the behavior, and increase the person's ability to function (see Chapter 2). This understanding of the nature of the brain damage—that it is not uniform, that it is usually progressive, and that, directly or indirectly, it accounts for most of the behaviors observed—is critical to improving the quality of life for carers and patients.

Extensive skills are required to identify spared and impaired functions, reduce problem behavior, alter the patient's experience of suffering, and support the carers of people with behavior problems. This is not an "unskilled" job. It can correctly be termed *treatment* of a chronic illness (i.e., it is not "custodial") because it reduces the disability associated with the disease and alleviates suffering.

Cognitive or Neurological Symptoms

During the early part of the illness, the individual often experiences memory loss and aphasia (problems using and understanding language). This is followed by apraxia (inability to carry out purposeful movement in the absence of motor or sensory impairment), agnosia (failure to recognize things or people), and other symptoms, such as loss of the ability to learn and loss of the sense of the passage of time. When all other conditions that might affect the person's performance are eliminated, these symptoms remain despite efforts to modify them (U.S. Congress 1987).

The cognitive symptoms profoundly affect the way the individual perceives the world and thus affect his behavior. Memory impairment means that the person may not be able to remember having just done something, having seen the carers before, or having moved to this residence. The person may become fearful, clinging to those recognized from the past, or may begin a desperate search for something familiar. One can imagine being in a strange place where the bathroom hides, the people are all strangers, and even one's clothing is unfamiliar. Undesirable responses may be appropriate in light of the person's inaccurate perceptions. Anger and resistance are understandable responses when one perceives oneself to be dragged naked into a closet by three or four strangers. This resistance is not an appropriate response, however, from the point of view of staff trying to give the person a bath.

With aphasia, the person may not be able to make needs known or to understand what others are saying. The patient may become angry at people who seem to be talking gibberish. The person may experience pain and be unable even to give it a name. Aphasia can affect only certain language skills, thus, a woman who can still make her needs known may forget the names of her close family.

Apraxia is usually progressive, beginning with the inability to do fine motor tasks and progressing to difficulty walking and frequent falls. Unlike a person who has a paralysis, the person with an apraxia will usually be unable to learn to use assistive devices. The methods of helping an apraxic patient are different from those needed by physically handicapped individuals.

Agnosia is a particularly devastating symptom for families. The

individual may be unable to recognize loved ones—but has not necessarily forgotten the relationship. Some people do not recognize
themselves in the mirror and get angry at the "woman in the bathroom." Others urinate in wastebaskets because they do not recognize
that a wastebasket is a wastebasket.

Impairments such as the inability to learn, disorientation, the
tendency to perseverate (get "stuck" on one activity), the tendency
to respond to the strongest perceived stimulus, the inability to perceive
a gestalt, and an impaired ability to plan or sequence often lead to
inappropriate behavior. Usually the person is not aware of the specific
impairment that is causing trouble and, as the patient cannot remember, explanations are not helpful. However, these impairments often
cause suffering for the patient; for example, the panic of being in a
strange place and being unable to find those one loves. Patients may
be angered by the inability to do simple tasks like tying shoes or
buttoning. They may not understand why someone must dress them.
Carers ask patients to do things, and patients may be afraid or embarrassed because they do not understand the request. Although
patients usually do not remember facts, affect may be stored differently, and patients may remember the pain of frequent failures.

Carers report seemingly paradoxical behaviors: a wife who can
play cards but does not recognize her husband; a person who can
remember anger at her sister but does not remember the sister's explanation; the person who can do something one day but not the
next. Careful examination of such behaviors will reveal that spared
and impaired functions or the fluctuating and incomplete disruption
of neurological function may explain these seeming paradoxes. It is
important to explain this phenomenon to those who care for the
patient to maintain a positive caregiving relationship.

The Ability To Do Normal Daily Activities

People with dementia gradually lose the ability to perform activities of daily living (ADL) and instrumental activities of daily living.
These losses are due primarily to the cognitive symptoms just described. As the disease progresses, the person will gradually need
increased assistance and eventually will become totally dependent.
The clinician identifies specific areas of spared and impaired function
and adapts activities so that the person can continue to perform some
part of them (see Chapter 3). These interventions solve many behavior
problems. For example, the person who brushes his teeth in the toilet

may be disoriented. Orienting cues and reminders may help. The person who wanders away during lunch may be responding to distracting stimuli. Offering meals in a less distracting setting may help. Enabling patients to function as well as possible often seems to increase feelings of purpose, self-esteem, and success. This, in turn, reduces some negative behavioral outbursts.

A Loss of Judgment/Need for Supervision

Carers report that measures of impairment in the ability to perform tasks of daily living do not accurately reflect the problem presented by these patients. It is the loss of judgment, need for supervision, and need for verbal or physical cueing (rather than the physical inability to perform ADL) that accurately reflect the care needed by these patients. Language reflecting this is being developed and may be used in developing future eligibility criteria.

Behavioral or "Psychiatric" Symptoms

Certain symptoms, including paranoia, hallucinations, delusions, depression, anxiety, severe agitation, and sleeplessness, are considered "psychiatric" and respond well to the judicious use of psychoactive medications (see Chapter 2). Although all symptoms of dementia are manifested behaviorally, symptoms that cannot be immediately ascribed to specific neurological loss are often called "behavioral" or "psychiatric." They include angry outbursts, violence, apathy, stubbornness, resistance to care, suspicion, accusations, wandering, incessant repeating of the same question, being awake and active at night, use of obscene or abusive language, talking to deceased relatives, rummaging through other patients' rooms, stealing, getting lost, urinating in unsuitable places, hiding things, confabulation, refusing to give up activities that can no longer be performed safely, wearing clothing inside out or in the wrong order, refusing to change clothing or to bathe—the list is long. It is these behavior problems, rather than the cognitive symptoms or the need for care, that often distress caregivers most. However, these behaviors are responsive to treatment and can be reduced, even though little change will be seen in the underlying cognitive symptoms.

The difference between behavioral and cognitive symptoms is arbitrary. A person suffering damage to nerve cells or changes in brain chemistry can be expected to show odd behaviors that result from the neurological damage, and some behavioral symptoms can now be linked with specific neurological loss. It is also reasonable that persons suffering such devastating disabilities might experience depression, anger, fear, or anxiety. Thus, these symptoms are not so much "psychiatric" as they are the behavioral result of the neurological illness.

Among the behavioral symptoms, *catastrophic reactions* are particularly common and distressing, both to the patient and to the caregiver. These are overreactions to minor stressors (Goldstein 1952) manifested as angry outbursts, refusals, tears, agitation, pacing, or, in extreme cases, hitting or striking out. Catastrophic reactions may occur occasionally or almost continually. The struggle to make sense of one's environment may be enough to overstress many individuals. For example, the person who perceives that "this is not my home" may experience continuous anxiety and fear. Increased distractions, confusion, or intellectual demands can quickly precipitate a catastrophic reaction. Unlike similar behavior in cognitively well persons, these behaviors are largely beyond the control of the individual. The person may be reacting to understandable stress in the face of limitations. Haugen (1985) noted that behavior described by others as aggressive may really be a reaction of fear or anxiety. My clinical experience supports this. These patients have also lost the ability to inhibit inappropriate behavior. Catastrophic reactions create major burdens for caregivers and can result in inappropriate sedation or denial of services. Commonly, they are misinterpreted and their symptoms are exacerbated by the carer. Fortunately, they often respond to environmental interventions without the need for sedation.

Personality and Premorbid Coping Strategies

It is generally assumed that behavior in normal adults is shaped by the individual's personality and that the person acts as he does because of his experience of life, particularly his childhood. The behavior of people with dementia can be interpreted within the same framework. However, our understanding of the etiology of behavior is changing with new information about the biochemical nature of mental diseases and about the role of genetics in personality. The study of the neurological diseases of the brain, such as Alzheimer's, is expanding our understanding of the way behavior changes when parts of the brain fail. It is beyond the scope of this chapter to debate the intriguing relationship between the mind and the brain, which has been discussed (McHugh and Slavney 1983) and illustrated (Sacks 1970) elsewhere.

We cannot assume that the psychodynamic theories apply to those with brain damage in the same way that they apply to those who are cognitively intact. Almost nothing is known about the extent to which a person experiencing massive organic brain damage can continue to maintain a lifelong personality style or use familiar defense mechanisms. The inability to comprehend or process information and loss of the ability to control emotions or to express appropriate emotions may greatly distort the relationship between observed behavior and personality or coping strategies, yet the person is not a robot wired with failing neurons. Patterns of past behavior styles may continue, although their expression may become inappropriate (Shomaker 1987). For much of the course of the dementing illnesses, a unique person can be observed who still has an idiosyncratic style and who has a history (even if much of that history has been forgotten). In fact, the tenacity of aspects of personality may help to sustain caregiving, when, in the face of massive losses, the patient is seen to retain evidence of "her same old self."

Thus, we face a dilemma: when do we assume that behavior is based on brain damage and when do we assume that it is a part of personality or of lifelong coping strategies? Our assumptions powerfully influence our behavior toward the patient. When we are wrong in our assumptions, we can cause unnecessary frustration for families and unnecessary suffering for vulnerable patients. One can easily imagine the pain of a person who is treated as if she were using an undesirable defense mechanism when in fact she is terrified by what is happening to her and cannot articulate her need for support and understanding.

The sequences and mechanisms of receiving and responding to stimuli are not completely understood. What follows is not a model but a greatly simplified way to aid the nonneuropsychologist in understanding the difficulties a person with dementia may have in remembering and thinking. We take our own mental abilities so much for granted that often we assume that the response of the person with dementia is supported by the same complex and automatic mental skills. In contrast, we know that the person who is visually or hearing impaired will react to what his senses tell him and not to what one really said or showed him. The confused person may not be able to receive or remember what was said, or other intellectual skills may break down—he may not understand the words he heard; he may be confused about who spoke to him; he may be unable to evaluate what was said in light of what he knows or of where he thinks he is. Chapter 3 describes many of these difficulties of cognition. When a cognitive function fails, the person's response may seem to be a change in personality, or he may appear to be using behaviors such as denial and manipulation.

For example, the severe memory impairment that occurs early in the illness precipitates many misunderstandings. When a person insists that there is nothing wrong with him—he can still drive, live alone, etc.—carers often suspect that this is "denial." However, the person is often unable to remember his own recent acts or to compare them to memories of past behavior. Therefore, he has no knowledge of the mistakes that are evidence of his illness and truly does not know that he is ill.

Personality may determine one's response to one's perception of a stimulus. Thus, incorrectly perceiving an insult, one person may react with anger, another with tears, and a third by withdrawing—all responses that bewilder the caregiver, who did not intend to insult.

Therefore, in helping a person with a dementing illness, we must determine as accurately as possible whether the failure of cognitive functions caused the faulty behavior before we can explain behavior as part of a personality style or coping strategy. We cannot assume that personality is the primary cause of the behavior observed. Neuropsychology provides a detailed understanding of the areas of spared and impaired function in a given person (see Chapter 3). This gives us clinical tools with which to assist the confused person and with which to recognize both personality and impairment.

Old habits or old personality traits can be useful in helping the impaired person. One person who did not understand that she got lost outside still responded to the lifelong dictum that you don't go outside without your shoes on. People who are friendly and social may do well in day care. Conversely, when a person has difficulty adjusting to the community life of a nursing home, recognition that he has always been a solitary and reserved person may help staff members to accept and permit his need for privacy and solitude.

Many of the coping strategies recognized in psychodynamic theory (manipulative behavior, denial, obsessiveness, passivity, etc.) require intellectual skills such as recognition, planning, and memory.

Often what we see in people with dementia seems to be old habits of behavior rather than defense mechanisms. Thus, the person who has a history of being manipulative who develops a dementia may merely be carrying out old habits of behavior. The coping strategies that people with dementia tend to use are (1) old habits and (2) strategies that are simple, straightforward, and immediate (e.g., if a person does not understand what is wanted, that person may simply decline).

Caregivers often wonder about the dementia patient's "motivation." Motivation has many definitions and is loosely and vaguely used in the context of dementia patients. What is often meant is, What will make the patient want to do something? or Why does the patient do that? This concept of motivation requires that the patient be able to understand a potential reward, remember the promise of a reward, remember past similar events, sustain an expectation, and understand the context or setting (e.g., understand that she is in a nursing home and that the nurse wants her to eat, rather than believing that she is in a restaurant where the food must be purchased). Certainly, we can make the patient want to do something, but the method must be immediate (so that he does not have to remember it) or he must be frequently reminded and the reminders must be compelling (so that they override other distractions), clear to the patient, and relevant to him as an individual adult. Often the problem is not one of motivation but of communicating the desirability of an action or of overcoming the patient's anxiety.

Affect

Loss of intellectual functions does not necessarily change a person's ability to experience a range of emotions. Many behaviors seem to be expressions of affect, such as fearfulness, anxiety, and irritability. In a controlled setting such as day care, interventions that increase the individual's experience of pleasure, success, humor, and security can be offered.

Both positive and negative affect influences behavior. The person who is acting angry or agitated is not comfortable. Such behavior first and foremost is a symptom of patient distress. Some individuals seem to feel anxiety, fear, confusion, anger, or embarrassment much of the time. They may be more likely to respond to these feelings than to other cues in the environment. Catastrophic reactions, stubbornness, searching, trying to "go home," clinging, withdrawal, and similar behaviors may reflect the negative feelings that result from being unable to recognize one's environment or from fear of doing something wrong. Many people with dementia are unable to suppress a response to the strongest stimulus (see Chapter 3). The presence of strong feelings may make it difficult to have patients attend to instructions or tasks or even accept reassurance. Because of the individual's cognitive impairments, affect may seem misplaced. A person who seems angry with a caregiver may in fact be frightened or may have misinterpreted the intent of the caregiver. The key to successful management is to interpret such situations correctly.

Much of the success of good congregate programs is their ability to reduce negative affect and help severely impaired individuals experience positive feelings, such as happiness, humor, affection, security, and self-satisfaction. Efforts to enable these feelings are rewarding both for humanitarian reasons and because comfortable individuals behave more appropriately. Although the balance of positive/negative feelings may be shifted, the person's response to confused sensory input and massive brain damage cannot be completely reversed.

Depression, anxiety, and emotional lability may arise from the brain damage, a prior condition, or as a response to a situation. Such mood states are common in people with dementia. Their presence in no way negates the need for treatment.

The Presence of Excess Disabilities

Excess disability has been defined by Kahn (1975) as more disability than can be explained by the disease alone. In dementia, excess disability is commonly caused by the presence of other illness, medication, psychiatric symptoms secondary to the dementia, sensory impairments, stress, fatigue, and anxiety. Whenever possible, excess disability should be eliminated or reduced to maximize cognitive function and improve behavior.

Even minor *illnesses, medication* reactions, or *pain* can further cloud mental functions in people with dementia. These individuals may be unable to communicate their discomfort verbally (see Chapters 1 and 2).

Psychiatric symptoms (such as hallucinations, delusions, depression, paranoia, anxiety, or extreme agitation) can be caused by the dementing illness, by other illnesses, or by medications. These symptoms may affect mood and behavior directly and often interfere with the patient's ability to attend to enjoyable activities.

Elderly individuals experience normal changes in *sensory function*, and many also suffer from disease processes that impair sensory function. Sensory deficits doubly handicap the person who cannot recognize their presence or learn to compensate for them. Sensory deficits can cause behavior problems when their presence contributes to disorientation, inaccurate perception of the environment, or confusion. Struggling to see or hear also adds to fatigue. Others must assume responsibility for locating mislaid glasses and replacing hearing aid batteries. Supportive devices should be introduced as early as possible to facilitate patient adjustment. The physical environment can be modified to support sensory impairment. (See Chapter 9.)

Stress, fear, fatigue, and anxiety, common for the person with cognitive impairment who is struggling to function in a confusing world, may actually reduce the impaired person's ability to remember, think, or reason, increasing the disability and making the person even less able to respond appropriately. Fatigue, stress, fear, and anxiety often precipitate catastrophic reactions. In the grip of an overreaction to stress, the person's cognitive functions deteriorate, exacerbating the reaction. Many significant stressors are created by the interaction between the cognitive impairment and the physical and interpersonal environments. These stressors often can be modified or reduced.

Physical, Interpersonal, and Internal Environments

The physical, interpersonal, and internal environments play key roles in enhancing sensory function and in decreasing excess disability. It can be theorized that, because individuals with dementia learn very little, *all* changes to enable improved function and decreased problem behavior must be in the environment.

The internal environment must not be overlooked. The impaired person may be unable to communicate the experience of the internal environment (pain, stomach ache, hallucinations) and even may be unable to recognize what is being experienced. Physical pain can be a potent distractor, often triggering undesirable behavior.

The physical environment is discussed in detail in Chapter 9. The physical and psychosocial environments can be modified to increase patient comfort and reduce behavior problems (Haugen 1985; Coons 1986; Miller 1977). Several factors of the physical and psychosocial environment must be considered: the reduction of stressors, the opportunity for social relationships, the presence of adequate stimulation, and the ability of the impaired person to control and predict the environment.

There is a close relationship between stress in the environment and patient behavior/function. Lawton (1981) found that dementia patients are highly responsive to reductions of stress in their environment. Hall and Buckwalter (1987) designed a conceptual model in which patients with dementia show progressively lowered stress thresholds. As the stress threshold is approached, anxious behaviors are exhibited; as the stress threshold is crossed, dysfunctional behavior occurs. Caregivers can use client anxiety as a barometer to determine how much activity and stimulus the person can tolerate at a given point.

Common stressors include multiple simultaneous signals or distractors, demanding multistep tasks, nonverbal messages of haste, demands placed on impaired areas of cognition, fatigue, illness, frustration, not being understood, not understanding, negative nonverbal messages, anxiety, fear, etc. The carer will need to explore carefully the specific sources of stress for a given individual.

The kinds of environmental stressors that overstress a person with dementia may appear idiosyncratic. One person may enjoy a full choice of foods on his plate, but another may be overwhelmed by this. Sources of stress may not carry over from one situation to another. A person may be able to tolerate a large group for singing but not for meals. Nevertheless, some phenomena such as giving multiple simultaneous demands or rushing someone will predictably stress most people.

Coons (1986) showed that the physical and psychosocial environments can be modified to alleviate stressors and reduce catastrophic reactions. In a planned environment, patient feelings such as anxiety, fear of failure, and feelings of being lost are reduced. Residents in such programs often look less anxious and appear more relaxed and happy. This reduction in general stress levels probably plays a significant role in reducing catastrophic reactions. (See Chapter 14.)

People with dementia retain (until late in the illness) a need for interpersonal relationships and the ability to use nonverbal communication. At the same time, the nature of the symptoms and the need for extensive physical care disrupts normal relationships. When the caregiver is exhausted, untrained, or overburdened with the physical tasks of caregiving, the impaired person may experience little touch and no meaningful social interactions and be unable to maintain relationships. In such a situation, the human interactions may all be negative. Such an environment probably encourages undesirable behavior, apathy, or withdrawal. Negative behavior may be the only response the person is capable of making in an attempt to invite interaction. A therapeutic human environment restores humor, affection, and mutual assistance in ways that the impaired person can handle.

The environment must do more than simply reduce noxious stimuli; it must also provide appropriate stimulation, rewards, pleasure, satisfaction, etc. Lack of such an environment and long hours of idleness are nontherapeutic (Roth 1986; Miller 1977; Burnside 1982) and probably add to stress, self-stimulatory behaviors, and unnecessary decline and withdrawal. People with dementia have little ability to initiate, plan, and carry out activities. When this lack combines with an environment that offers little appropriate stimulation, some individuals may develop behaviors such as screaming, masturbating, and pacing. Others will withdraw or become apathetic. (Such behaviors can have other causes as well.) These behaviors usually diminish when the person is offered appropriate activities to fill the otherwise long, empty hours. Too much activity however, can overstimulate the person. The degree of patient involvement can be graded; active watching or even criticism may be an appropriate level of participation.

Human beings need to be able to control and predict their environment. An environment that cannot be controlled and predicted may lead to demoralization and apathy. Because the person with dementia does not remember, even the physical environment becomes unpredictable. The bathroom may seem to shift from place to place. Control over one's own body and one's personal care is gradually lost. The damaged sense of time exacerbates the feeling of an unpredictable environment. Thus, the environment must provide opportunities for the damaged mind to regain some measure of control and predictability.

Untrained caregivers often present as a hypothesis for behavior the concept that "she could do it if she tried." More experienced providers may dress this idea up in psychodynamic terms. It is a sufficiently common idea to deserve attention. Patients often retain many aspects of their personalities and social functions for a long time. They may be able to conceal impairments so that casual acquaintances see nothing wrong.

The person often does not recognize that he is impaired, and he may be upset when inappropriate behavior is not regarded as normal. The uneven nature of the damage and the fact that skills flicker—the person can do something one time but not another—lead caregivers to suspect that the patient is more in control than is actually the case. Then the caregiver makes inappropriate demands, triggering stress in the impaired person.

Two daughters reported that their mother, who had a dementia, would use the dishwasher in one household but refused to use the dishwasher in the other household. They believed that this was because Mother had always preferred one daughter over the other. Careful evaluation determined that one dishwasher was new and the mother could not learn to operate it, whereas the other one was old and familiar to the mother.

Mace and Rabins (1981) pointed out that many behaviors that appear volitional are not under the patient's control. The lack of memory, inability to plan, loss of judgment, and other cognitive impairments that can be documented in a given individual argue that the individual lacks the intellectual capability to carry out planned or deliberate behaviors. *Whenever there is doubt, the patient and caregiver will be best served by the assumption that the impaired person is already trying hard.*

The Goals of Behavior Management

The first step in planning a successful intervention strategy is to identify the goals of behavior change.

Common Goals

- Ensure the safety of the patient, caregiver, or others. For example, people with dementia who wander, smoke, drive, or attempt to cook often create risks for themselves and others.
- Provide support or relief for the family or paid caregiver. For example, repeatedly asking the same question, pacing, or shouting, although not dangerous, places considerable stress on the caregiver. A person who is awake at night and requires supervision from a family member can severely threaten the informal caring system.

- Control costs. For example, it may be less expensive to stop a behavior than to allow it to continue.
- Meet quality assurance standards, marketing demands, or community expectations. For example, in a nursing home, patients may not be able to hoard food; disheveled or socially inappropriate patients may not be allowed in public areas.
- Protect other residents/participants from annoyance and harassment.
- Improve patient function, autonomy, quality of life, and satisfaction or alleviate patient discomfort.
- Make patient care easier. For example, it is easier and quicker to bathe a cooperative person.

Weighing Options

Weighing the options in terms of goals is helpful in the problem-solving process. Identifying the goal often influences the choice of interventions and determines the urgency of change. A dangerous situation may require more aggressive intervention than an annoying one. When the only available intervention involves risk for the patient, such as the use of neuroleptic medication, the goal should outweigh the risks of the intervention. Goals may be in conflict. For example, safety goals may conflict with goals of patient independence or pleasure. Identifying the goal may suggest additional options. Relief can be offered to the caregiver in the form of respite care or additional staff instead of by stopping a behavior with restraint or medication.

Unrealistic Goals

Some of the goals sought by families, paid caregivers, funding sources, or institutions are not realistic in light of the presently irreversible nature of primary degenerative dementia.

- Altering the course of the disease. The interventions now available will not reverse or halt the progression of the dementia. Certain measures of function may change, while others will not change.
- Enabling the person to learn or relearn material. The patient is unlikely to learn to change behaviors or to regain lost skills. Therefore, therapeutic activities designed for other impaired populations that attempt to improve cognitive performance are usually inappropriate for people with Alzheimer's disease and related

disorders. Such activities provide another experience of frustration and failure for the person with dementia. They may exacerbate problem behavior, and they are frustrating and demoralizing for caregivers.

- Stopping all behavior problems. It may not be possible to stop all undesirable behavior. Even with the best care, an ideal milieu, and skilled staff, some problem behaviors may remain. At best, problem behaviors are less frequent, less intense, and less disruptive.

- Producing permanent change. The behaviors will usually recur if the intervention is stopped. People with dementia depend on the environmental change to support function and, when it is withdrawn, they usually cannot maintain improvements. This is different from the goal of rehabilitation in other diseases, which assumes that a time-limited intervention will produce permanent change. Programs that rely on funding with this kind of requirement can be caught between conflicting goals.

The Assessment of Risk

People with dementia present a special set of risks: the risk of intervention may equal or exceed the risk of continuing the behavior. For example, the ambulating frail patient who is at risk of falling, fracturing a hip, and dying may be equally at risk of rapid decline as a result of being confined to bed or chair. In weighing such decisions, the clinician must obtain as many facts about the case as possible, compare the risk of each option for this individual, and, wherever possible, involve the family in making an informed decision.

Fear of liability or mandated safety policies can impede this decision-making process. A discussion of these issues is beyond the scope of this chapter. However, those who set policy must be well informed about the special care needs of people with dementia. Further research to confirm clinical observations is needed to support the development of appropriate policies.

Approaches to Management

This section summarizes the most frequently used approaches to behavior management. Interventions are of two types: those that attempt to change the patient and those that attempt to change behavior by changing things external to the patient.

The management of behavior in people with dementia is challenging. In many situations, it may be impossible to stop all problematic behavior. There has been little research to confirm clinical experience, and not all clinicians agree on the most successful interventions. Nevertheless, clinical experience brings great optimism to the management of behavior problems. Staff in many congregate settings in the United States and other countries report dramatic improvements in patient quality of life and reduction of problem behaviors.

The finding that these individuals are responsive to change in their environment is encouraging because it means that even partial interventions can result in patient improvement. People with dementia can be slow to respond to interventions. Programs have reported continued improvement five months after the institution of an intervention (Coons 1986). Families and staff will need support during this transition period.

Prevention

Experienced clinicians emphasize that preventing behavior problems is easier and more effective than stopping them after they begin. Staff members of good programs report that certain undesirable behaviors occur rarely, if at all. These programs keep the patient as healthy as possible, create a supportive environment, and provide rest and support for the carers—both paid and family. Providing positive and satisfying experiences for the person with dementia has a pervasive impact on care and patient behavior. A positive experience distracts the person from undesired behaviors, reinforces feelings of self-satisfaction, reinforces appropriate social behavior, reduces stress, and reinforces the caregiver's positive view of the impaired person.

The problems arising from overreactions to stress—catastrophic reactions—are much easier to prevent than to stop when in progress. The person's cognitive ability deteriorates under stress, and the person may not able to attend to the carer's interventions while in the grip of a catastrophic reaction. The caregiver's ability to problem solve is also usually better when not in the midst of crisis. Triggers of these episodes can be identified and avoided. Clinicians can assist families and paid carers to identify the events that precede the undesired behavior. Changes in the sequence of events will often reduce reoccurrences.

Interventions That Attempt to Change the Patient

Medication

Medication is an important tool in the arsenal of behavior management, but it is a two-edged sword. Sleep medications, minor tranquilizers, and neuroleptics are commonly used to reduce disturbed behaviors. These drugs are most effective for the treatment of specific symptoms (see Chapter 2). However, psychoactive drugs are often used for their sedative effect (to control symptoms such as wandering, restlessness, and irritability) at dosages that interfere with remaining cognitive function and at which side effects occur. There is little evidence that they effectively control behavior when used at levels that produce side effects (Butler et al. 1987).

Restraint

Families and institutions often restrain people with dementia; egress is controlled through locks, latches the impaired person cannot work, physical restraints, and chairs the patient cannot get out of. Although restraint is occasionally necessary for safety, its use in behavior control should be limited. The use of restraints as a substitute for adequate staff or to provide respite care for the caregiver may be necessary but it is not in the patient's best interests. Restraint limits needed exercise and may prevent activity that has meaning for the person. It increases feelings of helplessness, anxiety, and anger. Most successful dedicated dementia care units and day care programs report that they are unable to reduce greatly or eliminate the use of medications and restraints for behavior control (U.S. Congress 1987; Mace and Rabins 1984).

Techniques That Require Learning

Techniques that require learning, such as behavior modification, reality orientation (Folsom 1968), and similar techniques, have in common that they require memory and new learning. They are limited by the individual's grossly impaired ability to learn or remember. It is clear that people with dementia are able to learn under some circumstances, but their learning capacity is greatly impaired. Little is known about what these individuals are able to learn and under what circumstances.

BEHAVIOR MODIFICATION. Behavior modification is based on the observation that an organism will learn to repeat rewarding behaviors (such as food seeking) and avoid behaviors that produce a noxious response such as pain. Even invertebrates will learn these responses. In humans, social rewards are so important than an individual may tolerate unpleasant consequences to obtain even minor or negative social interaction. Little is known about behavior modification in people whose cognitive function is severely compromised. Among the issues to be considered are the following:

- What learning takes place—how, and when—in people with dementia?
- As these individuals are often fearful, angry, or anxious, do these emotions interfere with learning?
- When do the needs of the patient override the reward? For example, the person desperately seeking "home" may not respond to a reward of cookies for not wandering.
- When are caregivers' goals inappropriate to the needs of the patient and therefore confounding to efforts to modify behavior? For example, the staff goal of having the person sit quietly may conflict with the patient goal of alleviating intolerable anxiety.
- When do behavior modification interventions conflict with the patient's compensatory efforts? For example, withholding friendly conversation from a person who acts out is in conflict with supporting compensatory efforts and remaining social skills.
- The carer and the patient may perceive themselves to be in different worlds. For the staff, the context is a quiet bath. The patient may perceive herself to be in Dachau and being taken to the gas chamber "showers."

Efforts to use techniques that require learning often frustrate both the confused person and the caregiver. Experiences of failure or angry outbursts of frustration give the patient negative feedback. Positive rewards may be effective when they are used in addition to efforts to create a supportive environment and to reduce negative experience. If this approach is tried, rewards should be immediate, straightforward, socially appropriate, and appropriate to adult behavior. The issues listed should be taken into consideration. However, behavior modification should be used with caution until research has identified learning approaches that are compatible with the deficits in dementia.

REALITY ORIENTATION. Reality orientation, as originally described by Folsom (1968), simultaneously uses two approaches: around-the-clock orientation by all staff and formal reality orientation sessions. Formal reality orientation sessions used alone may be of limited value to people with dementia because little learning will carry over to the next session. However, British programs strongly support their use. Clinicians report that using multiple environmental and interpersonal approaches consistently to orient the individual in the setting reassures the person and probably supports orientation. Insisting on orientation with the person who is anxious or determined is rarely helpful. Further research is needed to determine the role of orientation for people with dementia.

PUNISHMENT AND COUNSELING. Interventions based on the assumption that the person is acting out learned defense mechanisms or manipulative behaviors rarely are effective in the care of these brain-damaged individuals. Interventions such as punishment, argument, explaining, counseling, or ignoring "bad" behavior are often frustrating to carers and are in some cases cruel to the patient.

Reduction of Excess Disability

Efforts to eliminate or reduce excess disability are one of the mainstays of behavior management. The most prominent symptoms of concurrent illness, pain, or drug reaction may be the onset of undesirable behavior. Psychiatric symptoms can lead to behavior problems. Sensory deficits increase disorientation and confusion and can lead to increased agitation. In these frail people, fear and anxiety almost always generate behavior problems as well as causing suffering for the individual. There is little point to introducing other methods of changing behavior in a person who is delirious, drugged, unable to perceive the environment, tired, or frightened. Eliminating excess disability requires an initial evaluation of the person and the setting and continuing reexamination and medical support throughout the illness. (See Chapters 1 and 2.) The person's functional level must be regularly reassessed, and environmental changes must be made to support continued function.

Interventions That Change the Physical or
Psychosocial Environment

Clinical experience and the wisdom of family caregivers indicate that changes in behavior are often the result of changes outside the patient. Thus, interventions that change the human or physical environment are important in patient care. Such interventions can be grouped into (1) concrete advice, (2) general guidelines, (3) problem solving, (4) support of the caregiver, (5) creation of a prosthetic environment, and (6) milieu therapy.

Environmental changes often result in improved behavior and psychosocial function but not in improved cognitive abilities or change in the course of the disease. Improvements can be observed when even minor changes are made in the interpersonal or physical environment. Lawton (1981) termed this *environmental press*. Thus, a program that makes some appropriate improvements will be rewarded by improved function and a decrease in problem behavior. Good programs report numerous changes. Although creating an improved environment is challenging, it does not have to be extraordinarily expensive, and daily care can be carried out by trained nonprofessionals.

It may not be possible to implement extensive changes in either the physical or the psychosocial environment when the person is living at home, particularly if the caregiver is not well supported. Changes in the physical environment may be costly and can increase the carer's anxiety. When a family member is carrying the burden of care alone or has limited emotional resources, there are real limits to the extent of change in the carer's own behavior that can be requested. Additional environmental interventions can sometimes be provided by adult day care or in-home respite.

When change is attempted, the changes the carer is asked to make must be weighed against potential gains. The interventions must be simple, and the carer must be well supported by the clinician. Support groups provide peer support, which helps carers to make changes in the home and in their behavior. Similar requirements apply to paid carers. They must be well supported and not overwhelmed or overstressed; they must understand the proposed change and its goal; and they must perceive that the benefits of the change outweigh the effort involved.

The interventions described have been loosely grouped by the demands that they make on the caregiver. There is considerable overlap between categories, and interventions from several categories are often used together.

Practical Advice

Practical advice is a concrete suggestion for changing the behavior of the impaired person. Such suggestions are found extensively in the newsletters of chapters of the Alzheimer's Association. Many suggestions of this type are given by Mace and Rabins (1981), Gwyther (1985), and Ballard and Gwyther (1988). As an example, for wandering one could:

apply child-proof locks;
escort the person around the building and invite him back in;
leave the person in bedroom slippers;
use restraints;
disguise exits;
hide the person's coat; or
use electronic devices to alert the carer.

This approach is limited by the considerable variability among persons with dementia, their caregivers, and their settings. The same behavior often has different causes and will need different interventions for different individuals or for the same individual at different times. For example, some possible causes of wandering are the need for exercise, a search for something familiar, agitation, the need to use the toilet, restlessness due to medication side effects, or boredom.

The more concrete such advice, the more limited its usefulness. However, these interventions are easy for burdened or untrained caregivers to use, and there is enough universality among causes of behaviors that many suggestions succeed. Such advice is easy to disseminate and, when it works, it meets the immediate goal of helping the caregiver.

General Guidelines

This approach moves beyond concrete suggestions to offer guidelines for the carer's behavior that have been found to be successful in caring for people with dementia. These guidelines are often presented in connection with concrete suggestions. Gwyther (1985), Mace and Rabins (1981), and Zgola (1987) offer such guidelines. Because they involve change in the carer's behavior, they are slightly more difficult to apply. The carer must not be so stressed that he or she is unable to change. A few carers are unsuited by temperament to accepting the need for change within themselves. In general, however, carers, both family members and paid, adapt well to these guidelines. Role modeling by other staff or by families in support groups is an excellent teaching tool.

Sample Guidelines

- Recognize that the person has an impaired ability to learn and to adapt and that he has little understanding of the impact of his behavior. Behaviors are rarely under the person's control. They are not deliberate, willful, or manipulative. (This blames the disease, not the person, for the behavior and removes the behavior from the relationship between the carer and the patient. It is also a more realistic understanding of what is happening.)
- Keep the person as healthy as possible.
- Simplify tasks; simplify the environment. Break tasks down into simple steps.
- Know the person's limitations. Do not push the patient beyond them. Schedule demanding tasks for the person's best time of day.
- Give only positive reinforcement. The person may not know what to do when told "do not . . . ." Tell the patient what *to* do.
- Compensate for the person's limitations. Do those parts of a task she cannot do. Supply a word when she is struggling to find it. Carers ask how to tell when they are doing too much and when they should do more. In general, the carer should allow the person to do for herself until the first signs of stress are observed. Then the carer should assist before a catastrophic reaction occurs.
- Avoid being too interpretive. The cause of the behavior is most likely immediate and obvious, rather than psychodynamic or hidden.
- Use familiar routines. Rely on old habits and skills. Determine how the person used to do things (such as the sequence in dressing) and try to repeat habits.
- Carers must be flexible, changing approaches and schedules when they observe distress.
- When an approach seems to confuse or upset the person, try alternative ways of doing the task.

- Avoid the problem. For example, give baths as infrequently as possible without risking skin breakdown. Use a bath stool and a hand-held nozzle. Give sponge baths.
- Make use of the person's compensatory behaviors. People with dementia develop simple compensatory behaviors. The answer "I already had my bath" may be a way to compensate when the person does not know what he was asked to do. This attempt to cope with the illness should be regarded in a positive light and supported as healthy.
- Make what you do as person-oriented as possible. Avoid focusing your behavior on getting the task done to the exclusion of the person's needs.
- People with dementia often retain a sense of humor and can show affection. Learn to relax and share these moments.

The Management of Catastrophic Reactions

- Recognize the early warning signs; do not press the person at this time. Wait, try later, relieve stress. Early warning signs include refusals, restlessness, flushing.
- If a catastrophic reaction occurs, consider what happened just before that might have triggered it. Avoid this trigger in the future. Keep a log to help identify triggers. Common precipitants include: misinterpretation of a request, misinterpretation of sensory information, cognitive overload, inability to perform a task, fatigue, inability to communicate needs, frustration, response to a demoralizing or infantilizing approach.
- Recognize that the behavior is not willful and respond accordingly.
- Remove the person or thing that upset the patient. The person may forget the incident quickly.
- Avoid arguing or restraining; be calm and reassuring. Compensate for the person's limitations.
- Combative behavior is almost always an extreme catastrophic reaction. Look for ways to avoid pushing the person this far.

Guidelines for Communication

Because people with dementia lose the ability to use and understand language, communication difficulties result in frustration for the patient and the caregiver. Below are general guidelines for communication:

- Make sure that the person heard you.
- Lower the pitch of your voice. A raised pitch communicates stress.
- Eliminate distracting noises and activities.
- Use short words and short, simple sentences.
- Ask only one question at a time. Repeat questions exactly.
- Avoid questions altogether, or give clues to the answer. For example, "Yesterday you told me that you like scrambled eggs. Is that how you would like your eggs today?"
- Give only one step of instructions at a time.
- Speak slowly and wait for the response.
- Patients often are better able to use and understand nonverbal communication than written or spoken language. Learn to read moods and express things with a minimal dependence on verbal language.
- Remain pleasant, calm, and supportive.
- Smile and express affection.
- Look directly at the person. Observe whether the person is paying attention to you.
- Point, touch, show, initiate a movement for the person.
- Use as many communication pathways as possible: vision, sound, touch, etc. If the person does not understand what you said, try to help the person *see* what is wanted.
- Trust your ability to read feelings in the person accurately, even when what is said does not make much sense.

Breakdown of the Tasks

Breaking tasks down into small steps the person can comprehend is an important part of reducing stress and avoiding problem behavior. This skill is described in Chapter 6, by Zgola (1987), and in the videotape "Helping People with Dementia in Activities of Daily Living" (Robinson et al. 1987). The carer thinks through each step in a task and then determines which steps the impaired person can do. Tasks can be broken down so that one person does them step by step, with the carer filling in where necessary (for example, dressing), or the task can be broken down so that different members of a small group do different steps according to their abilities (for example, making soup).

Caregiver Support (When the Carer Is Family, Volunteer, or Paid)

Caregiver support is discussed throughout this book. In some cases, a behavior can be allowed to continue if the caregiver can be well enough supported to be able to tolerate the behavior. For example, the impact of suspiciousness and making accusations depends on how the carer perceives the behavior—as deliberate and personal or as part of the illness. People with dementia often remain sensitive to the moods of those who care for them, and this awareness affects behavior. The tasks of providing care place huge demands on the carer—whether family, volunteer, or paid. An exhausted caregiver or one who does not feel supported elicits more negative responses from the impaired person. One study showed that a therapeutic program for patients and carers may slow behavior deterioration in patients. (Winogrond et al. 1987). Few of the interventions described will be successful when the caregiver is untrained, unsupported, underpaid, exhausted, or unhappy; does not understand the nature of the illness; or is not suited to such work.

Volunteers and paid caregivers should have a desire to do this work and a personality that allows flexibility, a tolerance for deviant behavior, a sense of humor, and the ability to experience and express genuine affection. Family members usually care for patients as long as possible, but those who are overwhelmed or unwilling to care should not be coerced by financial constraints to continue. Abuse can occur in such situations. All caregivers must be trained. They must understand the basic characteristics of the illness and how it affects behavior. They must have a repertoire of appropriate interventions.

Caregivers must have ongoing support. Zarit et al. (1986) pointed out the importance of support for family members, and support is necessary for staff members also. Family members, friends, family support groups, and professionals are all sources of support. Many families find support in written materials. Volunteers and paid providers must have the full support of administrators and supervisors. They make a personal commitment to a program to provide care successfully. [See Chapters 13 and 14 and Edelson and Lyons (1985).] Frequent staff meetings provide opportunities to ventilate ongoing training. Salary is indicative of the community value placed on the individual's work and is an important indicator of support. Volunteers and paid providers become attached to their charges and mourn transfer, decline, and death. They will need additional support during these times.

Problem Solving

In the problem-solving approach to behavior management, the caregiver endeavors to determine the reason for the patient's behavior and bases the intervention on this. The best of the materials explaining this approach also give the caregiver some idea of why the patient may be acting in this way. Much of the information shared in family support groups, books, and newsletters is a combination of practical advice and problem solving (Gwyther 1985; Mace and Rabins 1981).

Problem solving provides greater flexibility for addressing behaviors that are resistant to more concrete interventions. Problem solving requires more skill than other interventions and requires a well-supported, able carer. Clinicians can bypass caregiver difficulties by solving specific problems with the carer. Problem solving is an individualized intervention. Determining the probable cause of an individual behavior at a specific place and time and with specific people offers a much greater chance of successful intervention. Identification of the probable cause usually suggests an appropriate intervention. The goal and urgency of the intervention is considered. The first intervention tried should be the least aggressive/risky. The clinician reviews with the carer the causes of the problem and asks what events led to the behavior. Can it be prevented in the future?

The Six "R's" of Patient Care

This can be used as a memory device for carers.

- *Reassess* when change is observed or when an intervention no longer works. Do not assume that change is due to patient decline.
- *Restrict*: The most common method of intervention is to stop a behavior from occurring. When someone is at risk, restriction may be the fastest way to ensure safety.
- *Reconsider*: Consider the meaning of the behavior for the patient. From his point of view, is this a reasonable behavior? For example, the patient being put to bed at night by a staff member may be perceiving that a stranger is undressing him and may not understand that he is in a nursing home and unable to undress himself.
- *Rechannel*: Find a way for the behavior to continue in a safe and acceptable way. For example, give the person who is taking things apart a meaningful item to disassemble; give the retired nurse

who is attempting to "care for" the other residents a real task to do; give the rummager a box of meaningful items to sort.

- *Redirect*: Divert behavior that is leading to an outburst. Use distraction; take a restless person for a walk.
- *Reassure*: Reassure the person that she is safe, that you will see that she does not embarrass herself or get lost. If an outburst occurs, reassure her that you understood her distress.

Behavior problems often have different causes in different patients. Although uncommon, sexual behaviors are so upsetting to carers that they are used here an as example of the variety of causes of behavior. The reader may identify additional possible causes.

Possible Causes of Inappropriate "Sexual" Activities

- Need to use toilet.
- Infection, discomfort, itching.
- Boredom, effort to provide self-stimulation.
- Disorientation to place (masturbating in day room).
- Disorientation to person (approaching a nurse or daughter).
- Need for touch, companionship.
- Establishment of a relationship with another, willing patient. (This is not necessarily a patient problem. It can be viewed as a problem when it conflicts with the values of others.)
- (Probably rare) hypersexuality as a result of a brain lesion.
- (Rare) continuation of lifelong problem that the person can no longer conceal. (The clinician should be most cautious about posing this hypothesis.)
- An inept attempt to reestablish a masculine role. (Flirting with the nurses is socially acceptable for younger men; the confused person may be too blunt or choose the wrong words.)
- An inappropriate response to friendly staff behavior. (The point here is not whether staff "invite" such behavior. Affectionate behavior is common between younger carers and older patients. The same behavior may encourage "gentlemanly" behavior in another person. The issue is how to rechannel the behavior in this individual.)

Once a probable cause has been determined, appropriate interventions are usually obvious. They should be tried one at a time. If interventions fail, a different cause is hypothesized (Table 4.3).

Problem solving is more time-consuming to teach, and it requires

TABLE 4.3 Various Possible Causes of a Problem Behavior and Their Solutions

Causes of Wandering	Possible Solutions
Need for exercise	Take patient for brisk walks Offer calisthenics Provide interesting space for wandering
Restlessness	Provide errands Provide area to explore Provide exercise Provide physically active group activity
Looking for something	Identify and provide what is being sought or provide more orienting cues (that this is your house, etc.) Reassure, respond to feeling Provide role-appropriate tasks
Agitation	Treat as for catastrophic reaction
Need to use the toilet	Assist to toilet Use scheduled toileting

practice and role modeling. The caregiver must be well supported, not overly stressed, and intellectually and emotionally capable of this approach. Given the large population in need of care, these requirements become significant drawbacks. Not all family caregivers have the resources required, and nursing home staff turnover may be too great to invest the time required to teach this approach. However, nonprofessional staff and families can learn it. Programs report that trained staff have greater job satisfaction and lower job turnover (Sorenson 1988).

The Prosthetic Environment

The concept of the prosthetic environment is similar to the concept of milieu therapy. The prosthetic environment assesses areas of spared and impaired function in each person and supports remaining function while avoiding or substituting for areas of impaired function. The total environment (physical and human) is a prosthesis because it supports partial independence by substituting for or avoiding lost abilities. This enables the person to do as much as possible for himself, it relieves the person of unnecessary stress and anxiety, avoids frustration, enables positive feelings, and reinforces self-esteem.

Creation of a prosthetic environment requires an understanding of the nature of the cognitive deficits in the irreversible dementias. The prosthetic environment attempts to substitute as much as possible for the massive cognitive damage these people experience. A fully prosthetic environment would be a facility built for the purpose and with a highly trained staff. The responsiveness of people with dementia to their environment means that any environment can be modified to include highly effective prosthetic components.

Milieu Therapy

Milieu therapy holds that each of the environmental components in the milieu, "the program of activities which makes up the daily life of the individual, the staff, the physical setting, and other residents—has the potential for becoming a therapeutic or nontherapeutic agent in treatment . . . . The essential assumption underlying Milieu Therapy is that the total environment—the milieu—is itself a treatment agent and needs to be considered in planning programs and establishing therapeutic regimens" (Coons 1981). This approach considers behavior as a part of the patient or participant's total life and not as a separate or independent component. Improving behavior is secondary to the primary focus of improving the quality of the person's life. Milieu therapy emphasizes the importance of maintaining the person's sense of identity and dignity. It supports the maintenance of lifelong roles. Experiences of pleasure, humor, friendship, and success are regarded as therapeutically necessary. (See Chapter 14.)

All staff-resident interactions, the physical environment, the residents' health, etc., are considered therapeutic interventions that maximize function and reduce inappropriate behavior. This approach theorizes that, as the person's anxiety, confusion, and embarrassment diminish, the capacity for cognitive function is maximized and disturbed behaviors will also diminish. The goal is to create a milieu in which the person can experience pleasure, security, and personal worth on an existential, moment by moment basis. A prosthetic environment and individual problem solving are integral parts of this approach.

This approach has been dramatically successful in reducing or eliminating undesirable behaviors in a variety of programs worldwide, some working with the most severely behaviorally disturbed patients. There is little doubt that many ambulatory, midstage patients would be responsive to this approach. "There has been a decided reduction in incontinence . . . [and] by the fifth month most of the persons were sleeping through the night, patients have resumed old household tasks, become friendly and warm, wandering has been reduced" (Coons 1986).

Model projects have not been more expensive than other programs (Coons 1986). This approach is limited by the extent to which the milieu can be controlled or modified. An important part of the milieu is probably the social opportunities provided in a group setting in either adult day care or residential care. Perceived or real cost limitations, staff resistance to change, administrative resistance to change, a fixed physical plant, or the dynamics of a historically unsatisfactory caregiver-patient relationship can all significantly limit the extent to which the patient's physical and interpersonal environment can be manipulated to improve function or to decrease undesirable behaviors.

The demands of these latter approaches are considerably greater than those previously discussed. They require extensive training and support of caregivers. Caregivers must be intellectually and psychologically capable of implementing the interventions. In addition, the number and characteristics of people suffering from dementia who can benefit from milieu therapy is not known. Despite these limitations, this approach is exciting. It provides evidence that the quality of life for people suffering from dementia can be greatly improved, and it gives us the tools for successful intervention. In light of the demands of this approach, it is heartening that people with dementia will show improvement even when only some appropriate changes are made in the environment.

Conclusion

Problem behavior is evidence of suffering in the patient, it is a severe burden on the family, and it probably increases the national cost of care. This chapter has demonstrated that an extensive repertoire of successful interventions is available to alleviate behavior problems. There is no justification for the common position that drugs are the only behavior management resource available or that behavior management is "hopeless."

This chapter reviewed the theoretical causes of problem behavior in dementia: the role of the brain damage, the person's premorbid coping style, the person's feelings, the presence of excess disabilities, and the impact of the environment. The carer's assumptions about the cause of behavior influence the carer's behavior toward the ill person and the choice of interventions. The devastation of the disease process and its affect on the person's perception of the environment are believed to be the primary causes of behavior problems. Our knowledge of the validity of these causal theories is based on repeated clinical observation but needs further validation through research. Such research will light the way for a "second generation" of treatments that will be easier to teach, less costly, and more beneficial to the patient.

Identifying the goals of a specific intervention helps the clinician select the appropriate intervention. The clinician has a range of effective interventions from which to choose. The choice will be influenced by the goals of the intervention, its urgency, and the caregiver's ability to carry it out.

This chapter raises several ethical issues that are beyond its scope of discussion. Most important among these is the provision of interventions to change the behavior of individuals who cannot make their own wishes and needs known. This is done on the assumption that the brain damage is causing behavior and that the person would "prefer" not to act this way. No matter how beneficent such interventions are, the ethical implications still must be considered.

The care of people with dementing illnesses is not easy. This chapter does not offer solutions for each of the different problems facing clinicians. It does, however, offer a framework for thinking about behavior problems, guidelines for solutions, and the good news that we can help these individuals and their carers. It is hoped that this chapter provides a springboard for more optimistic patient care and for rigorous study of the behavior problems of dementia.

References

Ballard, E. L., and L. P. Gwyther. 1988. *In-home respite care: Guidelines for training respite workers serving memory impaired adults.* Durham, NC: Duke University Center for the Study of Aging.

Burnside, I. M. 1982. Care of the Alzheimer's patient in an institution. *Generations* 7 (1): 22–23, 50.

Butler, F. R., L. D. Burgio, and B. T. Engel. 1987. Neuroleptics and behavior: A comparative study. *Journal of Gerontological Nursing* 13 (June): 6, 15–19.

Cleary, T. A., C. Clamon, M. Price, and G. Shullaw. 1988. A reduced stimulation unit: Effect on patients with Alzheimer's disease and related disorders. *Gerontologist* 28 (4): 511–14.

Cohen, D., G. Kennedy, and C. Eisdorfer. 1984. Phases of change in the patient with Alzheimer's dementia: A conceptual dimension for defining health care management. *Journal of the American Geriatrics Society* 32 (1): 11–15.

Cohen-Mansfeld, J., and N. Billig. 1986. Agitated behaviors in the elderly. *Journal of the American Geriatrics Society* 34:711–21.

Coons, D. H. 1981. Milieu therapy. In *Topics in aging and long term care*, ed. W. Reichel, 53–65. Baltimore: Williams & Wilkins.

Coons, D. H. 1986. *A residential care unit for persons with dementia*. Contract report prepared for the Office of Technology Assessment, U.S. Congress. Washington, DC: U.S. Government Printing Office.

Cornbleth, T. 1977. Effects of a protected ward area on wandering and non-wandering geriatric patients. *Journal of Gerontology* 35 (5): 573–77.

Edelson, J. S., and W. H. Lyons. 1985. *Institutional care of the mentally impaired elderly*. New York: Van Nostrand Reinhold.

Folsom, J. C. 1968. Reality orientation for the elderly mental patient. *Journal of Geriatric Psychiatry* 1:291–307.

Goldstein, K. 1952. The effect of brain damage on the personality. *Psychiatry* 15:245–60.

Gwyther, L. P. 1985. *Care of Alzheimer's patients: A manual for nursing home staff*. Washington, DC: Alzheimer's Disease and Related Disorders Association and American Health Care Association.

Hall, G. R., and K. C. Buckwalter. 1987. Progressively lowered stress threshold: A conceptual model for care of adults with Alzheimer's disease. *Archives of Psychiatric Nursing* 1 (6): 399–406.

Haugen, P. K. 1985. Behavior of patients with dementia. *Danish Medical Bulletin* 32 (1): 62–65.

Hiatt, L. G. 1980. The happy wanderer. *Nursing Homes* 29 (2): 27–31.

Kahn, R. L. 1975. The mental health system and the future aged. *Gerontologist* 15:24–31.

Knopman, D. S., J. Kitto, S. Deinard, and J. Heiring. 1988. Longitudinal study of death and institutionalization in patients with primary degenerative dementia. *Journal of the American Geriatrics Society* 36:108–12.

Lawton, M. P. 1981. Sensory deprivation and the effect of the environment on management of the patient with senile dementia. In *Aspects of Alzheimer's disease and senile dementia*, ed. N. Miller and G. D. Cohen, 227–50. New York: Raven Press.

Mace, N. L., and P. V. Rabins. 1981. *The 36-hour day*. Baltimore: Johns Hopkins University Press.

Mace, N. L., and P. V. Rabins. 1984. *A survey of day care for the demented adult in the United States*. Washington, DC: National Council on Aging.

McHugh, P. R., and P. R. Slavney. 1983. *The perspectives of psychiatry.* Baltimore: Johns Hopkins University Press.

Miller, E. 1977. The management of dementia: A review of some of the possibilities. *British Journal of Social Clinical Psychology* 16:77–83.

Rabins, P. V., N. L. Mace, and M. Lucas. 1982. The impact of dementia on the family. *Journal of the American Medical Association* 48:333–35.

Reisberg, B. 1983. Clinical presentation, diagnosis, and symptomology of age-associated cognitive decline and Alzheimer's disease. In *Alzheimer's disease: The standard reference,* 173–87. New York: Free Press.

Robinson, A., B. Spencer, S. Weaverdyck, and S. Gardiner. 1987. *Helping people with dementia in activities of daily living.* Videotape unit distributed by Michigan Media, 400 4th St., Ann Arbor, MI 48109.

Roth, M. Letter to author, October 28, 1986.

Rubin, E. H., W. C. Drevets, and W. J. Burke. 1988. The nature of psychotic symptoms in senile dementia of the Alzheimer type. *Journal of Geriatric Psychiatry and Neurology* 1 (January): 16–20.

Rubin, E. H., J. C. Morris, and L. Berg. 1987a. The progression of personality changes in senile dementia of the Alzheimer's type. *Journal of the American Geriatrics Society* 35:721–25.

Rubin, E. H., J. C. Morris, M. Storandt, and L. Berg. 1987b. Behavioral changes in patients with mild senile dementia of the Alzheimer's type. *Psychiatry Research* 21:55–62.

Ryan, D. P., S. M. Tainsh, V. Kolodny, B. Lendrum, and R. H. Fisher. 1988. Noise-making amongst the elderly in long term care. *Gerontologist* 28 (3): 369–71.

Sacks, O. 1970. *The man who mistook his wife for a hat.* New York: Harper & Row.

Shomaker, D. 1987. Problematic behavior and the Alzheimer patient: Retrospection as a method of understanding and counseling. *Gerontologist* 27 (3): 370–75.

Smallegan, M. 1985. There was nothing else to do: Needs for care before nursing home admission. *Gerontologist* 25 (4): 364–69.

Sorenson, C. Personal communication, March 1988.

Teri, L., E. B. Larson, and B. V. Reifler. 1988. Behavioral disturbance in dementia of the Alzheimer's type. *Journal of the American Geriatrics Society* 36:1–6.

U.S. Congress. Office of Technology Assessment. 1987. *Losing a million minds: confronting the tragedy of Alzheimer's disease and other dementias.* OTA-BA-323. Washington, DC: U.S. Government Printing Office. April.

Winogrond, I. R., A. A. Fisk, R. A. Kirsling, and B. Keyes. 1987. The relationship of caregiver burden and morale to Alzheimer's disease patient function in a therapeutic setting. *Gerontologist* 27 (3): 336–39.

Zarit, S. H., P. A. Todd, and J. M. Zarit. 1986. Subjective burden of husbands and wives as caregivers: A longitudinal study. *Gerontologist* 26 (3): 260–66.

Zgola, J. M. 1987. *Doing things:* A guide to programming activities for persons with Alzheimer's disease and related disorders. Baltimore: Johns Hopkins University Press.

Zimmer, J. G., N. Watson, and A. K. Treat. 1984. Behavioral problems among patients in skilled nursing facilities. *American Journal of Public Health* 74:1118–21.

5

The Management of Urinary Incontinence in Dementia

JOSEPH G. OUSLANDER, M.D., AND JANE L. MARKS, R.N., M.S.

The Prevalence and Scope of the Problem

Urinary incontinence is a disruptive health problem that is common among the elderly population. It is defined as a condition in which involuntary loss of urine is a social or hygienic problem and is objectively demonstrated (Abrams et al. 1988). Although incontinence is not a normal process of aging, frequently it is not addressed as a problem by the older people. Incontinence is highly associated with cognitive and functional impairments in aged people and is frequently one of the most difficult management problems for caregivers of this population. It is imperative that health care providers include questions concerning incontinence in the assessment process.

The prevalence of urinary incontinence in the elderly population is influenced by the operational definition, the population, and the setting of various studies. Two studies in the community indicated that approximately 14 percent of the elderly have urinary incontinence (Vetter et al. 1981; Yarnell and St. Leger 1979). Another study of more functionally and cognitively impaired community-dwelling aged people found 53 percent to have urinary or urinary and fecal incontinence. Among this 53 percent, more than half had both urinary and fecal incontinence. Caregivers reported that care of incontinent elders was more tiresome and difficult to manage than the care of continent elders (Noelker 1987). Recognizing contributing factors, such as incontinence, that add to the burdens of caregivers is crucial for the successful management of the elderly at home.

In long-term care institutions, the prevalence of urinary incontinence is close to 50 percent. Cognitive impairment and functional limitations are strongly associated with incontinence in this setting (Ouslander et al. 1982; Jewett et al. 1981). Urinary incontinence, especially when combined with other functional disabilities, is a major precipitating factor in the placement of elderly people in long-term care institutions (Smallegan 1983). One study noted that elders admitted to nursing homes had multiple problems, with an average of four health problems and an average of one problem that had become acute within the last month. It was noted that 89 percent of the aged people received major care for urinary incontinence before admission and that incontinence was a precipitating factor (13 percent) for nursing home placement (Smallegan 1985).

In no matter which environment, urinary incontinence has a major impact on the elderly person, the health care provider, and the caregiver. People may experience adverse physical and psychosocial effects from urinary incontinence. They are more prone to developing skin irritations and breakdown. The patient may become isolated because of embarrassment, which may then lead to depression (Brink 1980). The caregiver may also experience the physical and emotional impact of incontinence. The care can demand a great deal of time and energy and is physically unattractive for community caregivers. In addition to the care, the financial aspect of managing incontinence can be overwhelming. The annual cost of incontinence in nursing homes is estimated to range from $500 million to $1.5 billion yearly (Ouslander and Kane 1984). The cost of supplies and laundry for an incontinent community-dwelling elderly person averages $2.50 per day (Hu 1986). Thus, to treat the incontinence successfully, the clinician must support the caregivers and understand their needs.

This chapter provides an overview of the physiology, assessment techniques, evaluation, and management of urinary incontinence in elderly. It focuses in particular on techniques that may be of value in treating patients with dementia who are incontinent in the community setting.

Anatomic and Physiological Considerations

Urination is a complex process that involves the kidneys, lower genitourinary tract, pelvic floor muscles, prostate gland (in men), local innervation, and central nervous system (Kane et al. 1989). The lower genitourinary tract consists of the bladder, the bladder outlet, and the urethra, which includes the internal urethral sphincter and the external urethral sphincter. The bladder is composed of the detrusor muscle, which can relax and allow urine to be stored or contract to empty urine. The internal and external sphincters are circular muscles that surround the urethra. The internal sphincter is located in the proximal portion of the bladder outlet at the bladder neck region and is autonomically innervated. It constricts while the bladder relaxes to store urine and relaxes while the bladder contracts to release urine. The external urethral sphincter is distal to the internal sphincter and is under voluntary control. The prostate gland is located below the bladder in men and surrounds the urethra (Resnick 1984; Kane et al. 1989). The pelvic floor muscles support the pelvic viscera and assist in sphincter control (Mandelstam 1980).

The lower urinary tract is innervated by the parasympathetic, sympathetic, and somatic nervous systems (Fig. 5.1). Parasympathetic cholinergically mediated nerves supply the detrusor muscle and causes it to contract. The pathway originates from the second to the fourth segment of the sacral spine. The sympathetic nerves supply the bladder and the internal sphincter. Originating from the thoracolumbar level of the spine, the sympathetic impulses cause the bladder to relax by inhibiting the parasympathetic signal for the bladder to contract and by relaxing the bladder dome, which is mediated by beta-adrenergic tone. Alpha-adrenergic sympathetic impulses also cause the smooth muscle of the bladder neck and the urethra to contract. The contraction of the pelvic floor musculature and the external sphincter is under voluntary control and is innervated by the pudendal nerve originating from the second to fourth sacral segments of the spinal cord (Ouslander and Elhilali 1987).

Higher levels within the central nervous system (including the cerebral cortex and the brainstem) have several effects on urination. The micturition center located in the pons coordinates detrusor contraction with sphincter relaxation. The central nervous system also has an inhibitory center that prevents detrusor contraction in response to bladder filling and can forestall voiding until appropriate (Resnick 1984).

Disorders at Different Levels

Disorders of the central nervous system at different levels have varying effects on the function of the lower urinary tract. Optimal

FIGURE 5.1   Innervation of the lower urinary tract. After Kane et al. 1989.

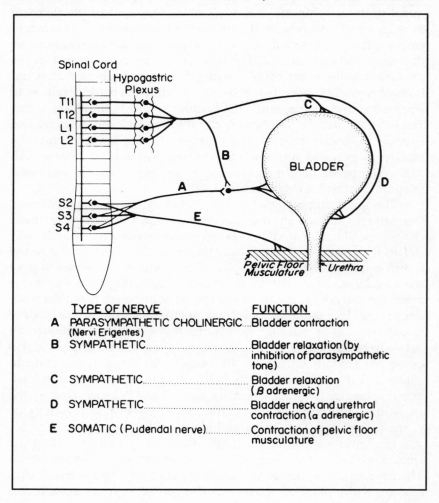

	TYPE OF NERVE	FUNCTION
A	PARASYMPATHETIC CHOLINERGIC (Nervi Erigentes)	Bladder contraction
B	SYMPATHETIC	Bladder relaxation (by inhibition of parasympathetic tone)
C	SYMPATHETIC	Bladder relaxation (β adrenergic)
D	SYMPATHETIC	Bladder neck and urethral contraction (α adrenergic)
E	SOMATIC (Pudendal nerve)	Contraction of pelvic floor musculature

therapy is often dependent upon identification of the underlying disorder. Cerebral disease such as stroke, primary degenerative dementias, normal pressure hydrocephalus, and Parkinson's disease may cause a loss of inhibitory influence, thus resulting in uninhibited or uncontrolled bladder contraction (detrusor hyperreflexia) (Staskin

TABLE 5.1 Requirements for Continence

Lower urinary tract function
Storage
    Accommodation of increasing volumes of urine under low pressure
    Closed bladder outlet
    Appropriate sensation
    Absence of involuntary bladder contractions
Emptying
    Bladder contraction
    Lack of anatomic obstruction
    Coordinated lowering of outlet resistance when bladder contracts

Adequate mobility/dexterity
To use toilet or toilet substitute and manage clothing

Adequate cognitive function
To recognize toileting needs and find a toilet or toilet substitute

Motivation to be continent

Absence of environmental and iatrogenic barriers
e.g., inaccessible toilets or toilet substitutes
        unavailable care givers
        drug side effects

Source: After Kane et al. 1989.

1986). A patient with a sacral cord lesion may present with a flaccid, large capacity, acontractile bladder, resulting in overflow incontinence. Suprasacral lesions between the micturition center and the sacral cord produce detrusor hyperreflexia with or without sphincter dyssynergia (Leach and Yip 1986). Detrusor/sphincter dyssynergia is defined as a detrusor contraction concurrent with an inappropriate contraction of the urethral and/or periurethral striated muscle (Abrams et al. 1988).

The Criteria for the Maintenance of Continence

For the maintenance of continence, certain requirements must be met (Table 5.1). The lower urinary tract must be able to store and empty urine appropriately. Adequate cognitive function to recognize toileting needs as well as to find a toilet is necessary. Patients with dementia may not sense a full bladder or may respond inappropriately to a full bladder. To reach the toilet and manipulate clothing to facilitate

TABLE 5.2   Causes of Acute Urinary Incontinence

"DRIP"

D — Delirium

R — Restricted mobility and retention[a]

I   — Infection,[b] inflammation,[b] and impaction (fecal)

P — Pharmaceuticals[c] and polyuria[d]

Source: After Kane et al. 1989.
[a]Anticholinergic and/or narcotic drugs and spinal cord compression.
[b]Acute symptomatic urinary tract infection and atrophic vaginitis/urethritis.
[c]See Table 5.3.
[d]Hyperglycemia and volume overload states (congestive heart failure, venous insufficiency.

toileting, one must have adequate mobility and dexterity skills. The environment must also be conducive to reaching the toilet. Any obstacles in the pathway to the toilet or toilet substitute need to be assessed. The bathroom should accommodate walkers and wheelchairs, if utilized, and should be recognizable for dementia patients. Devices such as grab bars may facilitate toileting. Last, the patient must be motivated to be continent. Psychological assessments may reveal factors contributing to incontinence. The presence of depression may inhibit cues from the bladder of the need to urinate and decrease the will to be continent, and expressions of anger and hostility can result in deliberate incontinence (Brink 1980; Orzeck and Ouslander 1987). Caregivers may foster incontinence by supporting this behavior.

Types of Incontinence

Urinary incontinence can be divided into two types—acute and persistent. Acute urinary incontinence has a sudden onset and is usually associated with an acute medical or surgical condition. It will often resolve with the resolution of the acute condition. If not identified, however, it may become irreversible. Persistent incontinence may result from an acute condition or from no clear contributing factor, and it continues, often worsening over time (Ouslander 1986a).

Acute and Reversible Forms of Urinary Incontinence

The acronym "DRIP" (Table 5.2) can be used to remember common causes of urinary incontinence. This is similar to an acronym described by Resnick for causes of transient incontinence, "DIAP-PERS" (Resnick 1986).

Delirium and Restricted mobility are common among acutely ill elderly persons. People with dementia are exceptionally vulnerable to delirium. If an acute problem occurs, the patient's behavior may worsen, possibly indicating delirium. Therefore, it is vital to recognize such episodes. Hospital staff may impose restricted mobility. Nursing home staff may restrict the mobility of people with dementia to reduce the risk of falls or to prevent wandering. Restricted mobility may decrease the patient's awareness of the need to void and ability to get to the commode or substitute, thereby causing incontinence. Resolution of the acute illness is likely to resolve the urinary incontinence (Kane et al. 1989).

Urinary retention with acute overflow incontinence may result from Immobility; anticholinergics, narcotics, and beta-adrenergic drugs (Table 5.3); or fecal impaction. Such incontinence may also be a symptom of spinal cord compression (Ouslander and Elhilali 1987).

Urinary incontinence can be precipitated by an acute Inflammatory condition of the lower urinary tract that causes frequency and urgency. Patients with dementia may be unable to report symptoms related to an acute inflammatory condition. Treatment of an acute cystitis or urethritis can restore continence. Fecal Impaction is common in the acutely ill elderly patient and is associated with transient urinary and fecal incontinence (Ouslander and Elhilali 1987).

Polyuria (increased urine volume) can result from metabolic conditions, such as poorly controlled diabetes, and volume overload states such as lower extremity edema from venous insufficiency with mobilization of fluid and polyuria at night. Treating the cause of polyuria during the day, when the patient may have better access to a toilet, may reduce nighttime incontinence. As with all symptoms in the elderly, a variety of drugs can contribute to or cause urinary incontinence (Table 5.3) (Kane et al. 1989).

Persistent Incontinence

Persistent incontinence can be classified into four basic types: stress, urge, overflow, and functional. The types, definitions, and common causes are shown in Table 5.4. Elderly incontinent patients may have two or more of these types of incontinence simultaneously (Fig. 5.2) (Ouslander 1986a).

TABLE 5.3 Drugs That Can Affect Continence Related to Bladder Function and Toileting Skills

Bladder Function	Drug	Potential Effect
I. Bladder filling	Diuretics Furosemide (Lasix) Thiazides (Hydrodiuril, Dyazide Zaroxolyn, others) Alcohol Caffeinated coffee, tea, colas	Increased urine flow (polyuria, frequency, and urgency)
II. Bladder storing	Antihypertensives Prazosin (Minipress) Methyldopa (Aldomet)	Bladder outlet relaxation (urinary incontinence)
III. Bladder emptying	Antipsychotics Haloperidol (Haldol) Thioridazine (Mellaril) Thiothixene (Navane) Others Amantadine (Symmetrel) Diphenhydramine (Benadryl) Disopyramide (Norpace) Hydroxyzine (Atarax)	Anticholinergic (urinary retention and overflow incontinence)
	Antidepressants Amitriptyline (Elavil) Doxepin (Sinequan) Imipramine (Tofranil)	Anticholinergic, as well as constipation, fecal impaction

TABLE 5.3 (continued)

Bladder Function	Drug	Potential Effect
	Analgesics (narcotics)	Bladder relaxation (urinary retention)
	Codeine	
	(Tylenol #3, #4)	Constipation, fecal impaction
	Hydromorphone (Dilaudid)	
	Meperidine (Demerol)	
	Morphine	
IV. Toileting skills	Sedatives/hypnotics	Sedation (diminished awareness of toileting needs)
	Alprazolam (Xanax)	
	Chloral hydrate (Noctec, others)	
	Flurazepam (Dalmane)	
	Lorazepam (Atrivan)	
	Temazepam (Restoril)	
	Triazolam (Halcion)	
	Antidepressants (see above)	
	Analgesics (see above)	
	Antipsychotics (see above)	Sedation as well as rigidity (diminished ability to get to and use the toilet)

Common Causes of Persistent Incontinence in Dementia Patients

Several factors may contribute to or cause persistent urinary incontinence in dementia patients. Patients with impaired cognitive function may not recognize cues from the bladder of the need to void (Brink 1980). In addition, they may not be able to inhibit urination until an appropriate time. As the urgency increases, the patient may

TABLE 5.4 Basic Types and Causes of Persistent Geriatric Urinary Incontinence

Type	Definition	Common Causes
Stress	Involuntary loss of urine (usually small amounts) simultaneous with increase in intra-abdominal pressure (e.g., cough, laugh, or exercise)	Weakness and laxity of pelvic floor musculature Bladder outlet or urethral sphincter weakness
Urge	Leakage of urine (usually larger volumes) because of inability to delay voiding after sensation of bladder fullness is perceived	Detrusor motor and/or sensory instability, isolated or associated with one or more of the following: Local genitourinary condition such as cystitis, urethritis, tumors, stones, and outflow obstruction Central nervous system disorders such as stroke, dementia, Parkinsonism[a]
Overflow	Leakage of urine (usually small amounts) resulting from mechanical forces on an overdistended bladder or from other effects of urinary retention on bladder and sphincter function	Anatomic obstruction by prostate, stricture, cystocele Acontractile bladder associated with diabetes mellitus or spinal cord injury Neurogenic (detrusor-sphincter dyssynergy), associated with multiple sclerosis and other suprasacral spinal cord lesions
Functional	Urinary leakage associated with inability to toilet because of impairment of cognitive and/or physiological functioning, psychological unwillingness, or environmental barriers	Severe dementia and other neurological disorders Psychological factors such as depression, anger, and hostility

Source: After Kane et al. 1989.
[a]When detrusor motor instability is associated with a neurological disorder, it is termed, by the International Continence Society, detrusor hyperreflexia.

FIGURE 5.2 Types of persistent urinary incontinence. After Kane et al. 1989.

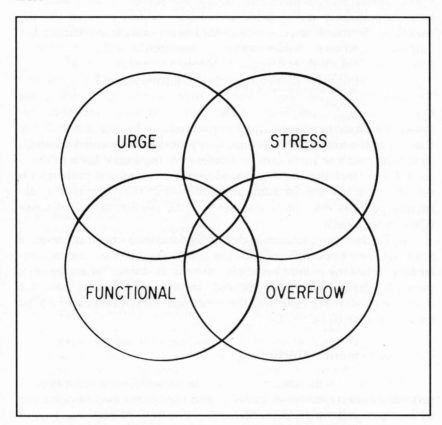

become anxious. Functional changes and limitations associated with the progression of dementia will affect mobility and contribute to incontinence. Patients with dementia may forget how to sit or position themselves to toilet (apraxia). They may try to get up before they are finished. Psychological factors may relate to behavioral incontinence. Patients with dementia may experience depression, and incontinence may result. Caregivers may foster dependency and reinforce incontinent behavior (Brink 1980). In assessing the causes of incontinence in dementia patients, one should consider carefully iatrogenic factors imposed by physicians and caregivers. Medications are often adjusted for behavioral management and should be assessed. Safety measures, such as restraints and geriatric chairs with tables, prohibit the dementia patient with impaired communication skills from seeking the bathroom. End-stage dementia patients are often bedridden and therefore dependent on their caregiver for toileting needs.

The environment plays a key role in contributing to incontinence. The inability to remember where the toilet is located, as well as the distance to and accessibility of the toilet may cause incontinence. Patients with dementia may not find the toilet or be able to see clearly the way to the toilet. They may use inappropriate receptacles in which to urinate, such as trash cans or flower pots (agnosia). Each of these contributory factors should be considered in the dementia patient with urinary incontinence. In addition to these functional problems, dementia patients may have another type of persistent incontinence (Ouslander 1986a).

By far the most common in dementia patients is urge incontinence with detrusor hyperreflexia (Staskin 1986). The bladder muscle contracts without the patient being able to hold the urine. When the urge presents, the patient needs to void. Incontinence results from the decrease in warning time and the functional limitations experienced by a patient with dementia.

The Assessment of Incontinence

All patients with urinary incontinence should have some type of (in)continence assessment. Patients and caregivers may be reluctant to mention incontinence problems for a variety of reasons. Health care providers should, therefore, include questions concerning continence in their general history and review of symptoms. The manner in which the subject is approached will promote disclosure of the problem and facilitate appropriate intervention. Use terminology the patient can understand (Brink 1980). Examples of questions regarding incontinence include: Do you have any trouble with your bladder or passing your water? Does your water come too frequently or too quickly? Do you ever leak urine in your underpants? Have you ever wet your underpants before getting to the bathroom? Have you ever gone to the bathroom and noticed that your pants were wet or damp from urine? Whether the incontinence is acute or persistent, all pa-

TABLE 5.5 Components of (In)continence Assessment

All Patients	
History	Past genitourinary conditions and surgery
	Active medical problems
	Medications
	Characteristics of incontinence
	Onset and duration
	Frequency, timing, and amount of leakage
	Sensation of bladder fullness/emptying
	Symptoms of urgency, stress, dysuria, hesitancy,
	etc.
	Fecal incontinence
	Patient's responses to incontinence
Physical examination	Mental and psychological status
	Mobility
	Abdominal
	Pelvic/rectal
	Neurological
Postvoid residual	Assesses bladder emptying
determination (PVR)	Identifies urinary retention and overflow incontinence
Urinalysis	Identifies urinary tract infection
Urine Culture	
Sensitivity	
Blood	Glucose, BUN, creatinine
Selected Patients	
Urological/gynecological evaluation	
Urodynamic tests	

tients should have a history, physical exam, postvoid residual, urinalysis, urine culture, and certain blood work (Table 5.5).

History

Obtaining a thorough history is an important component of the (in)continence assessment. The interviewer needs acute listening skills to obtain accurate information regarding incontinence. The interview may be lengthy and tiresome to the elderly person, and people with dementia may have a shortened attention span. When possible, allow for rest periods (Brink 1980). In assessment of the patient with dementia, the caregiver or nursing home staff can clarify information, or provide the majority of information. When possible, past medical records should be reviewed to augment the history. Active medical

TABLE 5.6   Clarifying Symptoms as to Type of Incontinence

Type	Question
Stress	Do you ever leak urine when you cough, laugh, sneeze, lift objects, or go from a sitting to a standing position?
Urge	Do you ever leak urine when you have a strong urge to urinate and can't make it to the bathroom?
Overflow	Do you ever have to strain to pass your water? Does your stream ever stop and start?
Functional	Do you have difficulty in managing toileting, such as walking to the toilet, undressing, and using the commode?

conditions and medications should be assessed for their possible contribution to incontinence. This includes present problems and past operations, evaluations, and findings. The history may reveal vital information related to incontinence (Ouslander 1986b).

In assessment of the incontinent, cognitively impaired patient, clarification of when the incontinence began in relationship to the dementia is important. The patient or caregiver may have successfully hidden or been able to manage the incontinence until the dementia ended the ability to do so. Perhaps incontinence antedated the dementia and therefore warrants further investigation of other contributing factors. If the incontinence followed the dementia, establish whether it is progressing parallel to the dementia. If the incontinence does not seem to parallel the dementia, what other contributing factors are elicited?

Clarifying the symptoms of incontinence is an important component of the assessment and may prove challenging with cognitively impaired patients. Symptoms in relation to the type of incontinence should be elicited from both the patient and the caregiver, if possible (Table 5.6). Aged patients may often have multiple voiding symptoms associated with incontinence. The predominant complaint among elderly patients is "can't get to the toilet on time" (urge incontinence). A mixture of urge and stress incontinence is common among women, whereas obstructive voiding symptoms (such as difficulty in starting urination or slow, interrupted stream) are common among men (Ouslander, Raz, et al. 1986). Once the symptoms have been identified, it is important to gain insight into the frequency of incontinence episodes.

Establishing the frequency of incontinence episodes can be difficult, but it is facilitated by the use of an Incontinence Monitoring Record (Fig. 5.3). Careful recording by the caregiver may clarify the patient's symptoms and help establish a plan of intervention (Autry et al. 1984; Demmerle and Bartol 1980). This record requires the willingness of the caregiver because it takes time and effort to complete throughout the twenty-four-hour period. It usually consists of noting every two hours during the day whether the patients are wet or dry, if they urinated in the toilet, and the amount. Night events should also be noted. Behaviors and other factors surrounding the incontinent episode should be recorded in the comment column. It is also important to assess the type and amount of fluids consumed as well as the time of consumption. This assessment can be obtained by having the caregiver chart the fluid intake. Modifying the Incontinence Monitoring Record (Fig. 5.3) to include fluid intake will augment this assessment. Consumption of coffee, tea, and colas acts as a diuretic and should be noted. A one- to two-week period of record keeping is important in establishing a voiding pattern for baseline assessment (Autry et al. 1984). Such monitoring provides a global assessment and a means to measure the effectiveness of the selected interventions (Demmerle and Bartol 1980). However, the duration of a baseline assessment must be individualized.

Physical Examination

The physical examination includes assessment of mental status and mobility and of neurological, abdominal, rectal, pelvic, and genital areas. It may be helpful to have another person assist by frequently reassuring the patient. The mental status and mobility capabilities must be assessed carefully because of their association with toileting skills (Orzeck and Ouslander 1987). Among dementia patients, incontinence may result from the inability to plan ahead for voiding, as well as from apraxia with toileting skills (Brink 1980).

The neurological exam focuses on the evaluation of previous neurological disorders and any potential problems. Identification of previous unrecognized neurological disorders and new focal findings might reveal the underlying cause of incontinence. These disorders include multiple sclerosis, Parkinsonism, and normal pressure hydrocephalus. The exam includes assessment of motor strength, tone, sensation, and reflexes (Ouslander and Elhilali 1987; Orzeck and Ouslander 1987).

FIGURE 5.3 Incontinence Monitoring Record. Copyright 1984. Regents of the University of California. Reprinted with permission.

INCONTINENCE MONITORING RECORD

INSTRUCTIONS: EACH TIME THE PATIENT IS CHECKED:
1) Mark *one* of the circles in the BLADDER section at the hour closest to the time the patient is checked.
2) Make an X in the BOWEL section if the patient has had an incontinent or normal bowel movement.

🖊 = Incontinent, small amount	∅ = Dry
⬤ = Incontinent, large amount	△ = Voided correctly

X = Incontinent BOWEL
X = Normal BOWEL

PATIENT NAME _____ ROOM # _____ DATE _____

	BLADDER				BOWEL			
	INCONTINENT OF URINE	DRY	VOIDED CORRECTLY	INCONTINENT X	NORMAL X	INITIALS	COMMENTS
12 am	● ●	○	△ cc _____				
1	● ●	○	△ cc _____				
2	● ●	○	△ cc _____				
3	● ●	○	△ cc _____				
4	● ●	○	△ cc _____				
5	● ●	○	△ cc _____				
6	● ●	○	△ cc _____				
7	● ●	○	△ cc _____				
8	● ●	○	△ cc _____				
9	● ●	○	△ cc _____				
10	● ●	○	△ cc _____				
11	● ●	○	△ cc _____				
12 pm	● ●	○	△ cc _____				
1	● ●	○	△ cc _____				
2	● ●	○	△ cc _____				
3	● ●	○	△ cc _____				
4	● ●	○	△ cc _____				
5	● ●	○	△ cc _____				
6	● ●	○	△ cc _____				
7	● ●	○	△ cc _____				
8	● ●	○	△ cc _____				
9	● ●	○	△ cc _____				
10	● ●	○	△ cc _____				
11	● ●	○	△ cc _____				
TOTALS:							

The abdomen is palpated for bladder distention. The rectal exam assesses perianal sensation, sphincter tone, prostate size, and the presence of fecal impaction. The pelvic exam encompasses visualization of the genital area for any skin irritations and inspection for large cystoceles and pelvic prolapses. Assessment of the vaginal mucosa for the presence of atrophic vaginitis is completed during the pelvic exam (Orzeck and Ouslander 1987). Signs of atrophic vaginitis include pale, friable, thin, and shiny vaginal mucosa and petechiae, loss of rugal folds, and vaginal erosion (Resnick 1986).

Postvoid residual determination, urinalysis, and urine culture and sensitivity should also be completed as part of the (in)continence assessment. Before obtaining a postvoid residual, have the patient void in a container when the patient has the "urge to go." This can provide some baseline data such as approximate voided volume. If the patient is not inhibited by your presence, you may also observe whether the patient strains to void or whether urine stream is slow or interrupted. Ideally within ten minutes, catheterization for the postvoid residual should be completed. This enables the examiner to obtain a sterile urine for culture and sensitivity, as well as being able to detect retention. There is no precise value, but if the postvoid residual is greater that 100 ml, referral for further evaluation should be considered.

The relationship of otherwise asymptomatic bacteriuria and pyuria to incontinence is unclear. It is reasonable to attempt to eradicate a urinary tract infection, especially if more than five to ten white blood cells per high power field are present, and then observe for any changes in continence status (Kane et al. 1989).

Certain patients may need to be referred to other specialists for further evaluation. These patients include those with urinary retention; a pelvic, rectal, and/or prostatic mass; severe pelvic prolapse; hematuria; recent genitourinary procedures; and urinary tract infection (Ouslander 1986b).

A select group of patients will benefit from further diagnostic evaluation. Urodynamic tests can identify specific dysfunctions of the lower urinary tract (Ouslander 1986b). Patients who benefit from such an evaluation include those with an associated neurological abnormality, incomplete bladder emptying with overflow incontinence; complex stress incontinence with urethral dysfunction, and/or failed attempts at recommended treatments (Leach and Yip 1986). The appropriate role for urodynamics in older patients, especially among those with cognitive impairment, is controversial. Evaluation of urodynamics generally requires a separate visit to a site with special equipment and personnel trained in its use and interpretation and requires that patient to be catheterized, which can be uncomfortable. In addition, the tests are relatively expensive. They can be especially difficult to perform and interpret with a cognitively impaired patient (Ouslander et al. 1987). However, Resnick and colleagues (1989) found that urodynamic studies are feasible and may lead to specific forms of treatment even in a very elderly institutionalized population. Patients with dementia may need to be referred for urodynamic evaluation if they present with symptoms or signs of obstruction or neurological disorders that suggest an acontractile bladder or detrusor sphincter dyssynergia.

The Treatment of Incontinence

Treatment for urinary incontinence encompasses specific and non-specific interventions. Specific interventions include behavioral therapies, pharmacological agents, and surgical procedures. Specific treatments are selected depending on the type of incontinence, the patient's medical history, and input from the patient or caregiver. Primary treatments for each type of incontinence are listed in Table 5.7 and are discussed in detail elsewhere (Burgio et al. 1985, 1986; Schmidbauer et al. 1986; Blaivas and Berger 1986; Ouslander and Sier 1986).

The goal of improving continence is to maintain the patient's self-esteem and dignity. The patient may feel embarrassed over the incontinent episode, be uncomfortable, or even be unaware of it. Toileting skills need to be encouraged, as long as the patients are able, to promote their optimal functional ability. The treatment plan should be specific for the individual. The clinician needs to have a thorough understanding of the patient, the caregiver, and the overall situation so that the optimal plan of care is developed for that patient. Obtaining information about the patient's habits, past interests, and occupation may be helpful in developing a specific plan of care.

In this chapter, we focus on treatment interventions for urge and functional incontinence, which are by far the most common types of incontinence among dementia patients. Considering the fragile or

TABLE 5.7 Primary Treatments for Different Types of Urinary Incontinence

Type of Incontinence	Primary Treatments
Stress	Pelvic floor (Kegel) exercises Biofeedback Alpha-adrenergic agonists Estrogen Bladder neck suspension
Urge	Pelvic floor (Kegel) exercises Biofeedback Bladder Relaxants Estrogen (if atrophic vaginitis/urethritis is present) Bladder and habit retraining Surgical removal of obstructing or irritation lesions
Overflow	Surgical removal of obstruction Intermittent catheterization Indwelling catheterization
Functional	Habit training/scheduled toileting Incontinence undergarments, pads External collection devices Environmental manipulations

Source: After Kane et al. 1989.

compromised state of dementia patients, behavioral therapies are probably the primary treatment intervention for urinary incontinence in this patient population. Pharmacological agents may also be incorporated, but the potential side effects must be monitored carefully by caregivers and health professionals.

Nonspecific supportive techniques are also important in the management of urinary incontinence. Environmental factors can play a key role in precipitating incontinence, and simple alterations often promote continence. Incontinence products such as diapers and padding are readily available for family caregivers. Their appropriateness depends on the incontinence evaluation, the patient, and the caregiver. Management of urinary incontinence by catheters is also possible.

The selected treatment depends on the patient's status and the caregiver's ability to manage the treatment. Support of the caregiver is vital. The health care provider must be realistic in developing a treatment plan. If one treatment is unsuccessful, the provider must not feel a failure. Follow-up visits are important to evaluate the selected treatment regimen and make adjustments.

Baseline Data

Before treatment is begun, a baseline assessment made by utilizing an incontinence monitoring record can be helpful in planning and implementing a treatment program, as well as in assessing the results of treatment (Demmerle and Bartol 1980). Figure 5.3 represents one example of such a record (Ouslander, Uman, et al. 1986). The incontinence monitoring record must, however, be easy to complete and not cause additional stress for the caregiver.

Adequate hydration is one of the basic, vital components in obtaining continence. The recommended daily amount varies from 1500–2000 to 2000–3000 cc depending on cardiac and circulatory systems (Demmerle and Bartol 1980; Wells and Brink 1981). Bladder fullness stimulates the need to void. Inadequate intake can result in incontinence and confusion (Wells and Brink 1981). Maintaining fluid intake among dementia patients can be quite difficult and can require considerable effort on the part of the caregiver. Incontinence monitoring records can reveal inadequate fluid intake, and adjustments can be made. Products such as Jell-o and Popsicles (if appropriate for the patient) can be incorporated to encourage fluid intake (Wells and Brink 1981). Spacing fluids or offering small amounts frequently may encourage intake (Spiro 1978). Positive reinforcement may augment intake as well.

Older persons excrete most of their fluid intake after 9 p.m. (Resnick 1986) and, therefore, may complain of the need to urinate throughout the night. It is often recommended to restrict fluid intake during the evening, especially of caffeinated beverages because they act as diuretics. This is a reasonable approach as long as an adequate intake can be consumed in a restricted time frame and its effectiveness is evaluated.

Bowel regularity is also a key factor in promoting urinary continence. Fecal impaction is related to urinary incontinence. Adequate fluid intake and adequate dietary intake of high-fiber foods promote bowel regularity. Toileting after meals, especially after breakfast, will take advantage of the gastrocolic reflex. Caregivers should make every effort to provide an atmosphere of privacy and, if possible, calmness to facilitate bowel evacuation (Wells and Brink 1981; Kane et al. 1984).

Nonspecific Supportive Interventions

Environment

Simply altering some environmental factors may assist with incontinence. A first step is to assess the location of the toilet. If the patient has difficulty with mobility, the distance may be too great to reach the bathroom on time, especially if it is located on the second floor. The patient may not have enough energy to travel to the bathroom (Brink 1980). The patient's warning time (when the urge to void is felt and how long the patient can hold) can be evaluated (Chalifoux 1980). The pathway to the bathroom must be clear and adequately lit to facilitate mobility. The bathroom facility should be assessed for its facilitation of toileting, including an adequate room size to allow assistive mobility devices, devices such as grab bars to promote transfer, and devices modifying toilet structure to promote comfort (Brink and Wells 1986). A bar placed in front of the toilet may act as a safety guard for patients with cognitive impairment and give them support to lean on while toileting; however, it should not be used as a restraint (Demmerle and Bartol 1980). Assessment of the patient's ability to manipulate clothing to facilitate toileting is necessary. To promote toileting, the atmosphere should be private, calm, and warm (Brink and Wells 1986).

Sometimes simple alterations to the environment may allow that extra safe time for reaching the bathroom (Brink and Wells 1986). Patients with dementia may not remember where the bathroom is located. Something to designate the way to the bathroom and the bathroom itself (i.e., visible signs and a colorful object on the door conspicuous from all approaches) may facilitate the patient's ability to locate it (Demmerle and Bartol 1980). Also, simple alterations in clothing may give the elderly person the independence and the added time necessary to manage toileting (Brink 1980). Sewing Velcro into pants and skirts rather than buttons and zippers and the use of elastic waistbands may make toileting much easier. It is important to keep patients with dementia in clothes to promote both continence and dignity.

Toilet Substitutes

Depending upon the (in)continence assessment, portable receptacles instead of toilets may be recommended, especially at night, when trips to the bathroom may be hazardous. It is important to promote privacy to facilitate toileting. Commodes, in various designs, are available. In selection, keep in mind comfort, safety, and feasibility. Cushioned seats and supportive backs aid comfort; full forward arms and adjustable heights promote transfer. Commodes with wheels may be hazardous (Brink and Wells 1986).

Bedpans may be utilized at night or at the end stage of dementia. However, they are awkward to facilitate bowel and bladder emptying, and they may be uncomfortable as well. Assist the patient to a sitting position by supporting the back with pillows, bending the knees, and positioning the feet to allow for the patient's comfort. Such positioning will facilitate toileting (Palmer 1985). Fracture pans may provide more comfort and less hip flexion (Brink and Wells 1986).

Urinals are small, portable receptacles to collect urine. In using male urinals, care must be taken not to allow the urine to spill out. Female urinals may require a sitting or standing position (Brink and Wells 1986). Women with dementia may be further confused by this practice of standing to void.

Absorbent Products

Numerous absorbent products are available. However, they should not be viewed as a treatment, but as an adjunct in managing incontinence. Patients should be evaluated before managing incontinence with such a nonspecific aid. Absorbent products include undergarments and pads. They are available in two forms: disposable and launderable. Launderable undergarments may have disposable inserts. Disposable undergarments are available with tab adhesive or with reusable elastic bands. Pads are used to protect clothing and furniture. The products include a surface layer to allow urine to pass through and a layer of highly absorbent polymers backed by a protective barrier. When utilizing absorbent products, it is vital to change them regularly and to provide good skin care. In selecting the appropriate product, the severity of the incontinence, comfort to the patient, appearance, and cost must all be considered. Often the family caregiver is so burdened that this is the choice of management. The health care provider must be supportive and instruct caregivers in proper use. Undergarments may promote incontinence by communicating to the patient that incontinence is acceptable. They should be used with discretion, especially when incorporating behavioral therapies (Ouslander and Elhilali 1987; Palmer 1985; Brink and Wells 1986).

Catheters

Three types of catheters are available: external, intermittent, and indwelling. Numerous types of external catheters for men are available. They generally consist of some type of condom that is connected to a drainage system (Ouslander and Elhilali 1987). They are held in place with an inner adhesive strip, an outside adhesive strip, or self-adhering condom catheters. The ideal external catheter has molding at the end to hold the device away from the penis and funnel urine in a large volume (Brink and Wells 1986). Condom catheters are available in one standard size, and several types come in different sizes to fit better. Skin care is crucial. Urine is constantly bathing the penis. It is important to watch for any skin breakdown or swelling of the penis. If any of these symptoms are noted, the catheter must be discontinued. It is usually recommended that the catheter be changed daily. Shave any hair that may stick to the adhesive. The catheters should be used to manage intractable incontinence of men who do not have urinary retention and who are extremely physically dependent. These devices can foster dependency among incontinent patients, so they should not be used as a matter of convenience. A female version of the external catheter is now available; its safety and efficacy are not well documented (Ouslander and Elhilali 1987). Confused patients may pull or tug at such devices (Palmer 1985).

Intermittent catheterization is a procedure that involves straight catheterization 2 to 4 times daily, depending on residual urine volumes. It is helpful in the management of a subgroup of patients with urinary retention and overflow incontinence. It is more feasible for women. Studies carried out in young paraplegics and elderly female outpatients should not, however, be extrapolated to an institutional or elderly male population. Catheterizing elderly men may be more difficult, and they may have anatomic abnormalities of the lower urinary tract that may increase the risk of infection from repeated catheterization. The practicality and safety of this procedure in long-term care have never been documented. Further studies are needed to substantiate the safety of this procedure in long-term care. In the home setting, the technique may be performed as a clean technique (Ouslander and Elhilali 1987).

Indwelling urethral catheters are indicated for chronic use in a certain group of patients, including those who have urinary retention that is causing problems such as persistent overflow incontinence, symptomatic urinary tract infections, or renal dysfunction due to hydronephrosis. If the retention cannot be treated, the risks of indwelling catheters outweigh the risk of chronic urinary retention. Another indication for chronic indwelling catheters is skin irritations that are being contaminated by urine. Terminally ill patients or patients who are severely impaired (i.e., patients with end-stage Alzheimer's disease or other types of dementia) may experience discomfort from frequent changing of bed linens. Therefore, a chronic indwelling catheter is appropriate to promote optimal comfort. Last, there may be a group of patients in whom more specific treatment failed or who prefer to use an indwelling catheter. Key principles in the care of patients with chronic indwelling catheters are listed.

- Maintain a sterile, closed, gravity drainage system.
- Avoid breaking the closed system.
- Use clean technique in emptying and changing the drainage system; wash hands between patients in institutional settings.
- Avoid frequent and vigorous cleaning of the catheter entry site; washing with soapy water once per day is sufficient.
- Do not routinely irrigate.
- If bypassing occurs in the absence of obstruction, consider the possibility of bladder spasm, which can be treated with a bladder relaxant.
- If catheter obstruction occurs frequently, increase the patient's fluid intake and acidify the urine if possible.
- Do not routinely use prophylactic or suppressive urinary antiseptics or antimicrobials.
- Do not do routine surveillance cultures to guide the management of individual patients, because all chronically catheterized patients have bacteriuria (which is often polymicrobial) and the organisms change frequently.
- Do not treat infection unless the patient develops symptoms; other possible sources of infection should be carefully excluded before attributing symptoms to the urinary tract.
- If a patient develops frequent symptomatic urinary tract infections, a genitourinary evaluation should be considered to rule out pathology such as stones, periurethral or prostatic abscesses, chronic pyelonephritis, etc.

Specific Interventions

Behavioral Treatment

Behavior is an act that a person does that is measurable (Maney 1980). Behavioral treatment (therapies) consist of various procedures to modify the behavior of incontinence through systematic environmental changes (Burgio and Burgio 1986). Behavioral therapies include patient-dependent procedures and caregiver-dependent procedures (Table 5.8). These and other similar techniques have been reviewed in detail elsewhere (Burgio and Burgio 1986; Hadley 1986). The most appropriate behavioral therapy for patients with dementia will generally be caregiver-dependent. This will require a commitment on the part of the caregiver. For the therapy to succeed the caregiver must recognize incontinence as a problem and be willing to expend the energy to promote continence (Maney 1980). The health care provider must reinforce the importance of the caregiver's role in the treatment of incontinence. At the same time, support of the patient is vital. When talking with the patient, speak slowly and distinctly; repetition may be necessary (Palmer 1985).

Toileting schedules such as fixed or flexible times are often incorporated as a behavioral treatment for dementia patients who experience urinary incontinence. When a toileting schedule is used, incontinence monitoring is important. In keeping the baseline data on the incontinence monitoring record, it is important to note behavior before and during an incontinent episode (Maney 1980). Patients with dementia may not communicate the need to void, but their behavior may indicate this (Palmer 1985).

Scheduled or timed toileting involves a fixed voiding schedule that remains unchanged (Hadley 1986). (See Table 5.9 for an example of scheduled toileting instructions.) Initially, an every-two-hour schedule is recommended. The patient is toileted every two hours during the day and evening and every four hours at night. The nighttime toileting may not be feasible for the caregiver at home. Therefore, a nonspecific aid such as an incontinence pad may be used. Scheduled toileting may be a challenge to initiate and maintain for some cognitively impaired elderly persons. They may not remember that they just voided on the toilet and may request to go to the bathroom within a short period. Reinforcement, support, and distraction to other activities may facilitate the scheduled voiding plan (Demmerle and Bartol 1980). However, an acute process such as an infection can cause fre-

TABLE 5.8 Examples of Behaviorally Oriented Procedures for the Management of Geriatric Urinary Incontinence

Procedure	Description	Use(s)	Comments
Patient-dependent Procedures			
Pelvic floor (Kegel) exercises	Repetitive contractions of pelvic floor muscles	Stress and urge incontinence	Requires adequate cognitive and physical function and motivation; may be done in conjunction with biofeedback
Biofeedback	Use of bladder and rectal and/or vaginal pressure or electrical recordings used in teaching patients to contract pelvic floor muscles and relax bladder	Stress and urge incontinence	Requires equipment and trained personnel; relatively invasive; requires adequate cognitive and physical function and motivation
Bladder retraining	Progressive lengthening or shortening of intervoiding interval, with adjunctive techniques;[a] intermittent catheterization used in patients recovering from overdistention injuries with persistent urinary retention	Urge incontinence Acute incontinence, e.g., poststroke, postindwelling catheterization	Goal is to restore normal pattern of voiding and continence; requires adequate cognitive and physical function and motivation
Caregiver-dependent Procedures			
Habit training	Variable toileting schedule with behavior modification and adjunctive techniques indicated[a]	Urge and functional incontinence	Goal is to prevent episodes; can be used in patients with impaired cognitive and physical function; requires staff/caregiver availability and motivation
Scheduled toileting	Fixed toileting schedule with behavior modification (may also incorporate prompted voidings) and adjunctive techniques if indicated[a]	Urge and functional incontinence	Goal is to prevent episodes; can be used in patients with impaired cognitive and physical function; requires staff/caregiver availability and motivation

Source: After Kane et al. 1989.

[a] Adjunctive techniques: (1) techniques to trigger voiding; (2) techniques to empty bladder completely; (3) alterations of fluid intake.

TABLE 5.9 Scheduled Toileting

Purpose: Management of Urinary Leakage by Toileting on a Schedule

1. Record baseline bladder record.
2. Begin the program by having patient try to urinate:
    a. as soon as he gets up in the morning;
    b. every ___ hours (even if he doesn't feel like he has to go); record results on Incontinence Monitoring Record;
    c. before he goes to bed;
    d. every four hours at night.
    e. When patient is dry and urinates in toilet, offer positive reinforcement.
3. If the patient has trouble starting to urinate at these times, try to:
    a. run the faucet;
    b. lightly stroke her inner thigh;
    c. gently tap on the suprapubic area.
4. After the patient urinates, to make sure the bladder is empty:
    a. press the lower part of the abdomen;
    b. have patient bend forward as far as he can for a few seconds and have him try to urinate some more.
5. If the patient experiences a desire to urinate more often than every two hours, try to increase the time gradually until she can hold the urine for at least two hours.
6. If the patient does not make it to the toilet on time and has an incontinence episode, you should:
    a. toilet him to try to finish urinating because the bladder may not be completely empty. Do not engage in a conversation with the patient at this time. Do what is necessary to clean the patient.
    b. note on the Incontinence Monitoring Record when the incontinence episode(s) occurred.
7. Avoid serving caffeinated beverages at or after dinner time.
8. *At night,* if the patient has trouble waking up and getting to the bathroom, use a urinal, bedpan, or bedside commode.
9. Record fluid intake on the Incontinence Monitoring Record.

---

quency or change in incontinence status. This should be ruled out. Prompted voiding may be incorporated into scheduled voiding.

Prompted voiding is designed to check whether the patient is wet or dry at specific times and then prompt the patient to see if there is a need to go to the bathroom. These checks should be carried out with dignity. Only if the patient responds affirmatively is he toileted (Schnelle et al. 1983). A patient with dementia may not understand

TABLE 5.10   Habit Training Program

Purpose: Management of Urinary Incontinence by Promoting Patient's
Pattern of Voiding

Phase I—Record baseline bladder record.
Phase II
  1. Begin the program by having patient try to urinate:
      a. as soon as she gets up in the morning;
      b. after each meal;
      c. every two hours between meals (even if she doesn't feel like she
          has to go). If the patient voids before the scheduled time, adjust
          the toileting schedule from the time that she voided. Record results
          on Incontinence Monitoring Record.
      d. before she goes to bed;
      e. every four hours at night.
  2. If the patient has trouble starting to urinate at these times, try to:
      a. run the faucet;
      b. lightly stroke his inner thigh;
      c. gently tap on the suprapubic area.
  3. After the patient urinates, to make sure her bladder is empty:
      a. press the lower part of the abdomen;
      b. have patient bend forward as far as she can for a few seconds and
          have her try to urinate some more.
  4. If the patient experiences a desire to urinate more often than every
      two hours, try to increase the time gradually until he can hold the
      urine for at least two hours.
  5. If the patient does not make it to the toilet on time and has an
      incontinence episode, you should:
      a. toilet her to allow her to try to finish urinating because her bladder
          may not be completely empty;
      b. note on the Incontinence Monitoring Record when the
          incontinence episode(s) occurred.
  6. Avoid serving caffeinated beverages at or after dinner time.
  7. *At night,* if the patient has trouble waking up and getting to the
      bathroom, use a urinal, bedpan, or bedside commode.
  8. Record fluid intake on the Incontinence Monitoring Record.

what is requested of him or be able to communicate the need to void
for example, the caregiver may need to show the patient the toilet or
be aware of certain behavior that the patient may demonstrate before
an incontinence episode. Antecedents are stimuli or events that immediately precede behavior and function as cues (Burgio and Burgio

TABLE 5.10 (continued)

Phase III
1. After three consecutive days, review the Incontinence Monitoring Record.
   a. Note the times the patient is continent and does not pass urine at the time of toileting for at least two of the three days. This time may be eliminated from the toileting schedule.
   b. Note the times of incontinent episodes that seem to have a pattern over the three days and alter toileting times to one-half hour earlier to try to prevent incontinence episodes. (If toileting is more frequent than every two hours, try to extend the time to every two hours gradually.)
   c. If no pattern presents at this time, continue for another three days with Phase II.
   d. Continue to evaluate episodes until a pattern of voiding is established.

1986). A patient with dementia may have antecedent deficits; he may be unaware of the urge to void, unable to find the bathroom, or unable to remember that he had just voided (Burgio and Burgio 1986). Caregivers also must be aware of the words or expressions used by the patient to indicate the need to void. The incontinence monitoring records can be reviewed to evaluate incontinent episodes, fluid intake, and the patient's desire to void. Adjustment of scheduled toileting intervals and fluid intake can be made based on these data.

Habit training involves a variable toileting schedule based on the individual's need to void (Greengold and Ouslander 1986; Clay 1978). (See Table 5.10 for an example of habit training instructions.) Initially, the patient is assigned to a toileting schedule (usually every two hours). The patient is encouraged not to void except at the scheduled time but may use the toilet if voiding cannot be delayed (Hadley 1986). The caregiver must be instructed to recognize behaviors that indicate that the patient needs to void. If the patient voids before the scheduled time, the toileting schedule is then adjusted from the time that she voided. Some type of incontinence monitoring records must be used to chart the time of incontinence episodes, fluid intake, and the patient's desire to void. The toileting schedule is then adjusted to fit the individual's voiding pattern. If the voiding intervals are shortened to less than the desired every two hours, attempts should be made to lengthen the intervals (Long 1985). If voiding or incontinence continues to occur more frequently than every two hours, it is more likely that the patient also has a component of detrusor hyperreflexia and might therefore benefit from concomitant drug treatment. If continence is maintained for two hours, the caregiver may attempt to lengthen the interval progressively by 15 minutes until obtaining a once every three-to-four hours toileting schedule that reflects the patient's voiding habits. Most patients void upon getting up in the morning, within a half hour after meals, and before bedtime; therefore, this should be incorporated into the schedule (Spiro 1978).

In either toileting regime, hygiene is important. If the patient is wet during the check or if an incontinent episode has occurred, the patient should be cleaned and dried. Good skin care will help maintain skin integrity and prevent further problems. Keeping the patient clean and dry reinforces continent behavior (Maney 1980; Burgio and Burgio 1986).

In both habit training and scheduled toilet therapy, it may be necessary to incorporate the use of maneuvers to initiate voiding or to empty the bladder completely. Triggering maneuvers to stimulate voiding in patients include running water, stroking the inner thigh, and/or suprapubic tapping. These maneuvers must be done in such a way that the patient does not become upset. To ensure that the bladder is emptied, one should assist the patient in bending forward after voiding or pressing on the suprapubic area. The patient with dementia may not realize that the urge is present or that he has not completely finished voiding. Toileting schedules, reminders to void, and assistance are stimuli that may cue the patient with dementia to toilet (Burgio and Burgio 1986).

Drug Therapy

Several different types of medications may be used in the management of urinary incontinence. The appropriate drug will depend on the type of urinary incontinence and the patient's medical status. In the elderly population, it is important to consider the potential side effects and interactions of a new medication added to what may already be a complicated medical regimen.

The medications used to treat urinary incontinence have been reviewed in detail elsewhere (Ouslander and Sier 1986; Ouslander et al. 1985). Among patients with dementia, by far the most common indication for pharmacological intervention is detrusor hyperreflexia. Examples of drugs used to treat detrusor hyperreflexia are given in

TABLE 5.11 Drugs Used To Treat Urinary Incontinence Associated with Detrusor Hyperreflexia by Promoting Storage

Drug	Dosage	Side Effects
Anticholinergic/Antispasmodic		
Dicyclomine (Bentyl)	10–20 mg t.i.d	Dry mouth
Flavoxate (Urispas)	100 mg t.i.d	Blurry vision
Imipramine (Tofranil)	25–50 mg t.i.d	Elevated intraocular pressure
Oxybutynin (Ditropan)	2.5–5 mg t.i.d	Constipation
Propantheline	15–30 mg t.i.d	Urinary retention
(Probanthine)		Gastroesophageal reflux
		Tachycardia
		Delirium
		Postural hypotension
		Cardiac conduction defects
		(Imipramine only)

Source: J. G. Ouslander and H. C. Sier 1986.

Table 5.11. All of these drugs have some systemic anticholinergic effects and can cause delirium, and may potentially cause other changes in mental status and cognition as well.

Because of these potential side effects, we generally attempt to use a behavioral approach first. If this fails and the patient's clinical history suggests urge incontinence with no elevation in postvoid residual, we would begin oxybutynin in half the normally recommended adult dosage (2.5 mg three times daily). Oxybutynin has both direct relaxant properties on the bladder muscle and anticholinergic effects. It is frequently effective at this lower dosage and, even at full dosage (5 mg three times a day), seems to have no significant effect on pulse, blood pressure, or intraocular pressure in older people—although it does cause dryness of the mouth in many patients. We have noted no prominent mental status changes in patients treated with this drug. Unless depression is coexisting with dementia, we avoid using imipramine because of the potential cardiovascular side effects. All of these drugs must be used carefully in patients with glaucoma (in which case they should have approval and follow-up by an ophthalmologist; they are contraindicated in patients with angle closure glaucoma), in patients who might be predisposed to urinary retention (men with prostatic enlargement, diabetics with neuropathy), and in patients with symptomatic esophageal reflux. Because dementia patients may not verbalize side effects, they must be specifically questioned, and clues to side effects should be watched for (such as increased fluid intake due to dry mouth or fecal impaction due to constipation).

Conclusion

Urinary incontinence in the elderly is a devastating problem, encompassing physical, psychosocial, and environmental domains. Urinary incontinence is prevalent among a diverse group of aged persons, but it is often associated with impaired cognitive function and impaired mobility. It has an adverse impact on the patient as well as the caregiver. Therefore, health care providers should integrate questions concerning continence status in their basic history taking to enhance patients' and caregivers' knowledge of the problem. A thorough (in)continence assessment is necessary before appropriate intervention can be recommended.

Dementia patients with incontinence are a challenge to clinicians. The (in)continence assessment must be completed before an appropriate treatment can be planned. It is important to relate the onset of incontinence to the progression of dementia. Caregivers can augment the patient's medical and incontinence history. Once acute incontinence has been ruled out, the type of persistent incontinence can be identified. Incontinence monitoring records will enhance the assessment. The appropriate intervention can be selected; however, success often depends on the availability and motivation of the caregiver. Time and energy on the part of the caregiver are required to promote continence. Therefore, support and understanding of the caregiver's needs are vital.

Treatment of incontinence is a team effort; the health care provider, the caregiver, and the patient must cooperate to promote continence. Continual assessment of the selected treatment regime is important, especially as the dementia progresses. Alteration in the regime may be necessary as a result of the evaluation. The individuality of the patient must be considered as the treatment plan evolves to promote self-esteem and dignity.

References

Abrams, P., J. G. Blaivas, S. L. Stanton, and J. T. Andersen. 1988. The standardization of terminology of lower urinary tract function. *Neurourology and Urodynamics* 7:403–427.

Autry D., F. Luazon, and P. Holliday. 1984. The voiding record, an aid in decreasing incontinence. *Geriatric Nursing* 4 (January/February): 22–25.

Blaivas, J. G., and Y. Berger. 1986. Surgical treatment for male geriatric incontinence. *Clinics in Geriatric Medicine* 2:777–87.

Brink, C. 1980. Assessing the problem. *Geriatric Nursing* 1:241–45.

Brink, C., and T. Wells. 1986. Environmental support for geriatric incontinence. *Clinics in Geriatric Medicine* 2:829–39.

Burgio, K. L., and L. D. Burgio. 1986. Behavior therapies for urinary incontinence in the elderly. *Clinics in Geriatric Medicine* 2:809–27.

Burgio, K., C. Robinson, and B. Engel. 1986. The role of biofeedback in Kegel exercise training for stress urinary incontinence. *American Journal of Obstetrics and Gynecology* 154:58–64.

Burgio, L., W. Whitehead, and B. Engel. 1985. Urinary incontinence in the elderly. *Annals of Internal Medicine* 104:507–15.

Chalifoux, P. 1980. Recognizing warning time: A critical step toward incontinence. *Geriatric Nursing* 1:254–55.

Clay, E. C. 1978. Incontinence of urine: A regime for retraining. *Nursing Mirror* 146:23–24.

Demmerle, B. and M. Bartol. 1980. Nursing care for the incontinent person. *Geriatric Nursing* 1:246–50.

Greengold, B. A., and J. G. Ouslander. 1986. A bladder retraining program for elderly patients post indwelling catheterization. *Journal of Gerontological Nursing* 12:31–35.

Hadley, E. 1986. Bladder training and related therapies for urinary incontinence in older people. *Journal of the American Medical Association* 256 (3): 372–79.

Hu, T.-W. 1986. The economic impact of urinary incontinence. *Clinics in Geriatric Medicine* 2:673–87.

Jewett, M. A. S., G. R. Fernie, P. J. Holliday, and M. E. Pin. 1981. Urinary dysfunction in a geriatric long-term care population: Prevalence and patterns. *Journal of the American Geriatrics Society* 29:211–14.

Kane, R. L., J. G. Ouslander, and I. B. Abrass. 1984. Incontinence. *Essentials of clinical geriatrics*, Chapter 6. New York: McGraw-Hill.

Leach, G. E., and C.-M. Yip. 1986. Urologic and urodynamic evaluation of the elderly population. *Clinics in Geriatric Medicine* 2:731–55.

Long, M. L. 1985. Incontinence: The way you react to your clients' incontinence influences their attitudes about the problem. *Journal of Gerontological Nursing* 11:31–40.

Mandelstam, D. 1980. Special techniques: Strengthening pelvic floor muscles. *Geriatric Nursing* 1:251–52.

Maney, J. 1980. Modifying behavior at home: A team effort. *Geriatric Nursing* 1:255–57.

Noelker, L. S. 1987. Incontinence in aged cared for by family. *Gerontologist* 27 (2): 194–200.

Orzeck, S., and J. Ouslander. 1987. Urinary incontinence: An overview of causes and treatments. *Journal of Enterstomal Therapy* 14:20–27.

Ouslander, J. G. 1986a. Commentary: Basic types and causes of geriatric incontinence. *Clinics in Geriatric Medicine* 2:711–13.

Ouslander, J. G. 1986b. Diagnostic evaluation of geriatric urinary incontinence. *Clinics in Geriatric Medicine* 2:715–30.

Ouslander, J. G., M. M. Elhilali. 1987. *The diagnosis and management of urinary incontinence.* New York: Clinical Medicine Research Institute, Clinical Real Life Studies Program, and UCLA Extension.

Ouslander, J. G., and R. L. Kane. 1984. The costs of urinary incontinence in nursing homes. *Medical Care* 22:69–79.

Ouslander, J. G., R. L. Kane, and I. B. Abrass. 1982. Urinary incontinence in elderly nursing home patients. *Journal of the American Medical Association* 248:1194–98.

Ouslander, J. G., R. L. Kane, S. Vollmer, and M. Menzes. 1985. *Technologies for managing incontinence.* Health Technology Case Study 33, OTA-HCS-33. Washington, DC: U.S. Government Printing Office. July.

Ouslander, J. G., S. Raz, K. Hepps, and H. L. Su. 1986. Genitourinary dysfunction in a geriatric outpatient population. *Journal of the American Geriatrics Society* 34:507–14.

Ouslander, J. G., and H. C. Sier. 1986. Drug therapy for geriatric incontinence. *Clinics in Geriatric Medicine* 2:789–807.

Ouslander, J. G., G. C. Uman, and H. N. Urman. 1986. Development and testing of an incontinence monitoring record. *Journal of the American Geriatrics Society* 34:83–90.

Ouslander, J. G., G. C. Uman, H. N. Urman, and L. Z. Rubenstein. 1987. Incontinence among nursing home patients: Clinical and functional correlates. *Journal of the American Geriatrics Society* 35:324–30.

Palmer, M. 1985. *Urinary incontinence.* Thorofare, N.J.: Slack Inc.

Resnick, N. M. 1984. Urinary incontinence in the elderly. *Medical Grand Rounds* 3:281–89.

Resnick, N. 1986. Urinary incontinence in the elderly. *Hospital Practice* 21:80c–80z.

Resnick, N. M., S. V. Yalla, and E. Laurino. 1989. The pathophysiology of urinary incontinence among institutionalized elderly persons. New England Journal of Medicine 320: 1–7.

Schmidbauer, C. P., H. Chiang, and S. Raz. 1986. Surgical treatment for female geriatric incontinence. *Clinics in Geriatric Medicine* 2:759–76.

Schnelle, J. F., R. Traughber, D. B. Morgan, J. E. Embry, A. F. Binion, and A. Coleman. 1983. Management of geriatric incontinence in nursing homes. *Journal of Applied Behavioral Analyses* 16:235–41.

Smallegan, M. 1983. How families decide on nursing home admission. *Geriatric Consultant* (March/April) 21–24.

Smallegan, M. 1985. There was nothing else to do: Needs for care before nursing home admission. *Gerontologist* 25 (4): 364–69.

Spiro, L. 1978. Bladder training for the incontinent patient. *Journal of Gerontological Nursing* 4:28–35.

Staskin, D. R. 1986. Age-related physiologic and pathologic changes affecting lower urinary tract function. *Clinics in Geriatric Medicine* 2:701–10.

Vetter, N. J., D. A. Jones, and C. R. Victor. 1981. Urinary incontinence in the elderly at home. Lancet ii (8261): 1275–77.

Wells, T. and C. Brink. 1981. Urinary continence: Assessment and management. *Nursing and the aged*, ed. I. Burnside, 520–48. New York: McGraw-Hill.

Yarnell, J. W. G., and A. J. St. Leger. 1979. The prevalence, severity and factors associated with urinary incontinence in a random sample of the elderly. *Age and Ageing* 8:81–85.

6

Therapeutic Activity

JITKA M. ZGOLA

Activity of some kind, whether it is work or play, active or passive, exciting or mundane, is, to most people, synonymous with living. It is the way in which each person defines himself and his role in society and exerts control over the world around him. People with Alzheimer's disease or other dementing conditions, who cannot remember or who do not understand their environment, can participate in few activities independently.

Although many persons with dementia express dissatisfaction with their inactivity and the ensuing sense of uselessness, many are also resistant and negative when activities are offered. This apparent indolence or lack of cooperation can be a persistent source of frustration to caregivers who try to enrich these people's lives by offering them the pleasures of being active and filling a significant social role.

This chapter describes an approach to activity programming that is intended to serve the needs of both persons with dementia and their caregivers. The term *therapeutic activity* usually suggests a rehabilitative process that results in improved function. With respect to persons who suffer from dementia, however, therapeutic activity aims to maintain maximal function, enhance the quality of life, and alleviate some of the caregiver's stress and frustration.

Consequences of Inactivity

Emotional Consequences

The person who cannot produce, either physically or intellectually, is stripped of identity, social role, and sense of purpose. Her control and mastery are threatened, and, no matter how well loved or cherished, that person is prone to being devalued, either by herself or by others.

By its effect on the individual's memory, insight, and problem-solving skills, dementia limits not only the ability to perform specific tasks but also the ability to adjust to and compensate for disability. It leaves one without control and without alternatives and makes one dependent on whatever activities others may offer. That is the tragedy of dementia. It even denies the individual the means of overcoming handicap. In this way, it lays a heavy responsibility on whomever plans and delivers activity programming for that person.

At one time, it was thought that those who suffer from dementia lack the insight that would lead to the perception of loss and, therefore, depression. Experience has demonstrated otherwise. We now know that depression has a neurochemical basis that is not dependent on insight. Depression is now diagnosed and treated successfully in many persons with dementia (Fisk 1983).

Intellectual and Cognitive Consequences

Current investigations into dementia support the notion that functional decline in persons who suffer from dementia is not due exclusively to brain damage. These investigations suggest that such decline is, at least partially, due to a vicious cycle of impaired recent memory combined with sensory deprivation and inadequate input from the environment (Woods and Britton 1985).

This disparity between the actual degree of dysfunction and the degree that the disease itself would warrant is called "excess disability" (Brody et al. 1971). It is an important concept because it supports the idea that the person's decline can be slowed by meaningful activity and stimulation. In this way, it offers caregivers some recourse at a time when the untreatable nature of the dementia is its most publicized characteristic.

References to inadequate environmental stimulation as a factor contributing to functional decline must not be taken solely as a reflection on the quality of the environment. Even the most stimulating and loving environment can be inadequate to the person who cannot process information accurately or who cannot interact with it purposefully. A program geared specifically to the individual's needs and abilities will offer stimulation that the person can access and use meaningfully.

The physical consequences of inactivity in terms of muscle wasting, loss of joint range, and cardiopulmonary and circulatory problems are well known. Less attention, however, is paid to the effects that inactivity has on the individual's perception of his own body. The person who is immobile or who is restricted in the care for her own body loses touch with its appearance and its organization. The resulting diffusion of body image further adds to cognitive decline and loss of function.

Social Consequences

The fact that dementia is an invisible disability has important social significance. The extent of the person's disability is not obvious and may be misjudged by the casual observer. Failure to perform even the most basic tasks of daily living can easily be interpreted as laziness or disinterest. Friends and family members who try to encourage the disabled person can make unrealistic demands. Such demands can cause the person to react negatively, either lashing out or withdrawing still further. On the other hand, when caregivers believe that the person is totally disabled, they may restrict activity to the point where the person is denied any opportunity to contribute and experience achievement.

Such misunderstandings may cause rifts among members of the person's family and community and may result in the loss of these vital support systems just at the time when they are needed most. A program of appropriate and socially valued activities is one way of demonstrating to friends and family what the person is still capable of doing when the proper circumstances are made available. At a time when the person's disability is the main object of attention, a therapeutic activity program can help to shift the focus in a more positive direction, that is, toward the person's abilities and retained skills.

Identifying Appropriate Activities

A Broader Perception of "Activities"

Traditionally structured activity programs tend to focus on recreational and diversionary activities. These are most appropriate for persons who are reasonably self-determinate and who need diversion and recreation. When the aim of a program is to enhance the overall quality of life for a person whose control and mastery are diminishing, the concept of activity must be broadened to include the full range of daily activities. The following exercise will demonstrate why.

On two separate pieces of paper, imagine yourself making two lists: one of exciting, recreational activities (skiing, bowling, bingo perhaps, arts and crafts, etc.) and the other of more mundane tasks (dressing and grooming, caring for home and belongings, preparing a snack and sharing it with a friend, looking through the paper). Now imagine yourself walking down the street with both lists in your pocket when, before you, appears the Grim Reaper. "My friend," he says. "Your time is up. But I will give you 20 more years if you give me one of those lists. Consider it carefully, though," he cautions. "You will never again be able to do the things on the list that you give me." Which list would you give up?

It is safe to assume that the list most people would keep consists of those activities that are, for them, the most valued. To most people, that would be the second list, the list of personal care activities. These are the activities that define the quality of our day-to-day lives. It is the loss of these activities that is most painful to the person with a dementing condition.

A program of therapeutic activity is unlikely to achieve its objectives unless it provides participants with opportunities for success in the simple, everyday tasks of daily living. Such activities address the individual's most basic psychosocial needs: the need for identity as defined by a meaningful social role; the need for control and independence that is derived from caring for one's own body, personal possessions, and immediate surroundings; the need for self-esteem and the esteem of others that comes from performing a socially valued service or producing an object that is valued by oneself and others; and the need for meaningful relationships and inclusion in a supportive and accepting group.

If these very important needs are frustrated, a person will have little energy or appetite for recreation or diversion. Examples of activities that can be used to help handicapped persons meet these needs are given.

- Serving tea and passing the tray of cookies reinforces the individual's role as host or hostess and gives the person an opportunity to practice well-preserved social skills that contribute to self-esteem.

- Recounting war stories underscores an individual's valued role in defending his country.
- Applying makeup, choosing nail polish, combing hair and other grooming activities, even if done with help, give the cognitively impaired woman a sense of control over her own body and reinforce body awareness.
- Sorting through a sewing basket, jewelry case, or tool box helps to reestablish that person's control over the immediate environment and reinforces a sense of possession.
- Setting and clearing the table, washing and drying dishes, or dusting, sweeping, and tidying, even if done with help or supervision, are important ways in which the person can contribute to the environment. These are tasks that are universally appreciated and for which the person can honestly be thanked.
- Discussions of things with which participants are familiar such as events in the distant past, the morals and etiquette of their youth, etc., when effectively moderated (even if they engender controversy), serve to stimulate social bonds and provide a forum for self-expression.
- Sing-alongs and dances support a sense of group participation.
- Sitting within a small group that is involved in a calm conversation, having one's hand held, and having attention directed at oneself in a positive fashion reinforce a sense of inclusion for even the most severely impaired person.
- Smelling vegetables as they are chopped and sautéed in the kitchen spurs important memories and provides valuable sensory stimulation for a person who can no longer actively participate in kitchen activities.

This list is by no means all-inclusive, but it does demonstrate that simple, even seemingly trivial, activities are powerful tools for supporting a positive quality of life for the cognitively impaired person. It also reinforces the fact that even the most severely handicapped person is entitled to and can benefit from involvement in a program of specially designed and graded activities and experiences.

Any consideration of the kind of activity that will be comforting to a person must also include an examination of that person's values and previous life-style. The concept of leisure time and activities to fill it is relatively new. Many people who are now being affected by dementia had little time for or interest in activities that were not productive or work-oriented.

Selecting Specific Activities

The choice of specific activities must be based on five very important criteria:

- Each activity must be relevant to the person's social status.
- It must be voluntary.
- It must have a purpose that is obvious and acceptable to the participant.
- It must offer the participant a reasonable chance of success.
- It must relate positively to the program objective, that is, to improve the participant's quality of life.

Relevance of Activities to the Participant

In view of the fragility of the cognitively impaired person's self-image, it is essential that all activities offered to that person not only *be* acceptable adult activities but also *be perceived* by that person to be adult activities. One lady objected vehemently to using Crayola markers to check off her bingo cards. Even though adults do use Crayola markers, to her they were reminiscent of kindergarten, and she refused to be treated as a child. One must never forget how desperately these people struggle to hold onto self-esteem and how vulnerable that self-esteem is.

When a person is very impaired and can do little in the way of obviously adult activities, a caregiver may be tempted to occupy him with children's toys and materials, such as kindergarten puzzles or play dough. Even though the person may seem unaware of the nature of the activity being offered and of the message that accompanies such an activity, no one can ever be certain what is actually going on in that person's mind. One needs to see the pain in the eyes of only one person who has been so affronted to realize that whatever creative effort is required to avoid such an error in judgment is well worthwhile.

A carpenter's adjustable square is as easy to take apart and is as interesting to manipulate as any children's toy and is far more appropriate for a severely impaired gentleman to handle. Gingerbread dough can be pulled, stretched, and kneaded just as well as play dough and will still bake up into an acceptable product. Even if the person with dementia is not aware of what he is being given to handle, the image projected by that person will determine how others respond to him. Others respond to the image of childishness. A person playing with a child's toy may be treated as a child; whereas a gentleman who is handling a carpenter's square is more likely to be treated as a retired craftsman.

Voluntary Participation

Participation in any program that aims to reinforce a person's self-esteem and sense of worth must be voluntary. Sometimes it is necessary to use a bit of coercion to help the person overcome inertia or fear of the unknown. No one should ever be forced into participating in any activity to which she objects.

Obvious Purpose

Every activity in which one is invited to participate must have a purpose of which one is aware and of which one approves. Making pompom toys, for example, becomes acceptable when the product is intended for sale at a fund-raising event. It may be necessary to repeat the purpose of such activities frequently. As the purpose is forgotten, the distaste for apparently silly or childish pursuits may well up again; participants need reassurance that they are not being demeaned.

There is something objectionable about sending adults off with armfuls of projects that they have made in an activity group. If a participant wishes to take a project home as a memento or as a gift for someone, this should be encouraged, even if the fund raiser is short, but the choice must rest with the participant, not with the caregiver.

Here again, activities of daily living, such as grooming and housekeeping, have an advantage. They have an obvious purpose of which most participants need not be reminded. They are also unquestionably appropriate for adults. The products of a cooking group can be eaten immediately for lunch or as a snack.

Some activities are done just for fun or the pleasure of doing them. We must remember, however, that the perception of fun is subjective. Humor is a valuable commodity and should be applied generously, but what is fun for one person may be silly and demeaning for another. A person who cannot abstract or whose insight is limited may have difficulty understanding jokes, witticisms, or puns and may become very uncomfortable in such situations.

We must also remain sensitive to the fact that people with memory deficits and perceptual problems spend much of their time feeling anxious, frightened, and apprehensive. No one can really have fun under such conditions. Unless able to relax and feel safe from embarrassment, failure, or emotional hurt, the cognitively impaired person will not enjoy any "good time" activity.

The Potential for Success

At a time when the person is vulnerable to failure on all fronts, a specially designed program of activities should be the source of as much success experience as possible. The first step to ensuring success is choosing activities that are most compatible with the functional strengths and limitations of the participants. The best guide in this matter is a thorough functional assessment of each individual participant, but some generalizations can be made.

Activities that have the following characteristics are generally the most successful with persons who are cognitively impaired:

- activities that consist of one step that is repeated over and over, such as drying dishes, or activities that can be broken down into individual one-step repetitive tasks, such as making apple tarts — peeling apples, chopping them, rolling pastry dough, filling tart shells, etc. Each step can be assigned to one person, and the group then produces something that no one individual could have done.
- activities that have a strong rhythmic component, such as music with a definite rhythm, rhythmic exercises, and dancing.
- activities that present little or no potential for failure, such as dusting furniture, damp mopping the floor, raking leaves. As long as the person is provided with the proper instruments and is given a safe area in which to work, there is no chance of failure. Chopping vegetables for a soup, sanding a block of wood for a chopping block, painting a clear acrylic finish onto a decorated wall plaque are other examples of activities that really cannot be spoiled by impaired judgment or poor motor skills.
- activities that use old, overlearned patterns of movement such as winding balls of yarn, sawing wood, straight knitting, peeling potatoes, putting a golf ball, throwing bean bags, dancing, kneading dough. Many complex activities comprise several steps, each of which utilizes such a familiar pattern. Staff members should

have information about the person's past so they can identify those patterns with which he is familiar.

- activities that give immediate feedback about success or failure. Throwing bean bags is such an activity because players can tell immediately whether or not they have scored.
- activities with a fairly rigid, predictable, and concrete step-by-step process. Such activities ensure that the person will not encounter any unforeseen contingencies or have to choose from among a number of alternatives. Creative activities such as clay modeling and painting lack this kind of structure and are, therefore, very difficult for more severely impaired persons.
- activities that engage the person directly. Slide presentations and movies are totally passive and, therefore, tend not to work well with this population.

The Relation to the Participant's Program Objectives

If a program is to be therapeutic and serve the needs of its participants, the activities must be planned with specific objectives. These objectives will determine not only the kind of activity, but also the way in which the activity is presented and the particular aspects of the activity that are highlighted to the participants.

The objectives of any planned activity can be grouped into three basic categories:

- physical—promoting or maintaining strength, flexibility, and cardiopulmonary function;
- affective—serving psychosocial needs such as social inclusion, identity, and self-esteem (included here also is the need to have fun and laugh);
- cognitive—maintaining alertness to the environment and providing sensory stimulation, orientation, and body awareness.

An especially important objective in activity programs designed for persons with dementing illness is to enrich sensory experience (Paire and Karney 1984). Sensory deprivation can be a serious consequence of dementia. It results from the person's inability to make sense of the complex stimuli within a conventional environment. Therapeutic activity aims to provide the kind of sensory experience that the person can appreciate. Complex visual and auditory stimuli (such as pictures, print, or spoken language) may be meaningless to a person who has severe perceptual problems. They must be interpreted accurately to be useful to the individual. More basic stimuli, such as color, texture, movement, taste, smell, and temperature, provoke sensations that are either pleasurable or noxious. They do not need to be understood to be fully and richly experienced.

A general rule of thumb for choosing activities in which the person is likely to succeed and from which that person is likely to benefit is: First, look to the person, determine what she can do well and what she needs to experience. Construct the activity around these strengths and needs. Then analyze the activity to be certain that each component of the activity meets the original criteria and objectives. The knowledgeable selection of activities for persons with dementia depends heavily on the caregiver's insight into the effects of the disease on the affected person's performance.

Dementia, Behavior, and Activity

General Considerations

It is sometimes difficult to remember that the impaired person's problems and anomalous behavior are organically based and are usually outside the individual's ability to control. This is especially true when even severely impaired persons can appear to be so intact.

Caregivers must also remain sensitive to the fact that the majority of people with dementia are, in whatever they do, trying very hard to maintain an appearance of competence. All of their efforts are already directed toward doing the best they can. The healthy individual may slack off, but the person who is gradually losing the ability to perform competently tries mightily to hold on to whatever is left. His integrity is on the line, and he will not give it up easily. Much of the "difficult" behavior that is attributed to cognitively impaired persons is actually the result of their efforts to maintain control and a sense of mastery.

A good deal of this negativism is also due simply to fatigue. Maintaining the appearance of competence in the face of what may be severe impairment is hard work. Given this premise, it becomes obvious that efforts to encourage the person to try harder or to correct errors will not only be ineffective but will, in fact, create new problems.

Common Areas of Dysfunction

Even though each person with dementia is an individual and will react to her disability differently, there are some fairly common characteristics and symptoms of which the caregiver must be aware. The four major areas of dysfunction in cortical dementias, of which Alzheimer's disease is one, are memory, organization of movement, perception, and language (Joynt and Shoulson 1985). Definitions and accurate descriptions of these deficits are still the focus of much debate among neuroscientists. The purpose of this discussion is to help caregivers understand these problems in practical terms, that is, how they affect a person's ability to socialize, follow instructions, solve problems, perform tasks, etc.

Memory

Memory for things that occurred minutes, hours, days, or even a few years ago is usually the first to be affected. This memory deficit is not the result of stupidity or carelessness, and the individual can do nothing actively to improve it. This kind of deficit will not be improved by exercises or any other form of training. The person with this disability becomes totally dependent on the environment to provide frequent, consistent, and accessible reminders of important information. In the absence of such reminders, the person may become anxious and disoriented, may confabulate to fill in memory gaps, and may feel persecuted when confronted with events for which she cannot account.

Anyone who is working with such a person must be prepared to repeat information and answer questions over and over again without expecting the person to remember from one time to the next. Information that is repeated in exactly the same way each time may eventually sink in and be retained. When this does happen and when the memory-impaired person can say, "Oh yes, I know now," all of those countless repetitions become worthwhile. If, however, information is given in a different way from one time to another, it is perceived by the person as something new each time. Learning does not usually occur under these circumstances, and the frustration seldom abates.

Impairment of recent memory also interferes with learning. This is an important consideration for the activity planner. Activities that require the acquisition of new skills or learning of new information will be frustrating.

Most persons with dementia have some awareness of their memory deficit and are especially gratified when they are able to remember something. Memory joggers, such as "finish the proverb" games played in a group, can be a lot of fun. The first few words of a familiar proverb jog the memory, and the participants experience the pleasure of remembering the rest of the saying.

By the same token, not remembering is a painful experience for the memory-impaired person. It is very important, therefore, to avoid open-ended questions and testing situations, such as "memory-strengthening exercises." These only expose the person's memory deficit and do nothing to remedy it. Among the most innocent yet painful questions asked of the memory-impaired person are: "Do you remember what we did last week?" or "You remember who I am, don't you?" Such questioning is to be avoided and substituted by information-giving statements such as: "Last week we all enjoyed our trip to the market. Here are some pictures of that day," or "Hello, Mrs. Smith, I am Mary and I really enjoy coming to see you each Tuesday. I haven't seen you since last week."

Memories of the distant past tend to be preserved the longest. They can be a wonderful source of programming ideas. Old knowledge and old skills can be used to underscore a person's value and remaining competencies. Many persons with dementia can relate, in striking and personal detail, the historical events that they have survived. One gentleman told proudly of the contribution of Canadian troops to the building of the road to Mandalay. A lady who could no longer recognize her married daughter took great pleasure in identifying the famous faces in Karsh photographs. Such activities form a link, for these people, with more stable times. They also help reinforce a sense of identity whereby each one can say, "I have a history."

Perception

Perceptual dysfunction (agnosia) interferes with a person's ability to interpret environmental stimuli accurately and reliably. It causes the person to misunderstand or misinterpret visual, auditory, and tactile cues. Consequently, it may become difficult for the impaired person to recognize familiar objects or persons, judge distance and direction accurately, and understand spoken or written language.

The person with perceptual problems will be able to achieve best if the information to which he is expected to respond is free of ambiguities and is presented to as many sensory modalities as possible. A person with a severe deficit may fail to recognize a common object, such as a knife or a spoon, when it is just on the table but may be able to use it appropriately when it is placed in his hand. Therefore, if it is appropriate, the person may be encouraged to touch, smell, or even taste items that are presented. This will help to supplement the information that would be obtained by visual examination only.

When speaking to a person who has difficulty perceiving language accurately, the caregiver must remember to keep sentences short and precise and to avoid metaphors and complex figures of speech. Body language should be an accurate reflection of what is being said. The spoken word should be supported with concrete demonstrations and objects whenever possible.

Although it is important that the activity area be pleasantly and appropriately decorated, the place in which a cognitively impaired person is expected to perform should be as free as possible of distracting and confusing stimuli. Background noise and extraneous movement are among the worst offenders.

Organization of Movement

The inability to organize movement [i.e., to perform specific movements or tasks on command (apraxia) or to organize the steps within an activity into a logical sequence] interferes with the person's function on all levels. It can make even a simple task, such as getting dressed, a confusing and perplexing experience. Clothes may be put on in the wrong order. The person may move about aimlessly when asked to do something, apparently knowing that something is wrong, but unable to perform.

The apraxic person needs to have any complex task broken down and presented in a step-by-step fashion. The degree to which the task must be broken down may vary markedly from one person to another. Steps that the average person takes for granted are easily overlooked. For example, a cognitively impaired person who is holding something may need to be reminded to put it down before picking up something else. The person may not be able to come to the table unless first told to stand up. This inability to "organize oneself into a task" is sometimes misinterpreted as reticence.

Just as memories of the distant past are relatively spared, so too are old, overlearned skills and patterns of behavior. These patterns usually require some outside trigger such as a familiar place (the washroom) and contact with a familiar object (a dish cloth and soapy water) to get them started. Under the right circumstances, even persons who are very impaired may continue to do things such as play the piano, knit, or dry dishes and may experience the pleasure of independent, productive activity.

These old, familiar skills often form the basis of the most successful activities. Many people with dementia depend on them to maintain some degree of independent function. These patterns tend, however, to be very rigid and very fragile. Once the pattern is started, it must run its course. The person cannot handle interruptions or change. The situation is similar to that of a pianist who, having been interrupted in the middle of a piece, must start again from the beginning, or that of the typist whose keyboard has been mixed up.

Because of their dependence on overlearned skills, people with dementia usually find new, unfamiliar activities (such as the novelty crafts) difficult and frustrating. It is painful to see a lady grapple with some new unfamiliar job. On the other hand, it is pure delight to watch that same lady deftly pinch a perfectly fluted edge on a pie crust. This is not to say that novelty crafts should never be used. Many craft projects can be successful if they can be set up to employ these old, embedded skills.

Language

Although many persons with Alzheimer's disease can articulate well, many have difficulty finding specific words that express their thoughts coherently. They may misuse words or talk around the issue in an effort to identify the object by its use, locations, or some other characteristic. These language disorders make communication difficult and frustrating for both the aphasic person and those around her.

Discussions and conversations are an important part of any activity program. It is a grave loss if the aphasic person is excluded or if that person, by participating, makes things uncomfortable for other participants. Sensitive and supportive group leaders or facilitators can do much to reduce the impact of these language problems and help participants to express their ideas, needs, and feelings.

The key in such a situation is to remain alert to the feelings that participants are trying to express. The emotional component of even the most severely impaired person's statements, as expressed through tone of voice, facial expression, and gesture, is real, no matter how bizarre the actual words may be. These feelings should always be addressed with empathy.

At times, it may become necessary for the facilitator to find some rational meaning in what seems to be a totally irrational statement.

This task can be made much easier if the facilitator has some knowledge of the participants' personalities, opinions, values, and past and current life situations.

The emotional component of communication is especially valuable when bridging the communication gap between participants. Emotion is often the only basis for communication among severely aphasic individuals. If participants feel secure and are encouraged, by the facilitator, to make contact with one another, some very strong and mutually supportive relationships can develop. It is wonderful to observe two severely aphasic people deeply engrossed in a conversation or a joint project. Despite the fact that the words may be totally incomprehensible, the body language and the emotions are all there.

The value of these relationships may be overlooked and their development may be impeded in a group where participants are heavily dependent on the facilitator. It is helpful if the facilitator, alert to the need for participants to interact with one another, encourages mutual contact through safe touching, through seating arrangements, or simply by, for example, asking participants to pass items such as tea and cookies to one another instead of doing it for them.

Other Areas Commonly Affected

Many persons who suffer from dementing illness have difficulty making appropriate judgments, abstracting concepts, inhibiting impulses, and sustaining an appropriate level of attention.

JUDGMENT. A deficit in judgment will make it difficult for the person to anticipate problems and to choose appropriately from a variety of alternatives. For example, the person may not be able to judge when he has added enough of an ingredient to a recipe. The person may not respond appropriately to a social situation.

Even if not fully aware of the nature of her mistake, the person is still acutely sensitive to negative reactions from others. Recurrent embarrassments have a devastating effect on the person's self-esteem and can eventually cause her to avoid all activities and social situations. Consequently, it is very important to shield the person from such events. This can be done by avoiding potentially embarrassing situations and by drawing attention away from errors when they do occur. Dealing with failure is an important part of activity programming.

ABSTRACTION. Difficulty forming abstract concepts may prevent the cognitively impaired person from being able to visualize objects or events unless concrete examples are available. Therefore, when Mrs. Albert is asked to make a cup of tea when no teapot is visible, she may, because she actually does not know what is expected, say "No." Later, however, in the kitchen, where all the necessary implements and visual cues are available, she may proceed to make a cup of tea without any problems. This is another example of perceived negativism, where the person is actually unable to participate rather than unwilling.

Another consequence of an impaired ability to abstract is difficulty understanding metaphors, analogies, and other figures of speech. Although these are often useful tools for explaining situations, they tend to confuse the impaired person and should be avoided.

THE CONTROL OF EMOTIONS AND IMPULSES. Disinhibition, or the inability to control impulsive behavior, is another frequent source of embarrassment for the person with dementia. Joy, displeasure, sorrow, and other emotions may be expressed in exaggerated, sometimes grandiose gestures that escalate out of the person's control and can bring an activity period to an abrupt and embarrassing halt. The caregiver who learns to identify such situations before they get out of hand can either redirect the person's attention or draw the person away from the attention of others. This is important, not only to preserve the individual's self-esteem, but also to maintain the comfort of the other group members.

ATTENTION. Disturbances of attention are demonstrated in a variety of ways. The person may have difficulty concentrating on a task to the exclusion of other, irrelevant stimuli. He may not be able to attend to any one thing for more than a few minutes before wandering off to something else. Another person may focus excessive attention on one small part of the task, ignoring all the other aspects of the activity. For example, a lady who has been asked to clear the table may persist in picking at one little crumb that is stuck to the tablecloth.

The person who is experiencing such difficulties needs the worker's help to stay on track until the task is completed. This can be done by providing frequent but simple and friendly reminders. Although this works for most people, others may find it irritating and may become angry or ill-tempered with this treatment. In these cases, the activity can be planned so that it consists of many short, quick steps with a prompt built into the beginning of each one. The following is an example of such a situation.

Mr. Smith is drying dishes. This is an activity that he enjoys, but he hasn't done it often and frequently loses track of his work. The caregiver is working close by and every once in a while says something like: "How are those dishes coming along, Mr. Smith?" Mr. Smith responds amicably and returns to his task. This approach suits him. The task and the reminder are, therefore, appropriate.

Mrs. Brown, however, in the same situation becomes snippy and disagreeable. She needs another approach. The caregiver may ask her to dry the dishes while someone else washes. As each dish is washed, Mrs. Brown's partner hands it to her for drying. Each time Mrs. Brown is handed a dish, she receives an automatic prompt that helps keep her on track.

Initiating and terminating activities also poses problems for many persons with dementia. They just cannot get started on a task. Despite an actual willingness to be involved, they are stymied by an inertia that must be overcome by some outside force. Once started, these same persons often find it difficult to stop. They may persist in an activity until, again, some outside force brings them to a halt. This problem has been compared to that of a car with no gear shift and no brake. The motor may start (i.e., the person is willing) but the car will not move without a push. Once the car is going, it will just keep going in the same direction until something comes along and stops it.

The person with this problem can usually do quite well if given specific prompts. Placing the person's hand into the dishwater is a good way to help him start washing the dishes. Asking him for the dishcloth and leading him away from the sink may be the only way to get that person to stop wiping the counter.

Volition versus Illness

It is not surprising that caregivers sometimes interpret the impaired person's behavior as being willfully difficult and contrary. Such misunderstandings usually arise from two common phenomena. One is the person's ability to cover up. Most people with dementia retain a good repertoire of social manners and phrases that can make them look quite competent in a short, non-demanding social encounter. Many continue, for a long time, to use socially acceptable, even clever-sounding, expressions that can hide a memory deficit or functional gap.

A lady who is asked her age may answer quite irately, "Young man, I am sure that that is none of your business!" And who would not permit her that prerogative? A gentleman who is invited to come to the table for lunch may respond with a flourish, "My dear, can you not see that circumstances do not permit me to do that right now?" In fact, his comment may be more accurate than we know. The disabling "circumstances" may be that, seated with his back to the dining table, he cannot see where he is expected to go and does not know how he will get there or whether he will be able to find his way. Rather than risk the unknown, he declines lunch altogether. His articulate answer masks the extent of his impairment. Most people would conclude that this gentleman just does not want any lunch.

The second factor that may cause people to attribute negative behavior to willfulness is the apparent inconsistency of the person's skills. Two examples that illustrate this point were mentioned previously: the person who could not recognize her own daughter but who could identify Winston Churchill in a book of Karsh photographs and the person who refused to make a cup of tea when asked to do so but who later made one for herself when she went into the kitchen and saw the teapot on the counter.

Residual Abilities

Despite these deficits, many persons retain some very important positive qualities that must be supported and nurtured in any effective activity program. First and foremost is the person's dignity as an adult. The vast majority of persons who develop a dementing condition in their latter years have led responsible and productive lives. The respect that they have earned during those years must be demonstrated and maintained through the types of activities in which they are invited to participate and by the way in which these activities are presented.

The tendency to retain old, overlearned skills and memories has been discussed. A program that aims to promote self-respect and highlight competencies should take full advantage of these abilities. Familiar household tasks, such as raking leaves, stuffing pillowcases, and folding towels, and the mechanical and repetitive components of more complex projects, such as sanding wood or crocheting squares, provide the impaired person with an opportunity to experience success and a sense of participation.

No matter how impaired, the person remains emotionally sensitive and retains the need to express emotions, to have a good laugh, to share a tender moment, or to work off some anger. Among the most gratifying and mutually enjoyable activities are visits with animals and babies. Negative emotions also need a socially acceptable outlet. This can be achieved through vigorous activity such as hammering, punching bread dough, and, in fact, many of the activities that healthy people use to work off negative energy. Care must be taken, however, to limit the choice of such activities to normal, socially accepted activities that participants will recognize as appropriate for adults.

Throughout this discussion, the person with dementia has been referred to in general terms. As important as it is for caregivers to be aware of the problems that impede the affected person's function and the ways in which function can be facilitated, it is equally important that they keep in mind the unique nature of each person and avoid generalizations, assumptions, and stereotypes. Each person must be considered as an individual.

Making the Program Work

When specific objectives for each participant in the program have been identified and the appropriate activities have been selected, the success of even the most appropriate activity depends on the skill of the caregiver in setting it up, initiating the participant's involvement, and supervising it through to completion.

Setting Up

Advance planning is essential. Once the activity is chosen, it is broken down into its individual steps. Each step is analyzed in terms of each participant's ability to perform it and is assigned to the particular participant who would most enjoy doing it. The kind of instructions or demonstrations each participant is likely to need, the kind of sensory experience the activity offers, and potential hazards or cautions are all identified. It is helpful if program staff and volunteers have an opportunity to discuss these matters beforehand. Any part of the activity that is deemed too difficult for participants can be done in advance by staff members or caregivers.

An appropriate location, be it the activity room, the kitchen, the bathroom, or the person's bedroom, is then identified and prepared. Distractions and interruptions are eliminated wherever possible, and all necessary materials and equipment are collected. It is important that only those articles needed at any one particular time are placed within reach or sight of the participants.

Introducing the Activity

The tendency of cognitively impaired persons to decline invitations has been discussed. It is sometimes necessary to avoid giving the person an option about participating at the start. A simple directive is often easier to handle. The person may need reassurance that she will be permitted to watch at first and gradually move into the activity as she becomes more comfortable. Assurance of help is also comforting to the apprehensive participant. Physical prompts may be necessary to help the person initiate a pattern of movement. The presence of a finished example of the project or some other concrete reminder of the goals of the activity is often helpful.

Of course, one must remember that, if the person seriously objects to an activity, it should never be forced upon him. In such an event, it is a good idea for staff members to review the task against the five basic criteria of meaningful activity and determine whether it is, in fact, suited to that individual.

Guiding Participation

Once the person has indicated an interest and a willingness to participate, the activity is presented in simple step-by-step terms. If necessary, the worker may start by demonstrating or guiding the person physically through the activity. Physical guidance should always be offered within the person's line of sight, with warning and with firm decisive movements. Light, "tickly" touch can be distracting and even unpleasant.

When verbal instructions are given, they should be simple, concise, and precise. If a phrase to which the participant responds well is identified, it should be used over and over again without alteration. For example, one very severely impaired gentleman was successfully engaged in dealing out cards by the repetition of the phrase, "Hit me again." He had lost all concept of playing a game, but the simple act of dealing the cards out one at a time to someone else formed a bridge to the only active social encounter that this gentleman experienced.

Once the person is comfortable with the task, it is best to avoid any further instructions or comments that may distract or confuse. Too much help can be as disconcerting as too little. If the person seems to be going off on the wrong track, the helper should wait to see whether the person is just proceeding in her own way before offering correction. It is sometimes difficult to avoid imposing one's own standards on the person whom one is helping. In doing so, one may also lose sight of the original objectives of the activity.

Focus on the Objectives

Unless the helper or caregiver remains aware of the objectives towards which the activity is intended, the benefit of the activity may be lost. Making Valentine's Day cards, for example, if presented without any specific objective, could be quite meaningless. It would be done by the participants with some help, perhaps, in cutting and pasting lace and red hearts onto a piece of construction paper. The product might be acceptable, but what would the participants have really gained from the experience? In fact, some people might find it childish and demeaning and then the experience would have been negative.

This same activity can, however, be planned with the following objectives:

- to help patients recall a happy and valued relationship;
- to help patients express sentiments of affection and appreciation to a special person; or
- to provide a pleasant sensory experience.

With these objectives in mind, the helpers will focus more on the process in which the participants are involved than on the actual construction of the card. The card will include a picture of the loved one for whom it is intended. The introduction to the activity will consist of a discussion of that photograph. The helper will assist each participant in composing a note that expresses his feelings about that person. The lace and tinsel decorating the card will be used to stimulate memories and encourage sensory exploration by the participants. Even a very impaired person, who may be able to do little toward the actual construction of the card, would benefit from this activity if it were presented with attention to these specific objectives.

Another example illustrates why it is so important for everyone assisting with the program to be aware of the objectives of the particular activity. A daily exercise routine should:

- provide a gentle cardiopulmonary workout;
- maintain muscle strength and flexibility; and
- give participants an opportunity to experience the pleasure of movement.

One person is not performing the routine accurately, but is moving and seems pleased with her performance. She is enjoying herself. A staff member who is not aware of the objectives may attempt to correct this lady, confusing her, and perhaps even causing her to withdraw from the activity altogether. On the other hand, the staff member who is aware of the real objectives of this activity would not interfere unless the lady herself indicated a need for help and would permit her to continue enjoying the activity in her own fashion.

Handling Failure

The easiest errors to handle, of course, are those that were anticipated and, therefore, never happen. If a participant does make an error, however, the helper faces an important choice: to correct or to let the matter go. For example, a gentleman who is eating potatoes with a spoon should be left alone to enjoy his meal, whereas one who is attempting to eat broth with a fork will never succeed and must, therefore, be given a spoon. In both of these cases, it must be kept in mind that the initial error was that of the helper who left the inappropriate utensil within reach.

When a project does go awry, it may take some fast thinking on the part of the helper to make the best of the mistake, cover it up, or at least share the blame and so protect the person from failure. Here are two examples of projects that went amiss. In each case, the real culprit was the worker who did not foresee a potential problem. In each case, the error was handled effectively, the participant was spared the feeling of failure, and a potential disappointment was turned into fun.

One lady was to make a cake. The worker, believing that the lady was capable of measuring out the milk, gave her a pint of milk, a measuring cup, and instructions to measure out one cup. Instead, the lady emptied the entire pint of milk into the bowl of cake mix. The very creative worker added two eggs and spent the rest of the activity period frying crepes while the lady ladled the very thin cake batter into the crepe pan.

During a home visit, the worker had set a lady up to chop some onion for a lunch of egg salad sandwiches. Not having anticipated how quickly this lady could chop onions, the worker left her with one large Spanish onion and went downstairs to fetch the bread. By the time the worker returned, the lady had chopped the entire onion and had mixed it with two chopped eggs and a ladle of mayonnaise.

They both agreed that the sandwiches were a little heavy on the onion and laughed at the reception that their husbands would give them that evening. Those "onion and mayonnaise" sandwiches became a little privately shared joke whenever they met for months thereafter.

If an activity that is not entirely predictable is being planned, it is best to warn the group that it may not work. The activity then becomes an experiment, and everyone is successful in finding out whether or not it works.

The joy of doing is far more important than the absolute quality of the product. Wherever possible, as long as a person is not embarrassed by the quality of her achievement, she should not be denied that joy. If Mrs. Smith does not mind sleeping on wrinkled sheets, who should stop her from making her own bed?

The only true measure of how successful this process has been is the quality of the participant's experience. No amount of effort will convince a person who is dissatisfied with his product that it is good. By the same token, a person who is pleased with his perhaps unconventional effort should be corrected only if his approach is likely to cause personal danger, serious harm to property, or complete failure of the activity. Care must be taken also that the participation itself is an enjoyable experience. The memory-impaired person cannot function on the basis of "present pain for future gain." Such a person lives for the present.

Staffing a Program

Throughout this discussion, we have referred to "workers," "helper," and "staff" as those who carry out and support activity programming. Who actually performs the program? Within the context of the broadened perspective on therapeutic activity that includes all activities of daily living, the perception of program personnel is also broadened. In institutional settings, aides and orderlies who help the residents in their daily care, cleaning and maintenance staff who maintain the patients' rooms and common areas, and dietary staff who serve the meals and snacks all have an important role to play in keeping the residents active and involved in their surroundings.

In the community, visiting homemakers, friendly visitors, and other home support workers can contribute as much to their clients' involvement in therapeutic activity as do the personnel in special day programs. Their roles are not merely to teach crafts or to clean house but also to enable a sense of mastery and competence in the clients whom they visit.

Many family members find that involvement in a program of therapeutic activity helps them view their loved one in a more positive light. They find that, as they learn to interact with the person in a productive way, the tensions between them tend to diminish. Many aspects of their former relationship are rediscovered, or they find new ways of interacting that are also positive.

On the other hand, many family members find it difficult or impossible to assume a new directive role with respect to a parent or spouse. They cannot realign their expectations and methods of interacting with the person. Under such circumstances, attempts to carry out the kind of program described in this chapter can become unsatisfying and frustrating.

The same holds true for members of the health care field and other supporting occupations. Working with people who suffer from dementia in the context of life-style management or activity programming is a skill that can be learned. It is also a calling, however, and, as with any calling, it is not suited to everyone. There is no shame in admitting that one is unsuited to this kind of work. The shame would lie only in a failure to identify the need for such programming.

Conclusion

If we accept the premise that therapeutic activity should include all activities of daily living and that these activities should be set up in a way that will promote an experience of success and mastery for the cognitively impaired person, we are really accepting the concept of life-style management through activity. This approach broadens the scope of activity programming beyond the traditional concepts of recreation and diversion and brings it into a much more exciting perspective. It places into the hands of everyone who is involved with cognitively impaired persons the tools with which they can contribute something positive and inject pleasure and fulfillment into a situation that is often quite bleak.

References

Brody, E. M., M. H. Kelban, M. P. Lawton, and H. A. Silverman. 1971. Excess disabilities of mentally impaired aged: Impact of individualized treatment. *Gerontologist* 11:124–33.

Fisk, A. 1983. Management of Alzheimer's disease. *Postgraduate Medicine* 4:237–41.

Joynt, R. J., and I. Shoulson. 1985. Dementia. In *Clinical Neuropsychology*. 2d ed., ed. K. H. Heilman and E. Valenstein, 453–79. New York: Oxford University Press.

Paire, J. A., and R. J. Karney. 1984. The effectiveness of sensory stimulation for geropsychiatric inpatients. *American Journal of Occupational Therapy* 8:505–9.

Woods, R. T., and P. G. Britton. 1985. *Clinical psychology and the elderly*. Rockville: Aspen.

Suggested Readings

Burton, J. E. 1982. Programming to meet the needs of the elderly in institutions: Part II. *Canadian Journal of Occupational Therapy* 3:89–91.

Coons, D. H., and S. E. Weaverdyck. 1986. Wesley Hall: A residential unit for persons with Alzheimer's disease and related disorders. In *Therapeutic Interventions for the Person with Dementia*, ed. E. D. Taire, 29–53. New York: Haworth Press.

Edelson, J. S., and W. Lyons. 1985. *Institutional care of the mentally impaired elderly*. New York: Van Nostrand Reinhold.

Mace, N. L. 1987. Principles of activities for persons with dementia. *Physical and Occupational Therapy in Geriatrics* 5 (3): 13–27.

Zgola, J. M. 1987. *Doing things: A guide to programming activities for persons with Alzheimer's disease and related disorders*. Baltimore: Johns Hopkins University Press.

7

Issues In Late-Stage Care
KATIE MASLOW, M.S.W.

The last stages of Alzheimer's disease and other diseases that cause dementia are both physically and emotionally stressful for caregivers. Patients usually require extensive physical care, yet they are increasingly unable to respond to or cooperate with their caregivers. Decisions about certain medical interventions may become extremely difficult—for example, whether to provide or withhold surgery for hip fractures, cardiopulmonary resuscitation, tube or intravenous feeding, or antibiotic therapy or even whether to hospitalize a patient for diagnostic tests or intensive monitoring.

There is an extensive and growing literature on legal and ethical considerations in decisions about medical care for people at the end of life, including people with dementia. In contrast, relatively little has been written about the clinical aspects of caring for patients during the last stages of dementing disorders. This chapter raises some questions about what patients are like in those stages and what constitutes "good care" for them.

What Are Patients Like During the Last Stages of Dementia?

In 1982, Reisberg et al. described seven stages of primary degenerative dementia, the last stage being "late dementia," in which "All verbal abilities are lost. Frequently there is no speech at all—only grunting. Incontinence of urine; requires assistance toileting and feeding. Loses basic psychomotor skills, e.g. ability to walk. The brain appears no longer able to tell the body what to do. Generalized and cortical neurologic signs and symptoms are frequently present." Also in 1982, Hughes et al. delineated a five-stage Clinical Dementia Rating

(CDR) scale in which the last stage—"severe dementia"—is described as:

- severe memory loss; only fragments remain;
- orientation to person only;
- inability to make judgments or solve problems;
- no pretense of independent function outside the home;
- no significant function in the home or outside the patient's own room;
- much help required with personal care and frequent incontinence.

Since then, researchers from Duke University (Heyman et al. 1987) have added two stages to the CDR to classify later stages of dementia that they say are frequently seen in nursing homes and other chronic care facilities:

- "profound dementia," in which patients have "severe impairment in language or comprehension, inability to walk unaided, and problems in feeding themselves, recognizing their family, or controlling bowel or bladder function" and
- a "terminal" stage, in which patients require "total care because they are completely uncommunicative, bedridden, vegetative, and incontinent."

Cohen et al. (1984) described six psychological stages of dementia, the last one being "separation from self": "At this point, individuals are capable of reacting to certain things that happen in their environment, but do not have the ability to be active in their environment. The family accepts the patient as greatly changed and a 'different person.' The major needs of the patient are to be comfortable and secure. During this period patients seem almost part of another world, unable to communicate or to act, yet they may still remain important persons in the emotional lives of their families."

These descriptions suggest that there is uniformity in patients' functional abilities during the last stage of dementia. On the other hand, clinicians and researchers have emphasized as a general principle the variable presentation of dementing disorders in individual patients and the heterogeneity of patients in terms of specific cognitive losses and deficits in functional abilities.

How Uniform Are Functional Deficits During the Last Stages of Dementia?

It is clear that many and perhaps most persons with dementia are unable to speak, walk, feed, or toilet themselves during the weeks or months before they die. Yet no data are available to determine how many dementia patients lose specific functional abilities or at what stage of their illness.

Anecdotal evidence indicates that dementia patients differ in their functional abilities, even near the end of their lives. For example, some individuals with dementia continue to be ambulatory until weeks or even days before they die. Anecdotal evidence indicates that some dementia patients continue to speak, although only in single words or repetitious phrases. Probably very few persons in the last stage of dementia feed themselves independently, but some can be hand-fed, whereas others are apparently unable to swallow effectively and choke or gag when hand-fed.

These differences may reflect variation in the pattern or rate of neurological deterioration in individuals with the same disease. Alternatively, they may reflect different diseases or different types of the same disease—for example, different types of Alzheimer's disease. Very little is known about the natural courses of most diseases that cause dementia or about the usual causes of death for people with dementia. Thus, it is also possible that the patients who, for example, continue to be ambulatory until just before their deaths actually die at an earlier stage of their disease than other patients with the same disease, that, in effect, such patients never reach the last stage of dementia, and that, if they had lived longer, they would have lost their ability to walk.

Without better information about the natural course of diseases that cause dementia and the physiological processes that lead to specific functional deficits, it is impossible to describe the last stage definitively. It is also impossible to predict with any certainty that an individual patient will experience a given functional deficit before death.

What Are the Effects of Caregiver Expectations and
Related Treatment Practices on Patient Functioning
During the Last Stages of Dementia?

Many persons with dementia spend the end of their lives in long-term care facilities where the staff's expectations about and responses to specific patient problems can have a strong influence on patient functioning. Two examples come to mind immediately. Residents of long-term care facilities who appear unsteady on their feet are frequently physically restrained to prevent them from falling. If the facility staff assume that all people with dementia inevitably become nonambulatory, they may physically restrain a resident with dementia at the first sign of unsteadiness and continue to restrain the individual indefinitely, without investigating reversible causes for the unsteadiness—for example, medications or weakness related to another treatable condition (Buchner and Larsen 1987). Once restrained for more than a few days, the individual may become permanently nonambulatory.

Similarly, residents of long-term care facilities who either will not eat or choke and gag while eating are frequently tube-fed. If staff members assume that all people with dementia eventually develop swallowing difficulties due to irreversible neurological losses, tube feeding may be initiated when a resident first stops eating and staff may fail to consider other possible causes for the eating problem— for example, an acute illness that causes loss of appetite. When tube feeding is continued beyond a certain point, an individual with dementia may actually lose the ability to swallow.

Similar situations may occur with respect to agitated or withdrawn behavior, incontinence, alterations in the patient's sleep/wake cycle, and other patient behaviors and characteristics; that is, staff members may assume that these conditions are caused by the patient's dementing disorder and are, therefore, inevitable. As a result, they may fail to consider other, sometimes reversible causes for the conditions.

Such situations may be less likely for patients cared for at home because family caregivers may have less firmly established expectations about what dementia patients are like near the end of their lives. On the other hand, family caregivers who are told to expect specific functional deficits and behavioral problems are unlikely to question the cause of these problems when and if they arise.

Given the current lack of information about the course of diseases that cause dementia, about how and why specific functional abilities are lost, and about the extent of individual variation in manifestations of these diseases, caregivers should be cautious about assuming that a patient's behavior or functional deficits are caused by dementia. "Good care" clearly requires that other causes be considered, even late in the patient's disease process.

What Principles Should Govern Medical Treatment Decisions for Patients in the Last Stages of Dementia?

Many people, including physicians, nurses, and legal and ethical scholars, agree in general that medical treatments may be withheld or withdrawn from people who are terminally ill due to any disease and who are expected to die within a short time with or without treatment. Public opinion polls indicate that about 75 percent of the public supports the idea that life-sustaining medical treatments may be withheld or withdrawn from terminally ill people, especially if the individual is suffering and the individual or family requests withholding or withdrawal (American Medical Association 1986; Malcolm 1984).

In addition, many health care professionals and others argue that the goal of treatment for patients in the late stages of any incurable disease is the patient's comfort and that treatment decisions should be made with this goal in mind. Hospice programs are structured around this goal, and some health care professionals advocate a hospice approach to the treatment of patients with dementia (Campion 1987; Lynn 1986; Volicer et al. 1986; Volicer 1986).

Finally, legal and ethical traditions in this country support the principle that patients' wishes about their medical treatment should take precedence over other considerations in treatment decisions. The courts have identified four societal interests that can in theory override a patient's treatment preference, (i.e., preservation of human life, protection of third parties, prevention of suicide, and protection of the ethical integrity of the medical profession). However, the courts have seldom ruled that these interests take precedence over a patient's treatment preference, especially in the case of a terminally ill patient.

These three general principles—that treatment may be withheld or withdrawn from patients who are terminally ill and will die in a short time with or without treatment; that the goal in caring for patients in the last stage of incurable diseases is the patient's comfort;

and that a patient's wishes take precedence over other considerations in treatment decisions—provide some guidance for people caring for patients in the last stage of dementia. However, many treatment decisions for these patients remain problematic because it is often unclear when dementia patients are terminally ill or what constitutes comfort care for them and it is usually impossible to determine their treatment preferences with any certainty.

When Are Dementia Patients "Terminally Ill"?

Lack of information about the course of diseases that cause dementia make it difficult to determine when patients with dementia are "terminally ill" (Rango 1985). Although some physicians, nurses, and others believe that they can often sense when patients are near death, anecdotal evidence suggests that patients with dementia sometimes "don't die when they should" or, conversely, die sooner than their caregivers expect.

Uncertainty about when dementia patients are terminally ill can lead to strong disagreements among caregivers about appropriate treatment decisions. Whereas most people agree that it is acceptable to withhold or withdraw medical treatments from individuals who are known to be terminally ill, there is much more disagreement about the appropriateness of withholding or withdrawing treatment from individuals who are severely debilitated but not necessarily terminally ill. As a result, even if caregivers agree in general that certain medical treatments can be withheld or withdrawn if a patient is "terminally ill" (and some people do not agree with this principle), they may still disagree strongly about whether treatment can be withheld or withdrawn from a dementia patient because they disagree about whether the patient is "terminally ill."

In 38 states, living will statutes allow individuals to document in advance their preferences about the use of life-sustaining treatments in case they become unable to make treatment decisions for themselves in the future. Most of these state living will statutes specify that an individual's living will can only take effect if he or she is terminally ill. If a patient's caregivers disagree about whether the patient is terminally ill when a particular treatment decision is made, they may also disagree about whether the living will should be honored.

What Constitutes "Comfort Care" for a Person in the Last Stages of Dementia?

Although the principle that patient comfort should be the goal of treatment for patients in the last stages of dementia may provide general guidance to caregivers, the implications of this principle are often unclear for specific treatment decisions because we know so little about what is comfortable for such patients. Consider, for example, a decision about whether to provide antibiotic treatment for a severely confused patient who has an irreversible disease that causes dementia and life-threatening pneumonia. On the one hand, if the patient is perceived to be suffering from the dementia even apart from the pneumonia, the principle would indicate that the patient should be allowed to die of pneumonia rather than live longer with antibiotic treatment. On the other hand, a severely confused patient may suffer from the fever and coughing associated with pneumonia (Lynn 1986). A patient with dementia cannot express his or her perception of the relative suffering associated with the two treatment approaches, and it is difficult for anyone else to make an accurate judgment about which approach will make the patient more comfortable. The potential for patient suffering due to invasive diagnostic tests required to identify the cause of the pneumonia and select an appropriate antibiotic further complicates the equation (Volicer et al. 1986). In this situation, some caregivers may choose to treat the symptoms of the pneumonia (e.g., the cough) and forgo the use of antibiotics.

Decisions about surgery for hip fractures, long-term tube feeding, and aggressive treatment of decubitus ulcers pose similar dilemmas. In each case, it is difficult to determine what treatment approach will maximize patient comfort.

Many basic questions about patient comfort associated with treatment or nontreatment remain unanswered, both in general and for the individual patient. In some cases, caregivers assume that they know the answers without even formulating the questions.

- What experiences, events, or situations cause suffering for a severely demented person?
- What is a severely demented person's experience of common medical and nursing procedures that the person is no longer capable of understanding—for example, being given medications or being bathed or turned?

- What is such a patient's experience of physical restraints that may be used to keep the patient from walking and perhaps falling or to keep the patient from pulling out tubes or catheters that are used for certain treatments?
- Is there a point at which conscious but severely demented patients cease to experience pain or certain types of pain? Do such patients suffer from hunger, thirst, and other such sensations?
- How should we interpret the moaning, crying out, or restlessness of a severely demented person? Should we consider these behaviors as manifestations of suffering as we would with a cognitively normal person?
- Is there suffering associated with just being alive for a conscious but severely demented person?

Answers to these questions either for severely demented people in general or for a specific dementia patient might allow caregivers to make treatment decisions in accordance with the principle that patient comfort should be the goal of treatment. We also need to know more about the relative risks of alternate treatment approaches for a specific patient, for example, the risk of falling versus the risks associated with being physically restrained for a prolonged period. Without such information, caregivers can only guess which treatment decision will maximize patient comfort on either a long-term or a short-term basis.

How Can a Dementia Patient's Treatment Preferences Be Determined?

Clearly, a severely demented person is not capable of making rational decisions about medical treatment. If the patient has ever executed a living will, that document expresses the person's treatment preferences. In addition, some people have signed a durable power of attorney that designates someone else to make treatment decisions for them if they are not capable of making decisions for themselves; if these people discussed their treatment preferences with the individual they designated as a surrogate decision maker, then that individual can express the patient's preferences when a decision is needed later on.

Most people have not executed a living will or a durable power of attorney, however. In the absence of such documents, caregivers sometimes rely on reports about patients' prior verbal expressions of their wishes. Alternatively, they may rely on an examination of the patient's previous life-style that may suggest a pattern of response in health care decisions—for example, whether the patient usually sought treatment for medical problems or routinely avoided doctors and hospitals and refused medical care.

Even with such indicators of a patient's treatment preferences, caregivers still face difficult questions about whether the preferences should be considered valid and applicable to the current treatment decision. Whether the condition to be treated is an inevitable consequence of the patient's dementing disorder, whether the patient is, in fact, terminally ill, and whether the patient will suffer more from treatment or lack of treatment are all relevant questions in determining whether a patient's treatment preferences expressed at an earlier time are applicable to the current treatment decision.

In summary, although the widely accepted principles for making medical decisions for patients at the end of life offer some guidance for caregivers making decisions for dementia patients, important questions remain unanswered. These questions are glossed over in much of the legal and ethical literature on this topic and in some of the published guidelines for decision making that are derived from the principles. Good care for patients in the last stages of dementia requires that caregivers acknowledge these questions and retain some skepticism about the automatic application of the principles in decisions for such patients.

Eating Disorders and Tube Feeding for Persons in the Last Stages of Dementia

A brief discussion of eating disorders and decisions about tube feeding for persons in the last stages of dementia illustrates the preceding points. Some people with dementing disorders stop eating, whereas others do not. It is known that some people with diseases that cause dementia—particularly Alzheimer's disease and stroke— have physical difficulty with swallowing (Castell 1986; Simmons 1986; U.S. Congress 1987b). The proportion of people with these diseases who have associated swallowing difficulties is not known, however, and there may be other reasons why some patients stop eating. Very little is known about how many or what proportion of dementia patients experience functional eating disorders at any stage of their illness, about what causes the disorders, and about how often tube feeding is needed or used for these patients.

One study (Siebens et al. 1986) found that 32 percent of the residents of one nursing home could not eat without physical assistance of some kind, including hand feeding. The need for assistance was correlated with swallowing disorders and was also correlated with low scores on a measure of cognitive ability—the Mini-Mental State exam (MMSE). None of the nursing home residents with a MMSE score indicating normal cognitive ability required assistance with eating, but 25 percent of those with scores indicating moderate cognitive impairment and 75 percent of those with scores indicating severe cognitive impairment required such assistance. Seven (9 percent) of the residents at this nursing home were tube-fed. Of these seven, the researchers were able to examine four, all of whom had severe cognitive impairment (H. Siebens, personal communication December 11, 1986). On the other hand, 25 percent of the residents with severe cognitive impairment were able to eat completely independently.

Although cognitive impairment was correlated with the need for assistance in eating, further statistical analysis revealed that the relationship did not hold up in the absence of swallowing difficulties. The researchers suggested that swallowing difficulties may be associated with only a specific type of dementia or a particularly severe form of dementia (Siebens et al. 1986).

Other researchers (Volicer et al., in preparation) have pointed out several possible causes of eating disorders in dementia patients other than loss of the physiological ability to swallow. These other causes include *swallowing difficulties* due to (1) pain from esophageal ulcers or other causes, (2) esophageal obstructions, or (3) overmedication that interferes with the swallowing mechanism, and *refusal of food* due to (1) dislike of the food that is presented, (2) failure to recognize edible objects as food, (3) loss of the sense of thirst or hunger, (4) loss of appetite associated with an acute illness or medications, (5) depression, or (6) a conscious decision to give up and die. Failure by caregivers to position a patient properly for eating can also cause problems.

Good care of patients in any stage of dementia, including the last stage, requires a careful evaluation of a patient's eating disorder and concerted efforts to treat reversible causes of the problem (Rango 1985). Caregivers should not assume that either swallowing difficulties or tube feeding is inevitable at any stage. When swallowing difficulties are suspected, even in the last stage of dementia, the patient should be evaluated by an expert in swallowing disorders, usually a speech-language pathologist.

If it is determined that a severely demented patient has an eating disorder that cannot be cured, a choice must be made about whether to tube-feed the patient. Usually such patients *are* tube-fed, although many clinicians and legal and ethical scholars agree that tube feeding may be withheld if the burden of treatment outweighs its potential benefit for the patient and if the family agrees that tube feeding should be withheld.

These decisions are extremely controversial, dividing families, health care professionals, and others involved in caring for a patient. The controversy focuses on two fundamental points: (1) whether tube feeding should be considered a medical intervention that can be withheld or withdrawn in certain circumstances like other medical treatments, or an essential component of caring for any patient who is unable to take in adequate amounts of food or fluids otherwise and (2) whether withholding or withdrawing tube feeding from a terminally ill or severely debilitated patient is killing the patient—because all human beings need food and fluids to live—or just allowing the patient to die of the underlying illness. In addition, providing food and water is a pervasive symbol of caring in this and many other societies, and failure to provide them, even when it involves tube feeding, is deeply troubling for many people.

Even if a patient's caregivers agree on these fundamental points, decisions about whether to tube feed a dementia patient may be complicated by questions about whether the patient is terminally ill, whether the patient will suffer more from tube feeding or lack of tube feeding, and how to determine the patient's treatment preference.

Claire Conroy, a severely confused elderly woman receiving tube feeding in a New Jersey nursing home, was the subject of two years of legal proceedings concerning withdrawal of the tube feeding (In re Conroy 1985). Ms. Conroy died early in the legal process even though it was not expected that she would die imminently and tube feeding had not been withdrawn. The case was continued after her death because the New Jersey court decided that the issues it raised were so important. However, if her caregivers had realized that she was terminally ill and would die with or without treatment, it is unlikely that her case would have been so controversial.

Some widely cited articles on tube feeding point out that terminally ill people often reduce their intake of food and fluids as death approaches; that people who are only hours or a few days away from death may suffer more if they are tube fed because the additional fluids can cause nausea, vomiting, abdominal pain, and pulmonary secretions that lead to gagging and choking; and that withholding or withdrawing tube feeding may improve the quality of the patient's last hours or days (Billings 1985; Zerwekh 1983). Ice chips, small amounts of water, or Vaseline (petrolatum) and a room humidifier are recommended to alleviate any discomfort due to thirst or dry mouth.

Although these articles specifically address the treatment of terminally ill patients who are expected to die imminently with or without treatment, they are sometimes cited to justify the same approach for dementia patients who are not known to be terminally ill. Yet virtually nothing is known about the effects of withholding or withdrawing tube feeding and the course of dying without this treatment for patients for whom death is not imminent. On the one hand, clinicians point out that some patients live a long time after tube feeding has been withdrawn and that malnutrition increases their susceptibility to infections and can cause deep decubitus ulcers that can be painful for the patient and demoralizing for caregivers (Mehr 1984; Pinchcofsky-Devin and Kaminski 1986). In addition, it is not known to what extent severely demented patients experience hunger and thirst.

On the other hand, demented patients may suffer as a result of tube feeding. Confused patients frequently try to and often succeed in pulling out feeding tubes. Some people believe that many of these patients are too confused to notice the tube and that pulling at it is just restless, meaningless behavior that is characteristic of some dementia patients. Others believe that confused patients try to pull out their feeding tubes because the tubes are irritating. Still others believe that some patients who try to pull out their feeding tubes may be expressing a preference to die. Clearly, a severely demented patient cannot indicate which of these interpretations is correct.

A further confounding factor is that confused patients who try to pull out their feeding tubes are frequently physically restrained; their hands are put in mittens and tied to the sides of their beds or chairs. How can caregivers determine how a severely confused person experiences being physically restrained for prolonged periods? And how should they factor this additional consideration into the decision about whether to tube-feed the patient?

With so many unknowns, caregivers must continue to proceed

cautiously in decisions to withhold or withdraw tube feeding from dementia patients who are not expected to die imminently with or without treatment. More research is needed on the relationship of eating disorders and dementia and on the impact of alternate treatment approaches for these patients.

One important clinical question is the relative merits of different types of feeding tubes for dementia patients. Many physicians believe that gastrostomy tubes (placed through the abdomen into the stomach), pharyngostomy tubes (placed through the neck, down the esophagus, and into the stomach), and jejunostomy tubes (placed through the abdomen into the small intestine) are more comfortable for long-term use than nasogastric tubes (placed through the nose, down the esophagus, and into the stomach) and that confused patients are less likely to pull out the former types of feeding tubes (Bucklin and Gilsdorf 1985; Lynn and Childress 1983; Major 1986; Meehan et al. 1985; Sriram and Pulac 1984). Gastrostomy, pharyngostomy, and jejunostomy tubes are used far less often than nasogastric tubes, however. This is partly because they are considered "invasive" by many health professionals because they require at least minimal surgery for insertion; nasogastric tubes do not require surgery and are considered "noninvasive" (U.S. Congress 1987a).

Because nasogastric tubes do not require surgery, many hospitals and nursing homes do not require formal informed consent from the patient or the patient's representative for their insertion. In contrast, health care facilities usually require formal informed consent for the insertion of gastrostomy, pharyngostomy, and jejunostomy tubes. Dementia patients are frequently incapable of giving formal informed consent for treatment, and many dementia patients do not have a formally designated surrogate decision maker. Ancedotal evidence suggests that, for such patients, a physician's choice to use a nasogastric tube rather than one of the other types of feeding tubes may reflect real or perceived difficulties in obtaining formal informed consent rather than a decision that a nasogastric tube is the best or most appropriate feeding method. Each type of tube presents certain risks, and research is needed to compare their risks and benefits in different patient situations. Moreover, changes are needed in institutional policies for informed consent so that these policies do not discourage the use of the most appropriate treatment (U.S. Congress 1987a).

Conclusion

This chapter has raised questions about good clinical care for people in the last stages of dementia. It has proposed that some of the commonly accepted descriptions of what patients are like in those stages are not uniformly applicable, that caregiver expectations and related treatment practices may determine patient functioning more than is generally realized, and that good care requires caregivers to consider reversible and treatable causes of functional deficits even in the last stages of a patient's illness. In addition, it is clear that uncertainty about when a dementia patient is terminally ill, about what constitutes comfort care for a dementia patient, and about how to determine a patient's treatment preferences makes it difficult to apply some of the widely accepted principles for making decisions about life-sustaining medical treatments.

A very important aspect of caring for people in the last stages of dementia that has not been addressed is treatment of the family. Chapter 8 discusses the care of the family in detail, and many of the points made in that chapter are as relevant to the care of families of patients in the last stages of dementia as to the care of families of patients in any other stage.

By the last stages of dementia, some family members may have detached from the patient emotionally and started new lives. Other family members may have grown closer to the patient than at any previous time. Most are somewhere in between. For each family member, the experience of the last stage of dementia and the death of the patient is unique—determined by a complex set of interacting factors, including the past and present characteristics of the patient; the history and emotional quality of the relationship between the patient and the family member; the characteristics, defenses, and coping skills of the family member; and the type and quality of care that the patient receives from formal caregivers. Formal caregivers should try to understand how a family member is experiencing this very difficult period and should refrain from unthinking judgments about family members who appear emotionally distant and "don't seem to care" or, alternatively, appear overly involved and "don't seem to have anything else going in their lives." All of these family members deserve support and understanding, not criticism.

Finally, changes in some policies and procedures of health and long-term care facilities that treat dementia patients could create an institutional environment in which patients in the last stages of dementia would be more likely to receive good care. Full discussion of these changes is beyond the scope of this chapter; they are mentioned here only to give a more comprehensive picture of the components of good care for these patients.

Many experts have emphasized the need to involve family members in decisions about withholding or withdrawing life-sustaining treatments for dementia patients (Besdine 1983; Cranford and Ashley 1986; Lynn 1986; Volicer 1986; Volicer et al. 1986; Winograd and Jarvik 1986). Families should be involved in decisions both about the overall goals of treatment and about specific treatments. As dementia patients frequently live in a long-term care facility for a prolonged period, there is often time for the staff and the patient's family to develop a relationship in which these difficult issues can be discussed openly. This important aspect of good care should not be left to chance, however. Health and long-term care facilities should develop formal policies and procedures for involving families in the decision-making process.

Patients should also be involved in treatment decisions if they are capable of participating. Unfortunately, when they are admitted to a long-term care facility, many dementia patients are already too confused to participate in treatment decisions. Nevertheless, institutional policies for decision making should specifically address the procedures that will be used to assess a patient's decision-making capacity and to ascertain a patient's treatment preferences directly, if that is possible. Such policies should also define procedures for reconciling differences of opinion among staff members about treatment decisions.

As stated earlier, some experts have proposed a hospice approach to the treatment of patients in the last stages of dementia. At present, hospices primarily serve terminally ill cancer patients. For a variety of reasons, few dementia patients are admitted to inpatient hospices: (1) their behavior may be disruptive to the atmosphere or typical routine of the hospice, or the hospice staff and administration may expect that it will be; (2) the inability of a dementia patient to give informed consent for withholding or withdrawal of treatment may be perceived by the staff and administration to increase their legal liability for decisions not to use certain treatments; and (3) uncertainty about how long dementia patients will live may raise concern about the ultimate cost of their care, as inpatient hospice care is more expensive than other forms of long-term care and the Medicare hospice benefit is geared to a six-month life expectancy.

The ideal institutional environment for patients in the last stage of dementia might be a setting based on the hospice concept that the goal of treatment should not necessarily be to prolong life but rather to improve the quality of the patient's life. However, implementation of this concept for dementia patients would require answers to many of the questions raised in this chapter. Most importantly, we need to know what constitutes comfort care for these patients, how the patient's treatment preferences can be determined, and how families and other informal and formal caregivers should be involved in setting treatment goals and making specific treatment decisions for these patients.

References

American Medical Association. 1986. *Public opinion on health care issues—1986.* Chicago: American Medical Association.

Besdine, R. W. 1983. Decisions to withhold treatment from nursing home residents. *Journal of the American Geriatrics Society* 31 (10): 602–6.

Billings, J. A. 1985. Comfort measures for the terminally ill: Is dehydration painful? *Journal of the American Geriatrics Society* 33 (11): 808–10.

Buchner, B. M., and E. B. Larsen. 1987. Falls and fractures in patients with Alzheimer-type dementia. *Journal of the American Medical Association* 257:1492–95.

Bucklin, D. L., and R. B. Gilsdorf. 1985. Percutaneous needle pharyngostomy. *Journal of Parenteral and Enteral Nutrition* 9 (1): 68–70.

Campion, E. W. 1987. Caring for the patient with Alzheimer's disease (letter to the editor). *Journal of the American Medical Association* 257:1051.

Castell, D. O. 1986. Dysphagia in the elderly. *Journal of the American Geriatrics Society* 34 (3): 248–49.

Cohen, D., G. Kennedy, and C. Eisdorfer. 1984. Phases of change in the patient with Alzheimer's dementia: A conceptual dimension for defining health care management. *Journal of the American Geriatrics Society* 32 (1): 11–15.

Cranford, R. E., and B. Z. Ashley. 1986. Ethical and legal aspects of dementia. *Neurologic Clinics* 4 (2): 479–90.

Heyman, A., W. E. Wilkinson, B. J. Hurwitz, M. J. Helms, C. S. Haynes, C. M. Utley, and L. P. Gwyther. 1987. Early-onset Alzheimer's disease: Clinical predictors of institutionalization and death. *Neurology* 37:980–84.

Hughes, C. P., L. Berg, W. L. Danziger, L. A. Coben, and R. L. Martin. 1982. A new clinical scale for the staging of dementia. *British Journal of Psychiatry* 140:566–70.

In re Conroy 98 N.J., 321, 486 A2d, 1209 (1985).

Lynn, J. 1986. Dying and dementia. *Journal of the American Medical Association* 256:2244–45.

Lynn, J., and J. F. Childress. 1983. Must patients always be given food and water? *Hastings Center Report* 13:17–21.

Major, D. 1986. The medical techniques for providing food and water: Indications and effects. In *By no extraordinary means: The choice to forgo life-sustaining food and water,* ed. J. Lynn, 21–28. Bloomington, IN: Indiana University Press.

Malcolm, A. H. 1984. Many see mercy in ending empty lives. *New York Times* (September 23) 1, 56.

Meehan, S., R. A. B. Wood, and A. Cuschieri. 1985. Fine bore enteral feeding and pulmonary aspiration. *British Medical Journal* 290:73.

Mehr, D. 1984. Feeding the demented elderly (letter to the editor). *New England Journal of Medicine* 311:1383.

Pinchcofsky-Devin, G. D., and M. V. Kaminski. 1986. Correlation of pressure sores and nutritional status. *Journal of the American Geriatrics Society* 34 (6): 435–40.

Rango, N. 1985. The nursing home resident with dementia. *Archives of Internal Medicine* 102:835–41.

Reisberg, B., S. H. Ferris, M. J. deLeon, and T. Crook. 1982. The global deterioration scale for assessment of primary degenerative dementia. *American Journal of Psychiatry* 139:1136–39.

Siebens, H., E. Trupe, A. Siebens, F. Cook, S. Anshen, R. Hanauer, and G. Oster. 1986. Correlates and consequences of eating dependency in institutionalized elderly. *Journal of the American Geriatrics Society* 34 (3): 192–98.

Simmons, K. 1986. Dysphagia management means diagnosis, exercise, re-education. *Journal of the American Medical Association* 255:3209–12.

Sriram, K., and B. Pulac. 1984. Nasogastric feeding in the elderly (letter to the editor). *Journal of the American Medical Association* 252:1682.

U.S. Congress. Office of Technology Assessment. 1987a. *Life-sustaining technologies and the elderly.* Washington, DC: U.S. Government Printing Office. July.

U.S. Congress. Office of Technology Assessment. 1987b. *Losing a million minds: Confronting the tragedy of Alzheimer's disease and other dementias.* Washington, DC: U.S. Government Printing Office. April.

Volicer, L. 1986. Need for hospice approach to treatment of patients with advanced progressive dementia. *Journal of the American Geriatrics Society* 34 (9): 655–58.

Volicer, L., Y. Rheaume, J. Brown, K. Fabiszewski, and R. Brady. 1986. Hospice approach to the treatment of patients with advanced dementia of the Alzheimer type. *Journal of the American Medical Association* 256:2210–13.

Volicer, L., B. Seltzer, J. Karner, and L. Herz. In preparation. Eating difficulties in patients with dementia of the Alzheimer type.

Winograd, C. H., and L. F. Jarvik. 1986. Physician management of the demented patient. *Journal of the American Geriatrics Society* 34 (4): 295–308.

Zerwekh, J. V. 1983. The dehydration question. *Nursing* 13 (1): 47–51.

II   THE FAMILY

8

Clinician and Family: A Partnership for Support

LISA P. GWYTHER, M.S.W.

"She seems like a giant skyscraper whose offices are being vacated one by one."—A daughter-in-law

"The handwriting is on the wall—why do I keep erasing it?"—A daughter

"I miss the mother I always knew, and I miss being my real self with mother."—A daughter

"Help! I'm running out of 'cope.' "—A wife
(Quoted by Lisa P. Gwyther in *Daughters of the Elderly*, 1988.)

"I can handle it—my wife has a mild case."—A husband (This is a composite written by the author.)

"Baby your mother as she babied you, back in your baby days."— Recited by an AD patient, Marie Siegle, who died in February 1987.

"The daily irritations are small, but like the constant dripping of water on a rock, they eat away at my love and patience."—A wife, Lois Ellert, Boulder, Colorado

"The outstanding memory I have is of being abandoned by the institutions I had formerly respected. I am not a nurse, just a human being with no choice in what is happening to me."—A wife (Sommers and Shields, 1987, p. 28)

"The logistics are easier than the planning. I still want to run away or be weak, but I have strength I never knew until I was tested."— A wife, Myrna Doernberg, conference presentation, October 1987

"One of my Grandmas gives me hugs and sends cards in the mail on my birthday . . . And sometimes, 'Just Because.' One of my Grandmas can't remember who I am or what day it is . . . So I give her hugs 'Just Because.' " — Kathleen Siegle

"I keep reading doom and gloom and all this negative talk. The positive side is I've still got her and continue loving her and remember how many wonderful years we had together. I go about doing what's necessary for her comfort. I approach it just as I approached going to work before retiring to be with her." — A husband, Glenn Fulton, North Carolina, letter to *The Caregiver* newsletter of the Duke Family Support Program

"Caregiving is like algebra — an equation with no constants." — A husband (Glenn Kirkland)

Why focus on the family? What's in it for the busy professional? The above family caregivers demanded professional attention. Their commitment to their relatives included a strong need to understand, to make sense of their situations, and to garner professional validation for their heroic efforts. We pay attention to families because they demand it. Families spend much more time with their relatives than professionals do. They have the capacity to effect changes in their relatives that professionals can only guide. Cognitively intact care-givers can remember and follow directions and suggestions. They can recognize and appreciate our efforts. They can learn, draw on experience, and problem solve. They can even share our caseloads by teaching others who follow. Best of all, they can apply our knowledge and experience and recognize and reward our efforts by effecting positive change in their situations. Families are our best measure of accountability — our most reliable indicator of effectiveness. Professional time spent with families is a cost-effective strategy from which everyone, including the patient, benefits. Consider the following encounter in a busy professional's day.

Scene: A Busy Family Practice Physician's Waiting Room

Dr. Peters leaves the examining room after a routine visit with Mr. Smith, a 67-year-old man with a diagnosis of Alzheimer's disease (AD) who cheerfully insists that he's there only at the insistence of a wife who can't tolerate an old husband. As Dr. Peters moves to the next examining room, he notices an agitated Mrs. Smith pacing the waiting room and disturbing others with her chain smoking. Wisely, he invites her into a private room.

Mrs. Smith doesn't wait for an invitation to launch her tirade, "I bet you believe him. Ooh, I feel so mean for saying that. He constantly tells me how much he loves me, but he behaves as no loving husband would. His last CT showed no atrophy—maybe he's just lazy or maybe he's manipulating me. Some days he really can do things right and I swear he understands what's happening. Other days, he knows just how to get me. He'll ask me 20 times if it's time to go. So I rush to finish my housework and the minute we get wherever we're going, he insists on going home. He used to try to help around the house when he saw how painful it was for me to move with my arthritis. Now he doesn't even notice or ask how I'm doing and he even accused me of stealing his jock strap—now why would I do that? If I could just get some rest. I do my housework during the day while he naps. But as soon as I get him in bed at night, he pops up. He constantly rechecks the locks or insists that I come to bed too. This is pointless— he's forgotten how to act like a man. As soon as I join him, he's up searching for the toilet, dressing in four layers to go to his old job, or struggling to have sex. He's very strong and he scares me—sometimes I think he doesn't even know it's me. Maybe he needs a sleeping pill, but I couldn't face turning him into a zombie. Maybe you could give me a sleeping pill?"

Common Themes in Family Encounters

Experienced clinicians recognize the common themes in this vignette. The patient rarely complains about symptoms, and he is generally puzzled or hurt by the family's insistence that something is wrong. The wife describes "good days, bad days scenarios" that are often the hallmark of early dementing illness. She attributes elaborate reasons, like manipulation, to the bad days without recognizing her husband's inability to plan and carry out such manipulation.

The misunderstood caregiver is universal—the patient often looks good in brief encounters, and it's the impatient caregiver in the waiting room who is most likely to draw attention to herself. It is frustrating to have no quantitative or visible disability to blame—somehow, even an abnormal CT scan would make this wife feel vindicated.

Patients become progressively more indifferent or unable to recognize the impact of their behavior or dysfunction on others. When patients are confronted about their uncharacteristic indifference, they frequently respond with hurt or surprise, or, even worse, with pathetic promises to try harder. All of these responses generate guilty feelings in caregivers, who inevitably lose patience with the constant need to repeat.

Dementia patients may love to be on the go or asleep, but short attention spans can preclude time-consuming outings. Time distortions are common; the person may believe that he has been out forever. Patients with dementia attempt to protect their constantly assaulted self-esteem by accusing those closest to them of taking things that they have misplaced. It is much easier for Mr. Smith to believe his jock strap was stolen than to confront his inability to care for his belongings.

Even sedentary activities like thinking will tire dementia patients quickly, and daytime napping leads to nighttime insomnia. Ideas often get stuck in AD patients' heads, and many patients check and recheck locks. It may be scary to be alone in a dark bedroom, removed from visual cues of security, comfort, and companionship. Dementia patients seem to fear abandonment, even briefly, in a world that no longer makes sense. It may be impossible for them to remember how long they have been in bed, and it takes longer for them to go from sleep to a waking state. Many patients jump from bed and act on a dream like going to work. Some men open closet doors to urinate or approach wastebaskets for the same purpose.

With night disorientation, there is a real risk that a man can overpower his more frail or smaller wife. Many spouses of dementia patients live in fear of the patient's viselike grip, particularly if the patient has forgotten appropriate intimate behavior or becomes frustrated and unable to perform. When families are at the end of their ropes, they often look to the physician for a quick fix, whether it's a drug or hospitalization. Neither of these alternatives may be possible or appropriate.

Guidelines for Professional Responses

What can a clinician offer when faced with a family caregiver like Mrs. Smith? There are a number of simple suggestions that will help her cope with her seemingly untenable situation.

First, it is helpful to acknowledge with her that the disease is causing her husband to behave in ways that he wouldn't ordinarily choose. This wife may be embarrassed to have a clinician think that she chose to marry such a man. A wise clinician can help her appreciate that his good days or protestations of love are probably genuine, and his apparent vigor is a tribute to his previous healthy life-style and her excellent care. At the same time, it helps to acknowledge with her what it took to get her husband to the office looking so well.

Dr. Peters can help her understand her husband's feelings. He can explain Mr. Smith's feelings of vulnerability, and how his damaged brain may make it more difficult for him to inhibit primitive defenses. Mr. Smith may be striking out at perceived threats, but that doesn't diminish the seriousness of the impact of his symptoms on his wife's health and well-being. It may, however, help her see the problem in a new, more manageable way. Her role is not entirely to keep these unpredictable outbursts from happening, but to prepare to handle her own reactions. If she can blame the disease, rather than him or herself, she is more likely to handle the symptoms appropriately.

A sensitive clinician can also help her put the patient's symptoms in the perspective of a degenerative or progressive disease. Change is the only certainty with such conditions, and she must prepare for changes in symptoms, some of which will seem easier and some harder as the disease progresses. It helps to acknowledge with her that this is not what they planned for their golden years. She has genuine feelings of anger, guilt, resentment, shame, and fear, which she should be able to express comfortably without attacking her husband. An Alzheimer's support group offers members an opportunity to be heard without long explanations, and the one-to-one linkages that develop in the group context can partially compensate for the caregiver's lost social life.

The clinician may help by pointing out ways for Mrs. Smith to conserve her rapidly waning energy. Many families need the validation or credible authority of a written prescription to take time off, lower housekeeping standards, hire help, or not entertain as frequently. Time off for this woman at scheduled, dependable, and convenient times may be much more supportive than sedation for her or her husband. There is good evidence that her perception of adequate informal support from friends or family will positively affect her well-being (George and Gwyther 1986). If friends or relatives offer to take Mr. Smith out, his wife may feel better supported and better able to tend to her own needs.

Some activities of daily living are more draining than others and should be scheduled at the patient's best time of day. For example, bathing and dressing may become battlegrounds, and it is usually helpful to get through them early and get out of the house for exercise. Exercise may help the person sleep better or avoid excessive daytime napping. The person may respond well to lots of nighttime reassurance, rather than arguments about when she joins him. Warm milk, back rubs, herbal tea, dim lights, soft music, or a chance to sleep in the recliner may all help him to relax and feel more secure. A commode next to the bed may prompt him to use it appropriately, particularly if wastebaskets are removed.

It's helpful to remind this wife that her husband is ill but is still an adult who will feel better if he can feel useful and appreciated in spite of his disability. Many men need to retain a sense of being the head of the household, and their wives must be creative in finding ways to make this happen. Failure-free household tasks for which he is appreciated and thanked will help his self-esteem. For example, some men with dementia are proud to be asked to carry or move heavy objects for their wives. One wife found every opportunity to tell friends and relatives that she depended on her husband for "brute strength."

In spite of a predictable routine, frequent breaks, and lots of reassurance, the patient with dementia may still experience moments of aggression or loss of impulse control. This wife should be encouraged to distract, divert, or head off her husband's outbursts with calm, matter-of-fact responses. Her responses should not further catastrophize the incident. Nothing seems to work better than a suggestion about a trip to get ice cream.

Before Mrs. Smith leaves the office, it's helpful to remind her that it's possible and desirable for them to take time to have fun as a couple or family. Moments of pleasure create memories for other family members that will help them cope with the rough times. Taking pictures, celebrating family events and holidays, making tapes or saving little notes, cards, poetry, or scrapbooks of funny things they said or did help the family regard their time together as meaningful. Some patients retain a sense of humor. Reminding each other of funny things that happened or funny things that were said helps all family members cope better with the more tragic elements of the illness.

What Do We Know About Family Caregivers?

American families are providing more care for more older, chronically impaired relatives than at any time in our history. The average married couple today has more parents than children and spends more years on parent care than child care (Brody 1985). Fuchs said that "demography is destiny" (Fuchs 1983). We know that the fastest-growing population group, those over 75, are at greatest risk of long-term functional impairments like dementing illness (U.S. Congress Office of Technology Assessment 1987). We also know that there is increasing labor force participation of those women most likely to assume caregiving roles—women between 45 and 65—although over one-third of caregivers are elders themselves (Stone et al. 1987). However, the family in late life continues to be a source of strength more often than of pathology.

The average American caregiver is a woman 57 years old caring for her mother or mother-in-law (Stone et al. 1987). Older persons first turn to a spouse, then a daughter, and then a daughter-in-law. Many women care for husbands in a final illness only to become the responsibility of their children when they too require long term assistance. Although caregiving is a normative experience, it can be stressful, particularly for those with competing work, marital, or family responsibilities (Brody 1985). Employed family caregivers, both spouses and adult children, are often forced to quit or reduce work hours, and many report spending thirty-five hours per week in elder care in addition to full-time jobs (Petty and Friss 1987). The corporate costs in poor concentration, distraction, excessive use of the telephone, and absenteeism are leading to corporate caregiver education programs. Caregivers must often juggle competing responsibilities to job, family, elder, friends, and finally themselves. Most families have experience helping each other with short-term disability, but a progressive illness like Alzheimer's disease generally implies a permanent imbalance in the family's normal give and take.

Most families care for their own without identifying with the role of caregiver. Many care from a sense of family solidarity or reciprocity. "She was a good wife and mother," or "he would have done the same for me." They describe their care responsibilities variously as "doing what has to be done" or "what is expected of a daughter or husband." Most families, however, find the role of a primary caregiver necessary, efficient, and desirable. It is possible to have a primary caregiver and achieve an equitable, although not necessarily equal, division of family responsibility.

Research on family care consistently documents heterogeneity among dementia caregivers and care receivers (Gwyther and George 1986). People become more individual with advancing age and experience, and the experience of husbands versus wives and spouse versus adult child caregivers is qualitatively and quantitatively different. "For women, caregiving is an expected duty; for men, it is an unexpected expression of compassion" (Sommers and Shields 1987). In several recent studies of husband and son caregivers, these men reported much less subjective distress and better self-rated health than female caregivers. Sons did less than daughters, particularly in personal care, and their caregiving periods were shorter. There seems to be a distinct division of responsibility based on gender, perhaps because there are social taboos against sons providing personal care.

Many husband caregivers express personal satisfaction with the responsibility. They view it as an opportunity to replace a lost work role or repay a lifetime of spousal nurturing. Some husband caregivers see the new learning involved in caring as a challenge that can engage a lifetime of work experience. Men often report a reliance on old coping strategies like going fishing, drinking, or vigorous activity. Contrary to popular belief, one Duke study of Alzheimer's caregivers found husbands more likely to keep their wives at home longer, perhaps because of gender differences in physical size and strength (Colerick and George 1986). But these husbands also reported more assertive setting of limits, delegating, and taking of shortcuts like eating meals out. Caregiving men report much less subjective stress, although they are more likely than noncaregiver men to use alcohol to cope with stress. Husband caregivers are often reluctant to join support groups, although they may be more likely to join advocacy efforts or to attend professionally led seminars.

With increasing or changing dependency in any family member, feelings intensify and relationships become more complex. Most caregivers report less personal time and privacy. Social and emotional sacrifices may loom larger than financial ones. Balancing time, effort, and emotional commitment to the patient and other family and friends can become problematic.

Many families have idiosyncratic ways of determining who among several children will assume responsibility for a demented parent. Sometimes, these decisions are made at birth, but it is not necessarily the eldest, the only daughter, or the one who stays in town. Sometimes, primary responsibility is rotated among siblings, and sometimes it is assumed by the patient's sibling. Black families may call upon more extended kin, such as nieces, grandchildren, or in-laws, whereas white families are more likely to identify a child or spouse as primary caregiver. Each family member must assess his or her geographic proximity, financial resources, time, other emotional demands, and degree of commitment before assuming a primary or secondary caregiver role. There is good evidence that secondary caregivers or caregivers of nursing home patients can be equally at risk of decrements in well-being, and there is often less community support for these caregivers (Gwyther 1988). Family conflicts often emerge with perceptions of inequity in responsibility.

For many families, the care of an older relative precipitates their first experience with asking each other or outsiders for help. Although only about 20 percent of family caregivers use any formal services, predictors of service usage are emerging. Younger, adult child caregivers are more likely to use services in parent care, particularly those caregivers with higher income and more informal social support. Informal support from secondary family caregivers may link the primary caregiver to available service options. Contrary to popular belief, there will never be a substitution of services for family care, but the demand for caregiver support services and institutional care is destined to increase. Although minorities are underrepresented in more expensive skilled nursing homes, this may represent discrimination in access, lack of financial resources, or cultural taboos against institutions. Minority members tend to be overrepresented in less expensive settings such as rest homes, board and care, and foster care. Many families have trouble deciding what help is needed, how to seek or evaluate that help, or even how to ask each other for help. If their perceptions of the patient's disability and needs differ, conflicts are likely to arise. Helping families accept services that may strengthen their continuing capacity to care is an important professional service. For example, one Duke study found that families using limited in-home respite services had modest benefits in the increased time and satisfaction with social and recreational activities (George 1986). They had some increase in positive moods, and, most important, they developed comfort in using supplementary help. In fact, they used more appropriate community services as a result of this positive experience. This timely use of community services may prolong the family's capacity for preferred home care while enhancing the effectiveness of that care.

Responding to caregiving demands, whether or not it is one's first experience, requires adaptation but does not, ipso facto, lead to stress or family pathology. What is most remarkable in the research literature is the evidence of family solidarity, strength, and resourcefulness in responding to caregiving with so little outside help. Often, it is the helping professions that do the greatest disservice to caregiving families. There are risks in well-intentioned overromanticizing or overpathologizing of people assuming the caregiving role.

The severity of the patient's illness or symptoms rarely determine the extent of caregiver burden. The critical variables in predicting caregiver burden are often gender, residence, and relationship between the primary caregiver and the care receiver (George and Gwyther 1986). The caregiver's perception of the problem and the adequacy of help available from family members have a significant impact on the subjective experience of burden. How much help one gets is not as critical as how dependable or adequate one perceives that help to be. However, there are certain unique aspects of dementing illness that put caregivers at high risk, particularly risk of decrements in mental health, well-being, and time for social, recreational, or leisure activities.

What Is Unique About Family Care for Dementia Patients?

For many families, recognition of the problem and the difficulty of obtaining an adequate evaluation are most problematic. Often the patient is reluctant to see a physician, the physician misses mental status changes, or the changes are too subtle to be quantifiable. There is no diagnostic test, and the early manifestations are often insidious changes in personality, mood, behavior, and function that may be attributed to stress, grief, family problems, or character flaws. Even with an adequate comprehensive evaluation, many families expect the patient to report accurately conclusions that he or she cannot remember or comprehend. The family may be given no help in interpreting the diagnosis in light of their relative's symptoms. Often, the time needed to ask questions and make sense of the explanations taxes the constraints of busy medical practices.

Families of dementia patients also face unique problems in planning. Often patients are unaware, indifferent, or suspicious of those who insist that they are ill. By the time that a working clinical diagnosis emerges, patients are often unable to participate in long-term planning. This can lead to lonely, guilt-inducing, and often conflictual decision making in even the closest family.

The ambiguity of a patient who looks well physically and functions well at times makes it even more difficult for families to convince other relatives or employers that the patient is disabled. The damage to the brain is real, but the fact that the radiological or psychometric evidence of that damage doesn't correlate with the severity of symptoms can cause heartache and confusion for well-meaning families. There is still a stigma attached to mental illness, and community members may be quick to blame the family or the patient's character for symptoms that are associated with psychiatric illness.

Another unique feature of dementing illness is its unpredictable rate and course. The family can only be told that the patient will need more help over time with very routine activities like bathing, eating, toileting, and dressing. Some patients may wander and become aggressive, but others become meek or submissive. Some progress rapidly, and others plateau or linger for years in relatively helpless conditions. Accidents and other illnesses may intervene. This means that it is difficult for families to plan. Many families are reluctant to spend money on outside help or services because they don't know if financial resources are sufficient for eventual long-term care. If they do seek outside help, many are disappointed to find that services aren't designed for or accepting of their relatives. In group situations, patients with dementia are often frustrated or demeaned by higher-functioning, physically frail clients. There is no reimbursement system to help families cover the personal care costs of dementing illness, whether at home or in the nursing home. Often, desired services are unevenly available or inequitably distributed, particularly in rural, suburban, or poorer areas.

Throughout dementing illness, the patient may have questionable competency and frequent insightful or lucid moments. The ambiguity, unpredictability, and variability among patients and even in the same patient over time create unique hardships for families seeking professional guidelines or for those eager to do "what is right for Momma." For the professional faced with the family of a person with dementia, it is helpful to start with some assumptions about family care.

Dementia care involves a number of common decision points or dilemmas for families. These include recognizing the problem or seeking help, deciding how much to tell whom, taking away responsibility for driving or handling money, taking on the patient's household roles, preliminary grieving over loss of intimacy or recognition, providing personal care to a previously dignified spouse or parent, deciding to bring help into the home, deciding that the patient cannot safely be left alone, and making a range of terminal care and life-sustaining technology decisions. If families have a knowledgeable primary care physician, access to information about normal aging and the effects of dementing illness, linkage to support groups and information from the Alzheimer's Association, and a supportive community, they are better prepared for long-term care.

Assumptions About Family Care

The caregiving family is alternately ignored, glorified, declared a clinical crisis, or treated as something fragile, natural, and therefore off-limits to professional tampering. All of these exaggerated responses do a disservice to families and to professionals concerned about serving them. It is helpful to remind ourselves and the families we serve of the following:

1. A family facing care for a demented elder has a problem in living. The family, in and of itself, is not necessarily the problem.

2. Given the heterogeneity of families affected by dementia, there is no one right way to care. Dementia patients respond positively to a variety of approaches.

3. There is also no one right place for a dementia patient to live or to receive care. Many families fear that social workers were put on this earth to put everyone in nursing homes or that doctors are here to remind them that the best place for sick people is at home. No good case can be made for either naive assumption.

4. There are no perfect saints or martyrs. Most people lose patience with a demented relative at some time. There are few persons whose sole aim in life is to martyr themselves for another. There is much less neurotic rescuing or manipulation than there is unmet realistic dependency needs of dementia patients. There is more underreporting of burden and underutilization of helping services than the reverse.

5. There is probably no perfectly fair, equal division of caregiving responsibility. Caregiving in a degenerative illness implies a perma-

nent imbalance in the normal give and take of family relationships. That does not mean that more equitable sharing of family responsibility is not a desirable goal.

6. There are no bad defense mechanisms. There are only defenses that don't work for the individual in a given circumstance. Family members may pejoratively accuse each other of denial. Some people need to deny the inevitable outcome to provide hopeful, consistent care on a daily basis.

7. There is no perfect control in a dementia caregiving situation. Even in the safest, most stimulating, and most reassuring environments and with the most informed, nurturing providers, some behavioral disturbances are inevitable. Rather than work on achieving perfect control of all possible situations, caregivers are better advised to work on their reactions to stressful situations, particularly those situations most detrimental to their mental health and capacity to function. Even in ideal care situations, contingency plans are necessary and wise.

8. Although a primary caregiver, particularly at home, is efficient and preferred, no one can do it alone. Primary caregivers need breaks, backup people, and services to supplement their individualized care.

9. Few incentives (financial, religious, or cheerleading) will make an unwilling family assume care for a demented relative. The corollary is that few, if any, disincentives will keep a determined family from honoring their commitment to care. Many children are shocked and saddened to realize that their well parent is prepared to risk his health and well-being to provide care. These adult children may react with anger and sadness to the risk of losing both parents to one's illness, but few are successful in opposing the competent parent's wishes.

10. Many families can mobilize easily for acute short-term illness or disability. Different coping strategies are required for a long-term, progressive illness. The critical variable in coping with a dementing illness is often the family's flexibility in modifying and adjusting expectations of themselves and the patient to fit realistic dependency needs and limits of family capacity.

11. Successful coping with dementia care usually involves a combination of strategies to change what can be changed and palliative strategies directed toward coping with one's reactions. Information gathering, direct action, and intrapsychic tricks are particularly successful. Intrapsychic strategies often involve cognitive restructuring. ("My husband is difficult but not nearly as difficult as the relatives of

others in my support group," or "I look on the bright side—tomorrow will be better.")

12. Most successful caregivers sum up their coping strategies with some combination of a sense of humor, a strong religious faith or belief system, ingenuity, practical problem solving, and the support of friends. A strong religious faith often provides explanations for the unknowable and a promise of future rewards. A church community or a group with similar beliefs can function as a support group. Religious or group rituals may provide a time-out or a reassuring break just like that provided by meditation or progressive relaxation. In recent Hopkins studies of caregiver coping, strong religious faith and the support of friends were most predictive of adaptive outcomes (Rabins 1987).

13. A family's knowledge of an available service, need for that service, and even desire for that service do not necessarily lead to appropriate or timely utilization. Service requests often do not correlate with need or professional prescription, and in general families use many fewer services than professionals would recommend for them (Stone et al. 1987).

What Do Families of Memory-Impaired Patients Want?

Families differ in their expectations of professionals based on age, education, socioeconomic status, and cultural, religious, racial, and ethnic background. For example, younger adult caregivers responsible for widowed parents are more likely to seek and use professional services. Sometimes, expectations are tied to previous experience or culture. Some families are insulted if their relative is not seen by several consultants and subspecialists in the context of an evaluation. Others are put off by bills from subspecialists whom they never see, believing that their contract was with the primary physician. In general, most families of dementia patients express the following criteria for evaluating services:

1. They want active treatment, in spite of their relatives' poor prognosis for recovery. That treatment includes both medical and social support services to enhance functioning and quality of life. Families want to learn how to become more effective and competent in providing care. Their enhanced confidence in the quality of their care may buffer the negative consequences or burden of caregiving.

2. They want expert skilled staff, not necessarily specialists, but

persons knowledgeable about the demands posed by their relatives and the resources available to meet their needs. They appreciate professionals who do not require long explanations about why the patients cannot respond to questions on their own, and they want professionals who have experience with a variety of practical approaches to symptom management. Ironically, some of the most respected care providers are those hands-on helpers with minimal formal training. These people can become expert in what works with specific patients or with your family—in essence, "a specialist in you." Many families learn through trial and error that the patient and family feel more secure with some care providers based on their age, gender, race, body build, philosophy, or disposition. These unrelated characteristics may remind the patient or family of another trusted helper.

3. Families want validation from professionals that they are doing the best they can in an often untenable situation. They want professionals to acknowledge their personal loss without becoming as overwhelmed and helpless as the family may be.

4. Families want reassurance, primarily reassurance of continuity. As their relatives deteriorate, they want established relationships with trusted professionals.

5. They want information to make sense of their experience and to provide some avenues for creative problem solving.

6. Families want to retain control of their situations and their relatives' care. Families generally ask professionals for guidance, information, suggestions, and validation of their decisions, but most families are reluctant to turn over responsibility for a beloved relative to an objective professional. Families often ask for support or advice in making difficult, lonely decisions, but they prefer to reserve the right to take or leave the professional's suggestions or to change their minds.

7. It is helpful to remind families that there is no perfect love or security. Time forces changes in deathbed promises, even with the best of intentions. Illness and dependency do not necessarily make people grateful or lovable, but even dementia patients appreciate opportunities to give back to those who care for them. One man said that he never would have had the opportunity to hear his father say he loved him if he hadn't assumed some responsibility for his father's personal care.

8. Families want more choices in services and payment options. No ideal services, housing options, or reimbursement options meet

all the needs of such a diverse population. Many families become frustrated because there are no choices in where to look for help or how to pay for it. There are policy-induced inequities in access, distribution, quality, and cost of services, which have become the major thrust of Alzheimer's Association advocacy efforts.

What Do Families Expect or Want from Individual Providers?

Again, families differ in their expectations. For many families, the only acceptable provider is a physician, even when they need information about services unfamiliar to most physicians. Some families will accept help only from ministers or religious leaders. Others prefer to rely totally on friends, relatives, or co-workers. In general, however, families state both personal and knowledge- or skill-based criteria for helping professionals.

Personal Characteristics

Families want professionals whose sustained availability is assured. They want professionals who are flexible, tolerant, and willing to take a fresh look at a familiar situation. Each family has idiosyncratic limits, and these limits must be respected. Families further appreciate professionals who are creative and practical in suggesting alternative problem-solving approaches. Professionals familiar with Alzheimer's support groups learn firsthand that there are many ways to cope with a familiar problem like taking away the car keys. A professional familiar with the family's limits or idiosyncracies can suggest several equally viable alternatives consistent with the family's values and beliefs.

Creativity is important here. A reasonably successful care plan for a lawyer who insisted on going to the office rather than an adult day center meant encouraging the family to keep employing the lawyer's secretary to screen calls and keep him busy with mail. Families also appreciate professionals who retain a sense of humor. Laughing with a family breaks down some barriers and helps keep them from becoming overwhelmed and immobilized by the hopelessness of their situation. Finally, families appreciate professionals who have nurtured excellent working relations with other relevant service agencies or professionals. A physician who has a dentist friend willing to see her most agitated dementia patients is in a much better position to assist that patient's family. A social worker who volunteers to train adult day center staff about Alzheimer's disease is more likely to help his dementia client and family with a successful referral.

Knowledge and Skill Base

Families want knowledgeable, skilled providers. They want physicians, nurses, and social workers to understand not only dementia but also the principles of geriatric medicine. Dementia patients may deteriorate rapidly with the onset of an infection. Symptoms of an infection like pneumonia may be atypical. Responsible providers must know more than dementia and its effects to assist both patients and their family caregivers.

Families rank information and interpretation high on their lists of needs. They want written materials and explanations individualized to fit their situations, brief to fit available time, and repeated often until they can integrate it. Much of this repetitive learning takes place in support groups, but a professional's teaching and translation skills become critical in clinical work with families. Many families misinterpret public awareness messages in frightening ways. A professional must be able to pick up distortions, find the source, and help families correct these distortions in dignified ways. For example, one executive read an article on "preventing senility" and immediately assumed that he was responsible for his wife's dementia. He concluded that the demands of his business life on his wife kept her from mental jogging or reading current events. Gentle reminders of what is known and not known about the etiology of dementia relieved him enough to have him care for her with less anxiety.

Crisis intervention skills are critical in work with dementia families. Most families do not request professional assistance until there is a family crisis—an incident of wandering, a patient losing his job, a family caregiver's acute illness. At a time like that, it is difficult to do a comprehensive family assessment or even to get all family members together in one room. Professionals who are skilled in telephone counseling or hotline work have a distinct advantage in engaging families in therapeutic relationships once the crisis is temporarily resolved.

Creative family counseling skills are also invaluable. Many families have never come together to make decisions like those necessary for dementia care. Engaging and supporting family strength, cohesion, and capacity are critical to the success of family counseling. Most families accept counseling better in the context of an interpretive session or a session on managing problematic symptoms. The focus on the identified patient helps individual family members come to terms with their own reactions and needs. It takes skill and experience to know when and how to include or exclude the patient without exaggerating the patient's fears or suspiciousness.

Finally, clinicians skilled and knowledgeable about grief and bereavement are well prepared to work with families of dementia patients. This degenerative disease, with its attendant insidious loss of the person as he or she was, inevitably leads to prolonged anticipatory grief. "It is so different with the slow agonizing piece-by-piece loss of the mother I knew and loved." Society does not provide families with appropriate mechanisms or rituals for grieving in anticipation. This preliminary grief does not, however, minimize the impact of death or the need for grief work or bereavement at the time of death. Professionals are urged to adapt hospice materials on grief and bereavement (Ballard 1989). They are excellent guides, although the patient dying of cancer may be more involved in aspects of grief work than a patient with dementia.

Many clinicians mistake appropriate preliminary grief reactions for clinical depression in Alzheimer's caregivers. In these situations, supportive counseling and education are more effective than medications with all their attendant side effects.

What Types of Services Are Needed over Time for Dementia Families?

A service chronology is a helpful memory jogger for professionals working with Alzheimer's families. Not all families come in at the beginning of an illness, and these services are often needed simultaneously or not specifically in this order. The listing is offered just to remind providers of generic service needed:

- Diagnostic services/functional assessment of patient's and caregiver's abilities and disabilities.
- Interpretive session for patient and family together or separately.
- Primary medical care: Establishing a primary physician to monitor both patient and caregiver over time and to manage acute and chronic illnesses.
- Acute hospital/emergency room care: This is necessary for both patients and caregivers. Planning in selecting a physician with privileges at the hospital of choice is well worth the investment.

Hospital emergency room staff and inpatient staff may be ignorant of the characteristics of dementia patients and their special language and behavioral problems.

- Information/referral services: Most communities have telephone information services through county health departments, councils on aging, or Alzheimer's Association Helplines. Many states have toll-free access to listings of state service providers and available nursing home beds, although the quality, comprehensiveness, and timeliness of these listings may vary.

Counseling Services

Counseling services are available on a peer or voluntary basis through Alzheimer's chapters or support groups. Traditional family, marital, or individual counselors must be familiar with dementing illness, especially its potential effects on caregiver well-being, personal time, mental health, stress symptoms, and family conflict. Experienced counselors recognize that caregivers run risks similar to those encountered by Type A personalities. Often the most harmful effects of Type A personality patterns are due to the person's distrust of the environment or of people. Type A people are forced to be hyperalert and hypervigilant and believe that they must plan ahead constantly to avoid disaster. Dementia caregivers must often think and plan for two and be hyperalert or vigilant in anticipating or heading off the unpredictable behavioral outcomes of their relatives' poor judgment. The cardiotoxic effects of this stressful full-time responsibility are only beginning to be explored.

Professional counselors must often address a family's barriers to the use of needed services. These barriers include cost, but it is more likely that the fear of future costs rather than the present service cost will keep a family from accepting timely service recommendations. Some families question the training of the providers, the convenience of the service, or the stigmatizing effects of the bureaucratic red tape associated with eligibility determinations. The Alzheimer's Association's Social Security Disability Log helps families frame their problems and needs in a helpful way. Some families just distrust strangers, especially families who fear that no one will have the personal investment that they have. There are rural/urban and cultural differences in the acceptability of various services or providers. Sometimes, the only available service option is too intense or at an inappropriate level for the patient. In reviewing services, it is helpful for the counselor and family to assess whether they are:

available (waiting list?);

appropriate (timely, level of care fits patient);

acceptable (meet family's criteria);

accessible (transportation and/or escort);

coordinated (provider will work with other professionals serving this family);

convenient (if it takes too much energy to get there, family will decline service);

dependable (there are too many other unpredictable issues in care—real help must be available as scheduled);

dignified (patient and family are treated as adults entitled to appropriate services);

equitable;

flexible (meet changing needs of patient and family);

family centered;

professionally directed;

safe and secure.

Mutual Support Self-Help Groups

These groups are an invaluable complement and supplement to professional or formal services. It is generally assumed that participants in these groups gain information, outlets for advocacy, coping models, and emotional support. Studies at Duke document that participants in support groups know more about dementia and more about available services, and, indeed, participants feel less lonely and better understood and supported than nonparticipants (George and Gwyther 1988). Interestingly, that knowledge among participants about the illness and services did not differentiate them from nonparticipants in their appropriate use of those services.

The focus of most groups is on mutual helping and strengthening, not "misery loves company." Often the group functions as a new extended family or a replacement society generating self-respect and self-confidence in members who recognize, in helping others, their success in coping. Caregivers have learned how to problem solve by gathering information, listening to experienced friends, and seeking models as well as professional expertise. All of these coping strategies are possible in the context of open-ended support/educational groups.

The emphasis is on keeping the group small, informal, local, immediate, and practical. The group gives individualized helping without the stigma of weakness or a dependent client status. The knowledge gained from support groups is personalized, nontechnical, and generally unavailable in libraries. Much of the shared wisdom is based on intuition, experience, spontaneous authenticity, and common sense. There is an absence of professional jargon and an emphasis on a variety of communication strategies including telephone, social visits outside the group, newsletters, and letters.

Many groups affiliate with a credible organization like the Alzheimer's Association or a health institution to legitimize and support their activities. The access to reliable information adds to the value of the group's activities. Groups that affiliate with national caregiver organizations gain advocacy outlets for their frustration and advance the dignity and public awareness of the critical role of family caregiver. The group generally decides where, when, and how often they want to meet. Consistency or dependability of time and place are more salient than when and where the meetings are held.

Support groups can function as a vocal constituency and ally to professional services. Many professionals believe that participation in a support group helps potential clients use professional services more appropriately. Support groups are responsive to current criticism of formal services, but Alzheimer's support groups are not antiprofessional. The intimacy and size of a support group can be an antidote to bureaucratic or costly, depersonalized services, which may be viewed as ineffective, overly regulated, or poorly accountable. Support groups are particularly effective for those who fear the dependency of client status or those who respond with greater energy to involved consumer roles. Many families recognize their needs for support as a bottomless pit and realistically assess the limits of professional time and availability. At a minimum, families respond positively to the presence of caregiver models of self-confidence, perspective, and hope.

The focus of mutual support groups is on adaptation and social reinforcement of positive coping. The group context is a safe environment in which to experiment with coping. Support group members are particularly knowledgeable and effective in suggesting hints for successful travel, holiday celebrations, or ways to handle the conflicting perceptions of out-of-town relatives. Cognitive restructuring is practiced when support group members remind themselves that forgetting is sometimes a blessing. The support group can be a source of new, more appropriate behavioral norms or ways to define one's identity. The graphic openness among members can be cathartic and an antidote to the isolation of caregiving. Alzheimer's support groups developed a Caregiver's Bill of Rights (see the sample at the end of this chapter), a uniquely empowering strategy to teach family caregivers that it is moral and ethical to consider their own needs. The rituals, traditions, individual recognitions, and fellowship provided in groups compensates for activities lost to the demands of caregiving.

Support groups offer caregivers an opportunity to rediscover a sense of community, in this case, a community of persons affected by dementing illness in a relative. This doesn't mean that natural support groups, like church circles, wives' club, carpools, or study groups cannot meet the informal support needs of family caregivers. In fact, some experts believe that the underrepresentation of minorities in mutual support/self-help organizations may indicate their greater reliance on more traditional informal support from churches, social organizations, or extended family. For many families, there is enough emotional support available within their existing informal networks. They turn to support groups for information and validation.

Most groups focus on learning skills that help caregivers regain a sense of control. The new peer group can become a social outlet, while it normalizes or universalizes the caregiver's feelings or experience. Families eventually come together to celebrate their strengths and survivorship. The groups provide a safe outlet for the intense feelings of guilt, anger, shame, and doubt that easily overwhelm the most committed caregivers. Often the relationships that develop among or between group members become a life preserver for isolated family caregivers.

Most groups develop an ideology, promote charismatic leaders as spokespersons, and articulate a value system that dignifies not only dementing illness but also family commitment to care. Meeting rituals like introductions, confessions, testimonials, evangelism, or absolution provide a variety of avenues for a diverse membership to find solace and strength. Families attending a group for the first time are often patient-focused—they want to achieve some adaptive competence, which often occurs through the progressive reciprocal strengthening of self-help organizations. Most committed families are pleased to learn that they are not pariahs in their desire to help their relative, and many are pleased to find a variety of altruistic outlets. Whether they help other group members, write their stories, talk to community groups, or donate to or participate in research, all recognize that meeting their altruistic needs helps them summarize, draw meaning, and survive intact.

One daughter summed up her family's experience with an Alzheimer's support group with the following lessons:

1. We made it this far. We wouldn't have believed we would make it through intact.
2. We're a closer family and appreciate each other more because we've been there for each other.
3. We should not take our life and health for granted.
4. We should not place our happiness in the hands of others.
5. We should enjoy and make the most of each day.
6. We must appreciate the little things in our lives.
7. We have grown in our understanding of others facing difficult situations.
8. We have some satisfaction that we have helped others.
9. We have had the opportunity to meet the most special, caring and wonderful people.

Diane Wilkins, Des Moines, Iowa

Another caregiving daughter learned these important rules in the context of a support group.

1. Accept help when it is offered. Your patient will be none the worse and you will replenish your energy and patience.
2. Don't be afraid to ask family or friends to keep you company if you can't get out.
3. Don't expect to accomplish all the things you did before.
4. Tune out objectionable parts of your relative's behavior. Leave the room and return when you're calmer.
5. Don't hate yourself if you should yell. The patient will forget, and your pent-up emotions need release.
6. Be sure to rest.
7. Keep your outside social contacts.
8. Remember you are entitled to pleasurable times, and little treats help you through the day.
9. It is OK to be upset with your situation. Your patient will get worse no matter what you do or how well you do it.
10. Join a support group.

11. Make a list of things you would like to do, and do at least one each week.

Ruth Rabyne, Chicago, Illinois

Self-help groups are based on a common problem in living that tends to break down all conventional barriers between people. Coming together empowers members who already are intensely involved and personally affected by their problem. They identify rather than empathize with each other, and they see themselves as consumers of services focused on their afflicted relatives. The open nature of most groups permits professionals or family members to observe, join, or align themselves in mutual concern about dementia care. Professionals can assume a variety of roles in relation to support groups. Ethical considerations must be respected, however, in exploiting the membership for practice-building motives.

Professional collaboration with support groups helps members redefine their problem in less pathologic terms, particularly if the professional has few preconceived assumptions about support group members' individual problems. Professionals can augment the group just by the value they attribute to the group's activities. Members become more secure when they feel supported and respected by collaborating or facilitating professionals. Professionals involved in support groups can help link individual members for support and assistance. The professional can function as educator, emphasizing the curative factors of the group such as universalization, inspiration, and hope. The professional can help members recall their precrisis success or identity and can reinforce their efforts to strengthen their coping skills or morale. The professional can also be sensitive to member fatigue and the need for respite. Family participants may appreciate a professional's reminder that there is often as much to be gained from a walk around the mall as from a support group meeting.

Professionals in both clinical and support group contexts help caregivers make sense of or take meaning from their experience. In the group context, a professional might point out the expectable regularities of reactions like puzzlement, uncertainty, or shame. Pointing out the role of humor in relieving group tensions may easily generalize to caregiving coping strategies outside the group. Professional giving or nurturing, even as concrete as helping with refreshments, helps replenish overextended caregivers. For a more explicit delineation between clinical and mutual support helping, see Table 8.1.

Respite Strategies

Once the patient cannot safely be left alone or when a patient becomes a caregiver's shadow because of clinging or dependency, it is time to consider respite options. Respite means time out or a break from the hyperalert vigilance involved in thinking for oneself and the patient. However, people define what's restful or relaxing in diverse ways. For some, it's an opportunity to be cared for by the household help; for others, it's a bridge game, a golf game, a chance to shop or visit unencumbered by the demands of a restless patient. Professionals should be sensitive to respite needs as well as the caregiver's criteria for suitable respite options. Respite can be provided by other family members, friends, or neighbors, in day centers, private homes, or residential or institutional settings, or by hiring trained help at home (see Chapter 10). All options may be appropriate over the course of a dementing illness, but there are often significant barriers (personal, familial, and institutional) that can be addressed by clinicians in ways that facilitate appropriate and timely use of services. At a minimum, a clinician should probe for potential personal barriers to taking breaks and help family caregivers review the costs and benefits objectively and subjectively. A glib suggestion to use the only available respite service in a community rarely leads to a completed referral.

Terminal Care Options

Most dementia patients survive to require some kind of terminal care, although even those families caring for the most terminal patients may report that the patient's death was unexpected (George 1984). Most private homes, with the competing professional and family demands on the caregiver's time, don't provide the economies of scale or the professional nursing for full-time terminal care. Yet more and more families are choosing to care at home, using a hospicelike approach, even after a period of nursing home placement. The professional should not assume that terminal care is necessarily more burdensome on the family. Families appreciate professionals who are familiar with the options and consequences of various care settings, but who support the family's wishes. Sometimes, a family feels better about trying terminal care at home before accepting the inevitability of placement.

TABLE 8.1 A Comparison of Helping Strategies

Mutual Support Group Helping	Clinical Helping
1. Focus on "afflicted"	Focus on "affliction"
2. Informal interaction between equals	Formal relationship between unequals
3. Helper is independent	Helper represents agency, profession
4. Helper is untrained, unsupervised, unpaid and has a subjective view	Helper is trained, supervised, paid, with objective view
5. Helper is unconditionally available	Helper has schedule of limited availability
6. Helper has no limits on numbers helped or limits on helping	Helper serves limited number of clients with agency or profession limiting
7. Helper keeps no records	Helper keeps records
8. Helper has authenticity of common life experience	Helper may have different life experience
9. Helper as role model, relationship based on identification	Helper develops empathy
10. Helping is "progressive reciprocal strengthening"	Helping occurs in nonreciprocal relationship
11. Helper expects to give and receive concrete and emotional help	Helper doesn't expect help and doesn't usually offer *both* concrete and emotional help
12. Helper is active, judgmental, supportive, critical, and talks subjectively	Helper is nonjudgmental, planned and listens objectively
13. Helper works at gut level—intuition, experience, common sense	Helper may work at more cognitive level
14. Helper emphasizes faith, willpower, self-mastery, appropriate behavior	Helper emphasizes insight, cognitive understanding, "symptom substitution"
15. Emphasis on day-to-day management	Emphasis on long term care
16. Helper has identifiable code of beliefs, practices, rules	Helper is nondirective re values, beliefs
17. Disclosures are shared with group, media	Disclosures are secret
18. Communication occurs through newsletters, letters, phone, and face-to-face	Helping occurs almost entirely face-to-face

Placement does not preclude the family's individualized contribution to the patient's care. Research consistently documents that families do not abandon demented relatives to nursing homes. There are losses and gains with all terminal care settings which are worth pointing out to families. Most families appreciate something to read on this issue, and the chapter on nursing home care in *Understanding Alzheimer's Disease* (Gwyther 1988) or *When Love Gets Tough: The Nursing Home Decision* (Manning 1983) may be helpful family reading.

Altruistic Outlets

Most families who commit five to twenty years of their lives to the care of a demented relative want to believe that the effort was worthwhile in spite of the inevitable death of their loved one. The family often recovers to the extent that they have altruistic outlets for their pain. Professionals must be sensitive to family needs, particularly in bereavement, to summarize and draw meaning from their experience. The family may appreciate a professional's suggestion or support for their reinvolvement with a support group or suggestions that the bereaved members use their teaching or public speaking skills to enhance public awareness. Other families may be encouraged to participate in or donate to research or to use their creativity in writing or art, leaving a legacy for other affected families and their own children about their experience and its meaning.

Summary: Assessing and Working with Families

Work with families of dementia patients has tremendous potential, but the goals, strategies, timing, settings, and knowledge base for family work must be modified to fit the unique problems posed by dementing illness. Family therapists serving dementia families should be thoroughly familiar with normal aging, dementing illness, and the impact of both on families. Often the first contact with a family is not for therapy, but for an interpretation of what is known about their relative's condition and prognosis. Educational approaches must be individualized. Communication must be adapted to the sensory losses of older family members or the ethnic, cultural, or racial experience of the family. Family sessions are generally less frequent, with more sustained telephone contact and more frequent contact at crisis or decision points. The focus of work with the family is on situational coping rather than correcting long-standing maladaptive family patterns. Sustained professional and family effort is required

to adapt to progressive losses in the patient. There are no ideal solutions for these families, and flexibility and creativity in problem
solving become most salient. The goals in working with the family
are to prevent excess disability in the patient (see Chapters 1 and 2)
and secondary disability in the caregiver(s). Therapeutic strategies
include individualizing information needs, crisis triage (the most troubling symptom approach), reinforcing adaptive coping, purposeful
ventilation and cartharsis, helping families equitably share responsibility, encouraging the use of appropriate formal and informal services, and helping families cope with grief, bereavement, and altruistic
needs.

The family becomes the client for the purposes of assessment,
and service is predicated on supporting and complementing the family's role in care. It is risky to make assumptions about who the family
is and what it can and cannot do. A structured assessment interview
or guide is also helpful, particularly if it includes input from the patient
and relevant family members. Any guide should provide structure
for an assessment interview, address feelings as well as facts about
social support, and organize information about the family in a systematic way.

Assessment should begin with basic demographic information,
especially educational and occupational history. A genogram provides
a pictorial review of the name, age, relationship, health, and frequency
of patient contact or assistance of relevant family members. The presenting problem and its chronicity or management until now, sources
of informal and formal help, and how helpers feel about what and
how much they are doing are all relevant to the assessment. The
combination of the genogram and the structured assessment often
helps the family clarify issues, note changes, and identify potentially
problematic illnesses or situations in the family's history. Often the
assessment helps to clarify relationships and feelings both inter- and
intragenerationally.

Housing and living arrangements are worth investigating. Many
people who presumably live alone have a variety of close-at-hand
relatives, neighbors, or friends who are not acknowledged for their
roles in discreet surveillance or informal support. Often, the problem
is not the dementia patient, but the fact that a spouse caregiver is
also caring for another ill, a retarded, or an alcoholic relative who
lives in the home.

It is a good idea to explore what other family members or friends know about the patient's problem. Some families are secretive and have made pacts not to tell the patient or influential friends or employers. More distant family members may have conflicting views of the patient's disability. If the illness is familial, the family will be influenced by their previous experience with dementia care. It is delicate but relevant to inquire about family difficulties with alcohol, chronic or acute mental illness, prescription drugs, or problems with the law. Most families will volunteer information about how close, distant, or dependent their relationships have been. "Pop will never be able to keep the books the way Mom did—he never went to school."

In summary, assessment and educational strategies may, of necessity, go hand in hand. To review the principles in this chapter, consider the following intentionally condensed encounter:

Scene: A Social Worker at a Memory Disorders Clinic Talks with a Daughter of a Nursing Home Alzheimer's Patient

Daughter: My brother, father, and I reached a stumbling block over my mother's care in the nursing home. She's been there a year now and I think she's given up. We all knew the move would kill her will to live, but with Dad hospitalized with his heart attack, we had no choice at the time.

Social Worker: The choices at that point in care are always equally unappealing. I'm sure if you had your choice, your mother would be well and back the way she was.

Daughter: (weeping) Oh, God, I miss her so much. She would have been so much better as a caregiver than I am—I've been in therapy all my life for agoraphobia. She's the strong one. But with all she's done for me, you'd think I could rally when she needs me. It takes everything I've got to leave my house and visit her regularly. I can't stand to see her this way. But my brother is three hours away and I feel so bad to have my dad there alone so much.

Social Worker: Is visiting the stumbling block you mentioned earlier? What does your dad expect of you?

Daughter: Oh, Dad would never complain about my visits. The problem now is her medicine. Dad thinks she's drugged and tied down so they won't have to watch her. He's fed up with the doctor, and he wants her medicines changed. But I have heard horror stories at the support groups about families who complained and were told to find another placement. She's so ill; I can't stand to see her moved again. My brother wants to charge in there on his white horse and rescue Mom and Dad, but he has no idea what goes on there and how hard we have worked to get the nurses to like us and to treat Mom nice.

Social Worker: Is there one sympathetic staff member there—one who seems to understand your family's feelings about the medicines?

Daughter: Don't get me wrong, she needed those medicines to calm her anxiety when she moved in and they did seem to help, but now she never really fights or screams. She probably doesn't have the strength. Dad just thinks she would be more responsive to him if she wasn't such a zombie. The nurse says it's risky to rock the boat when she's doing well on this regimen. She says dementia patients don't tolerate change well. But my friends in the support group say all nursing homes are self-serving and I should advocate for Mom as a prisoner of the system. I just want to do the right thing and not let my family down any more than I already have.

Social Worker: There is no right way in dementia care. Each patient's situation is different. Needs change and symptoms or problems change as the disease progresses. Your family has a right as her protective kin to represent your mother's wishes. You may certainly question and expect reasonable rather than expedient responses. Does the facility have regular patient care meetings on each patient?

Daughter: As a matter of fact, they do send Dad regular notices and he is invited to attend. He just got some notice about next week, and I think that's what has him riled up again.

Social Worker: Would you be able or up to going with him? This is an excellent opportunity to talk with the staff in a nondistracting environment. Don't accuse or draw conclusions about the staff's motivation. Just state your concerns about your mother's progressive deterioration, her change in problems, and let them know how important it is for all of you to have her respond to your visits. If they are uncertain how to proceed with changes in her care, they are welcome to call one of our consultants for suggestions. Our pharmacist has some excellent materials on medications, but it would be important to review her situation as well. We could send the general information to her physician or the pharmacist at the nursing home.

Try to talk to the staff in a way that you join them or align with them in your mutual concern with her care. Be sure to show your appreciation for what they are doing well or what has been achieved. But, as your mother's representative, be sure you make your wishes and those of your father very clear.

I'm impressed with your family's commitment to her and to each other. That commitment will give you the strength or resolve you need to do it. Please let me know how it all works out. If it's a bust, there are other approaches you can consider.

Daughter: Thanks. I'll try it. Maybe my brother can come too. Somehow it helps just knowing I can come back if it doesn't work. It's been hard dealing with so many people around Mom's care, and so many of them leave before we get to know them.

Be Careful: You Might Learn Something

My husband's condition has deteriorated greatly since I wrote "The Agony of Fear." Now he spends his time hunting for his wife, for he thinks I am his sister who has been dead nine years. Needless to say, my life is spent almost entirely in our home, but I have learned *so* much.

Things I Am Learning (As I Care for My Husband Who Has Alzheimer's Disease)

One of my favorite sayings is, "Be careful; you just might learn something new." I once thought that meant that you could learn from people you met, towns you visited, or places you worked. Now I know that you can learn really important things when your life does a complete U-turn and your priorities have to change.

1. I am learning to be HUMBLE.
   For years I thought the world would stop (or at least slow down a little) when I got off. But it hasn't. Someone else teaches my English classes; someone else has taken over my jobs at church and as a volunteer. That makes me humble.
2. I am learning to be PATIENT.
   I listen to the same old stories and answer the same questions almost twenty-four hours a day. A person with Alzheimer's has no control over his memory, so all the explaining does no good. When I get impatient, we are both in trouble.

3. I am learning to be CALM.
    Our kids call it "being laid back" or "rolling with the punches."
    I know that I can't make everyone I love happy or healthy or
    rich—all the time. So now when something goes wrong, I just
    say to myself, "So what?" This is really not me, but I am trying.
4. I am learning to LAUGH.
    My husband has a great sense of humor, at times. One day when
    he was disgusted that he couldn't remember how to do simple
    tasks, he said, "You can't even trust me to feed the dog." When
    I reminded him that we didn't have a dog, he said, "I know; he
    starved to death." We both had a good laugh over that.
5. I am learning to find JOY—in little things.
    Sometimes it is in a telephone call or a hug from a friend; often
    it is in a new recipe; many times it is just the good country smells
    as I go to the mailbox. Recently it has been the snow and the
    birds at the feeder. There is much to enjoy when you have the
    time.
6. I am learning to be STILL (something I have never been before in
    my life).
    The Psalmist says, "Be still and know that I am God." John Milton,
    in his poem "On His Blindness," says, "They also *serve* who only
    stand and *wait*."

I *hope* I am *serving*. I *know* I am *waiting*. What am I waiting for? I have
no idea! But, in the meantime, I am learning every day.

                          Nancy H. Choate, Morganton, North Carolina

Families of Dementia Patients: A Chronological Approach

S-O-A-P

Subjective:	Families' requests for help phrased in their own words (common requests, complaints used as examples)
Objective:	What the clinician observes about the family/patient's behavior (examples given)
Assessment:	Important areas to summarize and assess before making recommendations
Plan:	What to do with the family at this point

Families of Dementia Patients: A Chronological Approach

Early: **Diagnosis**

S: "How and how much should we tell the patient, employer, others?"

"I'm scared—she seems so withdrawn and indifferent."

O: Family seeks cures and multiple opinions, assigns blame, covers up for patient, or cheerleads for patient to try harder.

A: Premorbid family relationships and personalities

Available informal network—church, neighbors, friends, colleagues, family

Family's previous and concurrent caregiving experiences

P: Explain significance of informant history, testing, function, medications, and concurrent illness

Review rationale for "probable" diagnosis

Offer written materials and refer family to Alzheimer's Association for brochures and books

Correct misconceptions based on what family has read or heard

Prepare family for variation and ambiguities in patient function

Encourage family to inform relevant network discreetly

Prepare family to alter expectations of patient and for necessary role changes

Suggest legal/financial precautions (handling money, durable powers of attorney)

Offer hope, security of sustained availability of professional expertise and interest

Middle: **The Long Haul**

S: Caregiver complains of fear, crushed expectations, helplessness, frustration, anger, guilt, fatigue, grief.

O: Patient's poor judgment leads to safety risks. Patient exhibits behavior, mood, and sleep disorders. Caregiver seems depressed, isolated, and stressed.

A: Caregiver health and family tolerance for stress

Family conflict: differing information or perceptions of patient's disability/ability

Cultural, religious proscriptions/old promises

Available formal and informal support

P: Medical management of patient's most troublesome symptoms: medications for agitation, sleep, etc.

Routine primary care checks on other symptoms, illnesses

Support and validate family efforts to care

Ask about primary caregiver's health, symptoms

Suggest environmental/activity/safety modifications (e.g., help take away car keys!)

Prescribe respite and energy economies

Supportive counseling re family feelings and reactions

Provide additional information as needed

Help family *accept* and evaluate available help

Late: **Terminal Care**

S: "I can't make this decision alone—the devil (doctor) made me do it."

Family expresses feelings of failure, guilt, ambivalence, and grief.

"I feel married and not married at the same time—in a social limbo."

O: Family conflict, preferences, available care options, other commitments

A: Patient and family needs/priorities/competing demands

Losses and gains with institutional care

P: Family conference: use authority and expertise to validate timeliness of placement or terminal care at home

Begin to discuss ethical "what-if's" of terminal care decisions: feeding, infections, hospitalizations, etc.

Recommend facilities that provide good care for dementia victims and that are accessible to regular family visitors and preferred local physician

Help surviving caregiver cope with new free time, separation, future as single person

Help family find altruistic outlets, summarize experience, draw meaning, and say good-bye

Caregivers' Bill of Rights

In as much as WE, THE CAREGIVERS, devote ourselves and our internal and external resources to the maintenance and support of a loved one, we declare that we have basic inalienable rights. Furthermore, we recognize that we are not alone in our challenge to maintain a humane life-style for ourselves and our loved ones: NOW THEREFORE, we pledge our support to all who struggle with balancing the responsibilities of daily living. With this in mind, we mandate the following rights:

The right to live our own life to retain our dignity and sense of self.

The right to choose a plan of caring that accommodates our needs and the needs of those we care about.

The right to be recognized as a vital and stabilizing source within our families.

The right to be free of guilt, anguish, and doubt, knowing that the decisions we make are appropriate for our own well-being and that of our loved one.

The right to love ourselves enough to have the confidence to do the best that we are able.

With these rights, disabled and frail aged persons will be provided the highest and best care that we are capable of giving, and we may take pride in ourselves.

References

Ballard, E. 1989. *Managing grief and bereavement: A guide for families and professionals caring for memory-impaired adults.* Durham, NC: Duke University Center for Aging.

Brody, E. M. 1985. Parent care as a normative stress. *Gerontologist* 25 (1): 19–29.

Colerick, E. J., and L. K. George. 1986. Predictors of institutionalization among caregivers of patients with Alzheimer's disease. *Journal of the American Geriatrics Society* 34 (7): 493–98.

Fuchs, V. R. 1983. *How we live.* Boston: Harvard University Press.

George, L. K. 1984. *The dynamics of caregiver burden: A final report to the AARP Andrus Foundation.* Durham, NC: Duke University Center for Aging.

George, L. K. 1986. Respite care: Evaluating a strategy for easing caregiver burden. *Center Reports on Advances in Research* 10 (2).

George, L. K., and L. P. Gwyther. 1986. Caregiver well-being: A multidimensional examination of family caregivers of demented adults. *Gerontologist* 26 (3): 253–59.

George, L. K., and L. P. Gwyther. 1988. Support groups for caregivers of memory-impaired elderly: Easing caregiver burden. In *Families in transition: Primary prevention programs that work,* ed. L. A. Bond and B. M. Wagner, 309–31. Beverly Hills: Sage Publications.

Gwyther, L. P. 1988. Nursing home care issues. In *Understanding Alzheimer's Disease,* ed. M. K. Aronson, 238–62. New York: Charles Scribner's Sons.

Gwyther, L. P., and L. K. George. 1986. Symposium: Caregivers for dementia patients. Complex determinants of well-being and burden: Introduction. *Gerontologist* 26 (3): 245–47.

Manning, D. 1983. *When love gets tough: The nursing home decision.* Revised. Hereford, TX: In-Sight Books Inc.

Norris, J., ed. 1988. *Daughters of the elderly: Building partnerships in caregiving,* 153–70. Bloomington, IN: Indiana University Press.

Petty, D., and L. Friss. 1987. A balancing act of working and caregiving. *Business and Health* (October) 22–26.

Rabins, P. V. 1987. Psychiatry Department grand rounds. Hopkins study reported at Vanderbilt University, Nashville, TN, April 2, 1987.

Sommers, T., and L. Shields. 1987. *Women take care: The consequences of caregiving in today's society,* 28. Gainesville, FL: Triad Publishing.

Stone, R., G. L. Cafferata, and J. Sangl. 1987. Caregivers of the frail elderly: A national profile. *Gerontologist* 27 (5): 616–26.

U.S. Congress. Office of Technology Assessment. 1987. *Losing a million minds: Confronting the tragedy of Alzheimer's disease and other dementias.* OTA-BA-323. Washington, DC: U.S. Government Printing Office. April.

Suggested Readings

AAHA. *The nursing home and you: Partners in caring for a relative with Alzheimer's disease.* Alzheimer's Association Triad, P.O. Box 15622, Winston-Salem, NC 27113. $4.50. 32-page paperback.

AARP. 1986. *Coping and caring: Living with Alzheimer's disease.* Free single copies from Fulfillment, 1909 K St., NW, Washington, DC 20049.

AARP. *Miles away and still caring: A guide for long distance caregivers.* AARP, 1909 K St., NW, Washington, DC 20049.

Advice for adults with aging parents or a dependent spouse. Newsletter. Helpful Publications, Inc. 310 W. Durham St., Philadelphia, PA 19119-2901. (215) 247-5473.

Alzheimer's Association. 1988. *Understanding Alzheimer's disease: What it is, how to cope with it, future directions,* ed. M. K. Aronson. New York: Charles Scribner's Sons. Available from Alzheimer's Association chapters.

Alzheimer's Association, Atlanta. 1985. *Understanding and caring for the person with Alzheimer's disease.* 3120 Raymond Dr., Atlanta, GA 30340.

Alzheimer's Association, Eastern Massachusetts. 1988. *Family care guide.* One Kendal Square, Bldg. 600, Cambridge, MA 02139.

Brunette, M., and M. Fowler. 1988. *The yankee caregiver . . . if you care for someone with Alzheimer's.* Alzheimer's Center, 152 Dresden Ave., Gardiner, ME 04345.

Caregiving. Newsletter of Family Caregivers of the Aging, a program of the National Council on the Aging, 600 Maryland Ave., SW, West Wing 100, Washington, DC 20024.

Caring: A family guide to managing the Alzheimer's patient at home. 1985. New York City Alzheimer's Resource Center, 280 Broadway, New York, NY 10007.

Cohen, D., and C. Eisdorfer. 1986. *The loss of self.* A family resource for the care of Alzheimer's disease and related disorders. New York: W. W. Norton

Doernberg, M. 1989. *Stolen mind.* Chapel Hill, NC: Algonquin Press. Paperback.

Duke Family Support Program, Box 3600 Duke University Medical Center, Durham, NC 27710. (919) 684-2328; in North Carolina (800) 672-4213. A North Carolina central information point for families and professionals caring for memory-impaired elders. Complimentary general and specific information packets sent on request; newsletter, *The Caregiver,* published quarterly; linkage to support groups; and a telephone hotline for questions on research, diagnosis, and management of chronic illness or memory loss in later life.

Gwyther, L. P. 1985. *Care of Alzheimer's patients.* Published by ADRDA and the American Health Care Association. Available from Alzheimer's Association chapters in paperback.

How to hire helpers: A guide for elders and their families. Church Council of Greater Seattle, 4759 15th NE, Seattle, WA 98105. (206) 525-1213.

Jarvik, L., and G. Small. 1988. *Parentcare: A commonsense guide for adult children.* New York: Crown Publishers, Inc.

Kushner, H. 1982. *When bad things happen to good people.* Paperback, available in popular bookstores. Reassuring, compassionate.

Levin, N. J. 1987. *How to care for your parents: A handbook for adult children.* Paperback. Storm King Press, P.O. Box 3566, Washington, DC. (202) 944-4224.

Mace, N., and L. Gwyther. *Selecting a nursing home with a dedicated dementia care unit.* 1989 booklet available from Alzheimer's Association chapters.

Mace, N., and P. Rabins. 1981. *The 36-hour day.* Baltimore: Johns Hopkins University Press. Best guide to coping with early Alzheimer's disease and other memory disorders. Available from Alzheimer's Association chapters in paperback.

Manning, D. 1985. *When love gets tough: The nursing home decision.* Revised paperback. In-Sight Books, Inc., Drawer 2058, Hereford, TX 79045. A minister reflects on his decision to place his mother in a nursing home.

Norris, J., ed. 1988. *Daughters of the elderly: Building partnerships in caregiving.* Paperback. Bloomington, IN: Indiana University Press.

Noyes, L. 1982. *What's wrong with my grandma?* Alzheimer's Association, 207 Park Ave., Falls Church, VA 22046.

Parent care: Resources to assist family caregivers. Newsletter. Gerontology Center, 316 Strong Hall, The University of Kansas, Lawrence KS 66045. Rural focus.

Shelley, F. D. 1988. *When your parents grow old.* New York: Harper and Row.

9

Design of the Home Environment for the Cognitively Impaired Person

LORRAINE G. HIATT, PH.D.

It has been estimated that many more older people with mental impairments dwell at home, with families or alone, than in nursing homes. Several recent publications on designing environments for cognitively impaired persons in institutions have appeared (Hiatt 1987a, 1987b; Caulkins 1987), but little has been published on designing environments for cognitively impaired older people outside of institutions.

The following recommendations regarding the environmental design of dwellings for older people are based on research of a few dwellings and many institutions that was performed on-site. These recommendations should guide us only until we obtain more comprehensive firsthand information on their successes and limitations in the community.

The goals of this chapter are: (1) to identify characteristics of memory impairment that may combine with other illnesses or normal sensory changes of aging to create a need for special environments; (2) to suggest priorities for environmental evaluations; (3) to offer ideas for correcting common environmental limitations or problems; and (4) to suggest how the environment might better support mental functioning.

The environmental comments are focused on noninstitutional settings, with special reference to households where people live alone, family residences, senior housing serving mentally impaired people, and day care centers. However, many of the same principles are applicable to nursing homes and other congregate settings.

Why Turn to the Environment?

The environment provides special advantages and possibilities for older people and for their caregivers. The environment is there, twenty-four hours a day. Consequently, we need to understand its possible influences and use it to extend our efforts.

For people living at home, the environment is usually familiar. As one's memory for remote experiences or past environments may be better than one's capacity to learn how to react in strange, new, or unfamiliar settings, a familiar environment may support function. A few people become so severely disoriented that their sensitivity to the world diminishes. They may show little awareness of the larger environment or world, but may focus on some detail such as a slipper, a door handle, or the flow of water. Awareness may also differ in the same individual by the day, hour, or week. However, the majority of cognitively impaired people are probably far more aware of some aspects of their surroundings than others may realize. It is worth the effort to think through the influence of the environment and to use it as a part of a repertory of interventions or responses to mentally impaired persons.

Environments may support appropriate behavior. Sometimes an otherwise confused person will respond in a completely acceptable way in certain places or in the company of certain people. By making cues simple and available, we support behavior. A plate of good-smelling food set on the table says, "Eat." Environmental cues may also trigger negative responses. A wastebasket may become a toilet because it has attributes of familiar location, height, or dimensions. Familiar objects may be comforting: unfamiliar objects may add to confusion.

Although the average person may seem almost oblivious of the environment, taking minor noises or clutter for granted, the person with cognitive impairments may attend to details to the exclusion of the whole. The person's impaired ability to focus may be improved when such distractions are eliminated.

To identify places, cognitively impaired people may use realistic, three-dimensional, familiar objects more successfully than abstract features or symbols. This is why many people do not respond to color coding or graphic symbols but may respond to a barber pole as a signal of a barber shop, a door handle as a symbol of freedom, or a lock as a symbol of incarceration.

How Might We Use Environmental Design?

Support of Attention Span

By increasing the likelihood that the confused person will be able to complete a train of thought, the environment may serve to increase the ability to use residual mental capacities. Features that distract attention include noise, crowding, and nuisance features like glare, foul odors, and unrelated action or activity. Noise interrupts the thought process for all of us, especially as we age. Energy is required to tune it out. Noise-free environments facilitate attention span and make it easier to follow conversations. The problem is magnified when one experiences mental impairment. A person who is moderately impaired may respond to noise, glare, crowding, or unpleasant odors by withdrawal (closing the eyes), emotional outbursts, verbalization (chatter), or efforts to escape, such as flight or wandering.

Support of Social Interchange

In environmental design, one looks at both physical features (spaces and furnishings) and social considerations such as the presence of people and their impact on behavior. Crowding or density is one aspect of the social environment; group size is another.

Often groups larger than two to six will confuse people, but there are individual differences in how many people in spaces of what size confuse a particular person. Thus, it is necessary to know the individual and understand his or her former lifestyle. A person may effectively cope in small groups but seem more impaired in larger settings, particularly when several things are going on that are not unified by a common activity such as singing, liturgy, or exercise. This has implications for family meals, holiday celebrations, and taking a person shopping or to a doctor's office. The caregiver might plan smaller family gatherings or take the person shopping when the stores are least crowded.

Sensitivity to Personal Spaces

Some environments seem more crowded because the personal space available to each individual—the area that we define as our own territory—is encroached upon. People vary in how close to or how far from others they prefer to sit and in whether or not they are touched (Hiatt 1980b). A cognitively impaired person may feel crowded but be less able to move or respond verbally. The sense of being threatened, out of control, or socially violated may result in agitation and increased confusion. This may be why some people become flustered on day care buses or in waiting areas containing what they perceive as too many people. The fragile sense of command of a situation is lost when too many other people are present or when the people press too closely or place themselves too far away. The best way to learn about a particular person's reaction to personal space is to observe reactions and then adapt your behavior accordingly.

Few people can verbalize their territorial needs. When planning a day care center, it may be helpful to have clearly assigned spaces and furnishings: personalized chairs, storage areas, and places for display of one's personal items. People differ in their needs for territory; some may regularly "violate" the preferences and spaces of others, which makes it all the more useful to give each person familiar items to help mark out what is "yours" and "mine." At home, the caregiver might tell visitors that a certain chair is special to the confused person.

Maximizing Remaining Vision

As one ages, glare becomes more disabling. Glare may come directly from a light source, such as the sun or an unshielded light bulb, or be reflected from shiny floors, vinyl furnishing, or laminated table tops. Glare tends to be distracting. A flash of light or other startling stimulus may interrupt the thought process and stop a person from participating in a conversation or activity. We may be able to improve a person's attention by reducing glare (shading the lamp, relocating the light source or person, reducing the sheen or flashing, using window blinds or sun shades).

Uneven light (bright areas next to shadows) may also be confusing. The impaired person may see shapes in the shadows or perceive dark areas as holes.

As the eye ages, it needs more light to see well. Sometimes we can improve an impaired person's ability to do a task by improving the light. Good lighting and highlighting a focal point may help direct attention. Good lighting on the faces of participants at a group meeting around a table may hold people to the table and to the conversation. Good lighting must be even and constant. At no time should a bulb be harsh or visible like a spot or line of light.

Motivating by Aroma

Like glare, noxious odors may capture a person's attention, but the impaired person may not be able to follow through or respond appropriately. Aromas that are out of place (for example, the smell of a kitchen when no kitchen is visible) can increase confusion.

Meaningful aromas may be used to increase attention span. The smell of baked goods may reinforce an event or a meal. Clearly identifiable aromas may reinforce a sense of time (coffee and toast in the morning, detergent on wash days, shaving lotion in the area for toiletry, etc.). Aromas may have yet other possibilities, providing a source of pleasure (the scents of spring flowers or a holiday food) and offering a way to shift mood and the focus of attention from despondency to curiosity or elation. Not everyone is capable of recognizing all odors, and many have problems distinguishing or naming certain scents. Some odors may elevate anxiety, for example, strong tinctures that signify a clinic or hospital, ammonia, or smoke.

Supporting Hearing

Many people with dementia also have difficulty hearing. Some may be unwilling or unable to use a hearing aid. Reducing background noise and looking directly at the person when one speaks help the person to hear. Normal amounts of noise in some rooms can seem like a lot of noise and can add to the person's confusion. The addition of carpeting, noise-deadening (fire-proofed) wall hangings and furniture, or the use of smaller rooms, can make hearing easier for the impaired person.

Encouraging Motion by Design

Action becomes a focal point for people with dementia. Action, motion, or activity may serve as a source of interest. One of the problems with television for mentally impaired people is that the action is two-dimensional, too small, and too fast. By contrast, the comings and goings of neighbors, the activities of a dog or cat, the play of a single child, or the familiar motions of a spouse may be engaging. Exercise and motions such as rocking may "clear the head" or provide short-term benefits such as staving off emotional outbursts.

Watching too much action, however, may have undesirable effects. When there is little else to do inside a building (or little with which the person identifies) and a clearly visible roadway with some traffic or some bustle, the individual may be drawn to the outside. Some people who wander do not try to escape the home as much as they are enticed by or drawn to the flow of motion beyond. Some people become restless when they are in settings where motion is more vigorous or placid than to which they are accustomed.

Observing motion has many functions; activity and motion attract, repel, or stop a person. Direct participation in activities that engage the person in motion may provide an outlet for feelings. Sometimes, too much observation and participation leave the person overstressed and fatigued. The goal then is to become aware of how each individual's comfort level and attention span are influenced by motion, to be sensitive to the extremes, and yet to incorporate design features for safe levels of motion and participatory exercise.

Cuing Memory

Memory tends to be better when real and touchable objects or cues are used to reinforce thoughts. Objects, personal possessions, and stimuli such as sounds, images, and textures may all be more engaging to the person with dementia than are conversations about abstract memories. Although it is important to consider safety and personal injury, objects are usually an excellent way to stimulate memory and conversation (shells to remind one of a trip, childhood photos and music to reinforce a sense of past memories, the touch of pets or children to reinforce old emotions of joy and comfort). Because many people also have impaired vision, photographs should be large and clearly legible.

Although a person with a dementing illness may need a simple and safe environment, it should not be barren or stark. Interesting items include clothing, finger foods, or grooming and gardening supplies that the person can touch or manipulate. For some people, it is enough to have small items in view without fingering them, but other people need to take the objects in hand as well as look at them. Objects should be too large to be swallowed by mistake.

Objects can be a wonderful resource for shared activities and to trigger recollections. Objects comfort one who yearns for people and places that are unavailable. Brain-damaged people may respond somewhat differently from people with other forms of mental impairment. Some may not be able to tap into past memories, so familiar cues may be meaningless. It then becomes more challenging to create new connections between objects, features of the environment, and expected behavior.

The Use of Color and Pattern

Color

Color has sometimes been viewed as a "quick fix" for special populations, including people with mental impairments. There are no clearly established research-based data to suggest that color alone will shape behavioral responses for all or most individuals with cognitive impairments. In fact, there is no body of research to suggest that all humans react similarly to particular colors (Hiatt 1980a).

Research has demonstrated that responses to color are a function of many interacting attributes of the environment: the hue itself, lighting, the surface and texture, the amount of color, and the combinations in which it is used. Human responses to color are influenced by many factors, including exposure to various color schemes at different points in life, present-day memories and associations, and the tendency to be either environmentally aware or oblivious throughout life. What does this mean on an individual level?

A particular individual may react to some colors in certain ways. For many older people in general and for mentally impaired people in particular, color tends to be quite vague, abstract, and difficult to respond to.

Color should be considered part of a system of design resources that includes attention to texture, odor, objects, and sounds. Texture and odor may be more effective than color at eliciting responses or memory traces. Texture, color, objects, and pattern should all be used in concert to obtain an overall effect or impression.

The lens of the eye yellows with normal aging, so colors appear muddier or more drab to older people. It is more difficult to discriminate between colors of the same intensity and to name them accurately. Dark shades of socks or dark foods on a dark plate may be difficult to distinguish. Light tones may be equally perplexing: two toothbrushes of similar color and shape may be easily confused. Chicken, potatoes, and cauliflower on a white plate may be difficult to identify and unappetizing as well. This has caused some to suggest the use of very bright or primary colors for older people. This may work best for small objects that are easily confused or misplaced, but contrast may be more important than brightness.

The principle of contrast stipulates that the visibility of any color is improved when the focal object or feature is significantly darker or lighter than the background. Because many environments tend to be muted in tone, bright items stand out. Brightly colored pills, for example, will be more visible against a dull or light background. A room full of colors that are all bright may be just as disorienting as a design scheme based on all light or all dark colors. White plates may be easier to see on a dark blue placemat. Conversely, things that we do not want a person to notice can be made less conspicuous. An exit door, for example, may be painted to match the wall.

Color should be planned in terms of the goals for behavior. One would not paint a day care center in primary tones because it is not the walls that should stand out. Color should be used to emphasize what is significant, such as the objects in comparison to the back-ground wall, table, or floor surface.

The overall effects of color combinations may be more useful than the presence of one or two particular colors in reinforcing memory. Select a painting or fabric wall hanging that has several colors or a combination of colors that is appealing and then let the walls and other colors serve as a backdrop to the object(s).

Patterns

Patterns may suggest ideas or familiarity. Because the person with dementia may tend to see patterns as objects, however, consider the use of patterns that do not take on the appearance of objects. To test the effects of a pattern, stand as far away as one would in viewing the object or surface. Squint and look at the pattern. If it starts to waver (like diagonal lines or wavy stripes), "move" like the dots or patterns on some carpeting, or if it looks like a person or object, then the pattern may be too bold for everyday environments. Generally, a pattern will be more successful if it is identifiable and realistic, although some people are comfortable with abstract images.

How To: An Operating Plan for Using the Environment

Functional Characteristics of the Person

Designing for people with dementia should start from a realistic, functional profile of the population (Hiatt 1987a). Diagnosis typically provides information on health in terms of disease or condition labels

TABLE 9.1   Inventory of Environmental Factors

   I. The physical environment
      A. What environments does the person occupy? (Describe; include
         buildings such as home, grocery; spaces such as particular
         rooms, cars, elevators, and special chairs indoors and
         outside.)
      B. How large and small are these spaces? What is the person's
         reaction to size?
      C. What systems characterize these spaces? Systems include lighting,
         sound, communication systems, particular electrical/heating or
         cooling elements, etc.
         1. How does the individual react to or control these systems?
         2. What improvements might be made?
         3. What safety backups are needed?
  II. What is the nature of the person's social environment? To what group
      sizes and types of people does the patient react well? Poorly?
      How can social environments be optimized? How can confusion
      be limited?
 III. What is the person's psychological environment? That is, with what
      environmental images does the person seem comfortable? What
      preferences are expressed for places, spaces, objects, or
      conditions (lighting, sound, texture, odor)? How can enjoyable or
      nonthreatening stimuli be optimized and noxious stimuli be
      minimized?
  IV. A cultural environment refers to patterns, norms, and traditions.
      What rules and regulations seem difficult for the individual?
      What customs and traditions are helpful?
   V. Specifically, how can the environment be used to help the individual
      relax and thus facilitate wayfinding, sleeping, eating, bathing, or
      conversation?

(suspected senile dementia of the Alzheimer's type, cataracts, previous fracture, etc.). In designing, we need to consider the person in
terms of the interactive impact of these conditions on what the individual can or would like to do. Table 9.1 illustrates some of the
types of information that are helpful.

Life-Style

Once we understand the person, we then turn to information on
life-style and daily routine, which indicates how the environment will
be used and suggests some priorities for the setting. For example, if

the person spends a lot of time walking and used to do a lot of gardening, we might focus attention on spaces and design features that would support those interests.

Specific Disabilities

We can identify specific cognitive disabilities that the environment can help to minimize. For example, if the person has difficulty with time orientation, we can emphasize time-orienting cues such as the smell of food at mealtime and the arrival of darkness at evening.

Establish Some Goals

With information on the person and life-style, caregivers may then develop some goals. For example, the caregiver can:

- protect the person from hazards such as burning, errors in switch use, or falls by reducing the temperature on the water heater and removing throw rugs;
- improve the ability to focus attention on interpersonal activities, (for example, substitute one-to-one conversation for group visits);
- reinforce selective personal interests: pets, family life, grooming;
- increase the level of exercise, even passive exercise such as rocking on a platform rocker;
- surround the individual with some familiar symbols/objects for increased comfort: clothing, slippers, accessories, bed sheets, work implements, notebooks, etc.);
- develop cues for time: ticking or chiming clocks, regular television or radio programs, scheduled aromas (coffee in the morning, warm cocoa at night);
- provide information to assist wayfinding (make spaces more visible, add more cues);
- increase general function through improved lighting;
- provide comfort for sleep time, including features to aid relaxation: cozy coverlets, warm socks, soft nightwear;
- avoid inadvertent triggers of undesirable behavior;
- encourage better eating through positive use of food aromas to elicit natural digestion by using slow cooking methods rather than fast foods;
- provide external methods for diffusing agitation by offering opportunities to use familiar techniques such as digging, vigorous walking, or rocking;

- develop external, environmental methods for assisting with mood shifts (for example, try using fresh air to "clear the mind" when nothing else works to alleviate sadness).

This list illustrates many options. The goals appropriate for a particular person may be more limited, depending on particular needs. Goals must be planned on an individual basis and based upon good experience with the person.

Surroundings

The next step is to make an assessment of the household or setting itself. Noxious features should be minimized or removed; supportive features are developed. Priorities may be derived from the individual's goals. People and settings are different; features that are difficult for one person may not be particularly problematic for another. Trial and error are wholly appropriate.

The Social Environment

Thus, so far, the emphasis has been on the physical environment. Caregivers or companions who make up the social environment also play a key role in stabilizing behavior by:

- being alert to the potential impact of the environment on the immediate reactions or behaviors of the person;
- reflecting upon the individual's lifelong responses to environments and becoming more informed on the impact of environments on older or brain-damaged people;
- developing a repertory of environmental techniques for optimizing attention or communication;
- checking out environments for their possible negative effects and working to minimize factors such as noise, glare, and crowding (just as childproofing does not suggest that the child has been incarcerated, making a place safe for a person with dementia should be done to encourage freedom of movement and exploration);
- considering when particularly perplexing behaviors emerge (wandering, calling out, agitation, disrobing, etc.), whether there are features in the setting that cue or reinforce these responses for a particular individual (by looking at situations or settings through the person's eyes, we may begin to understand a chain of events

that elicit behavior that is dangerous, risky, unsuitable, or uncharacteristic);
- remembering that it is probably not possible that all behavior will
become normal, predictable, or manageable with environmental
manipulations;
- sharing ideas with others.

Conclusion

The environment is not the entire solution to the problems of
cognitive impairment, but spaces, their features, the impact of all of
the systems (such as lighting and color together) may affect behavior.
Design does not cause Alzheimer's disease, but it may contribute to
the confusion or competency an impaired person experiences.

References

Caulkins, M. 1987. Designing special care units: A systematic approach. *American Journal of Alzheimer's Care and Related Disorders and Research* 2 (2): 16–22.

Hiatt, L. 1980a. Touchy about touching. *Nursing Homes* 29 (6): 42–46.

Hiatt, L. 1980b. Color and care: The selection and use of colors in environments for older people. *Nursing Homes* 30 (3): 18–22.

Hiatt, L. 1987a. Environmental design and mentally impaired older people. In *Alzheimer's disease: Problems, prospects and perspectives*, ed. H. Altman, 309–20. New York: Plenum.

Hiatt, L. 1987b. Supportive design for people with memory impairments. In *Confronting Alzheimer's disease*, ed. A. Kalicki, 138–63. Owings Mills, MD: National Health Publishing and American Association of Homes for the Aging.

10

Respite Care: A Flexible Response to Service Fragmentation

DIANA M. PETTY

In an ideal world, many care choices would present themselves to the family and caregivers of a dementia patient. Peer groups and therapeutic programs for patients in the early stages, day care later on, home care whenever needed—even during nights and weekends—and care homes lovingly and practically designed; all of these would be available. And they would be paid for by insurance or a Medicare-type fund.

But for dementia patients and their families, this is far from an ideal world. In every community, either parts of the care program are missing or the ability to pay for adequate service is lacking. Respite care programming developed in the United States from two primary needs: to fill the gaps in America's care continuum and to support the family members involved in primary care. As agencies met with success in establishing and providing respite, the second reason, to help family caregivers, has become vitally important on its own. Few providers of service to dementia patients (or other adult patient groups) could now conceive of a service system without respite care as a component. More than one respite recipient has declared that the service "saved my life."

Defined most often as temporary, substitute care of a patient that occurs in or out of the home to provide a break from constant care demands for the caregiver, respite is an ideal service concept to be considered for families of people with dementia. Just as out-of-home day care is thought of as a service begun for children and disabled persons and later successfully adapted for frail elders, respite care (which includes day care) first appeared in the statutes of several states in the early 1970s as a component of services for developmentally disabled persons (Dickman and Warren 1981). Respite seemed a natural extension of crisis and shelter care services for children and adults with severe and multiple impairments. Respite care for older persons has evolved more slowly but is now being promoted throughout health and social service delivery systems (Pacific Northwest Long-Term Care Center 1982; Stone 1985). Many model programs exist, from voluntary church-sponsored day respite centers to resource centers for brain-impaired adults that broker respite services in many settings. Programs are funded by state and local governments, by private foundations and agencies, and with client fees (U.S. Department of Health and Human Services 1981).

One national advocacy organization, the Older Women's League (1983), sponsored model legislation in several states in the 1980s to encourage the development of statewide respite services for caregivers of frail and disabled adults. The Robert Wood Johnson Foundation (1987), in collaboration with the Alzheimer's Association, issued grant guidelines for respite centers to be operated by area agencies on aging or Alzheimer's Association-sponsored day care centers. These centers also received support from the federal Administration on Aging.

Increasingly, respite care is a mandated service in state-sponsored programs such as the Illinois Alzheimer's Disease Program, New York State's Expanded In-Home Services for the Elderly Program, and California's Alzheimer's Disease Institute (administered by the Office of Statewide Health Planning and Development) and regional resource centers for families and caregivers of brain-impaired adults (administered by the state department of mental health) (Illinois Department of Public Health 1986; Rabbitt 1986; California Health and Welfare Agency 1987). The question of whether respite care should be adopted for families of dementia patients seems no longer relevant. Instead, the questions of how, where, and how often are more frequently debated by clinicians, providers of service, and advocates.

The definition of respite care can still pose problems, however, particularly for government-sponsored programs. Although there is general agreement to define respite as services intended to provide temporary relief for the primary caregiver, there is debate about the elements of eligibility, duration, and service components. Problems over eligibility criteria include who the client is for purposes of service eligibility (is the patient, the caregiver, or a family unit the "client"?), what constitutes a "caregiver" (a paid or an unpaid person, relative or nonrelative, residing with the patient or elsewhere), and whether the patient's or the family's income—or both—should be a criterion.

With duration of service, problems arise over the definition of terms such as "temporary," "short-term," "intermittent," "time-limited," and "occasional" relief. Programs currently exist that fulfill every viewpoint on duration, but public policy makers and program administrators still struggle with the issue. Should respite care provision be limited to a specified number of hours or days per month or year? Should relief services be offered on a one-time-only basis, for a limited number of months within a year, or for the lifetime of the patient? California's Department of Mental Health has resolved the dilemma of duration for its regional resource centers for families of brain-impaired adults by prohibiting the cessation of respite after a prescribed period but allowing individual centers to set other limitations (i.e., hours per week or month) (California Health and Welfare Agency 1987). The most desirable amount of service is an important factor in designing a respite program and is discussed later in this chapter.

In defining what types of programs constitute respite care, policy makers and service providers may disagree about the individual program elements to include. For example, is round-the-clock companionship "respite" or full-time home care? Discussions over the term "substitute care" lead to a fundamental issue of long-term care policy, that is, should respite (or other long-term care services) support or supplant the family in its caregiving role (U.S. Congress 1987)? The way a respite service is defined and structured will cause one or the other philosophy to emerge. Most family members will argue for having their role supported and not replaced.

The term "respite" could be considered a formal name for what families, neighbors, churches, and other groups have always done when they helped a family in need or a disabled person who strives to live in the community or at home. Respite is the formal equivalent of "sitting with a friend," available to families that are already committed by emotion or necessity to keeping a loved one at home. Respite has the potential to be more helpful than informal assistance, however, because it can be scheduled and become part of a household routine (U.S. Department of Health and Human Services 1985).

Respite care differs from more traditional "in-home supportive services" by focusing attention on the caregiver's needs rather than only on those of the patient, although the patient actually receives the care or assistance provided. Many state- and county-funded home care services specifically prohibit clients' aides from assisting others who live with the client, but respite care specifically identifies the caregiver as equally significant in the care plan. The person who is responsible for round-the-clock care and decision making is thereby supported, not supplanted. Services provided to the patient usually consist of supervision, personal care, and activities designed for physical and mental stimulation.

If respite care was not a clearly demonstrated need of families before 1987, the U.S. Congressional Office of Technology Assessment (OTA) firmly established the need in its report that year, *Losing a Million Minds* (U.S. Congress 1987). In its inventory of services, the OTA asked those caring for dementia patients to assess the importance of various services. Of the top ten services rated as "essential or most important," six could be construed as related to respite care. These included the most often-cited need: "a paid companion who can come to the home for a few hours each week to give caregivers a rest," which literally describes respite. The fourth ranked service was a paid companion for overnight care. The other four respite-related needs were: personal care for the patient (i.e., bathing, dressing, or feeding); short-term respite out of the home in nursing homes or hospitals; adult day care; and nursing visits at home.

California's regional resource center program and the Family Survival Project's five-year demonstration project have consistently recorded respite care as one of the most-needed forms of assistance for caregivers of people with adult-onset brain impairment (Family Survival Project 1986–88; Petty 1981; Petty and Wolf 1982–85). Another study found that a significant number of caregivers of dementia patients spend more than forty hours per week in direct personal care (Ory et al. 1984). Researchers Linda George and Lisa Gwyther followed up on their Caregiver Well-Being surveys by designing a respite care project. The surveys revealed substantial burden in mental health, social, and recreational areas of the lives of dementia patient caregivers. Respite care was cited as the most desired but least available community service (George 1986).

Employed caregivers (i.e., those who work at regular paid jobs outside the home in addition to their caregiving role) compose a group ready for special attention, and respite could well be an employer-sponsored benefit of the future. In a recent study of working caregivers who care for brain-impaired adult relatives, those who hold down jobs more than part-time also spend another thirty-five hours per week giving care. This is in addition to an average of thirty-four hours spent at their jobs and thirty-six hours of additional paid care from an aide. This is not to say that nonemployed caregivers are not equally deserving of attention; in the same study, they were found to be providing eighty-four hours of direct care per week (Enright and Friss 1987; Petty and Friss 1987).

Benefits of Respite Care

Few completed rigorous studies have measured the benefits and outcomes of respite care. Anecdotal evidence and preliminary results, however, point to many positive aspects. In-home and out-of-home respite programs are believed to have reduced stress, prolonged the ability to care for a relative or friend at home, increased the ability to conduct necessary personal and family activities, provided flexibility in making respite an adjunct to other services, and augmented the pool of trained respite workers (Petty 1981; Petty and Wolf 1982–85; George 1986; Montgomery 1986).

In theory, the benefits of respite care also include the avoidance or deterrence of institutional placement, improvement in the caregivers' ability to maintain their health longer, and preservation of families' financial resources. Stretching of already limited community and agency resources and cost-containment of programs can occur (Petty 1981; Petty and Wolf 1982–85; George 1986; Schwartz and Dobrof 1987).

Avoidance or Deterrence of Placement

The OTA reviewed several studies and concluded that home care services do not generally substitute for nursing home care (U.S. Congress 1987). Over five years, the Family Survival Project discovered that the effectiveness of avoiding or deterring institutional placement fluctuated from year to year. A lower incidence of placement was reported in some years. Although the reasons for this variation were not investigated, it is believed that the age and overall health and cognitive status of both the patient and the caregiver have an impact on whether and how soon a patient is placed (Petty 1981; Petty and Wolf 1982–85). The Duke University Center on Aging Respite Care Project also found that higher service use by caregivers occurs shortly before placement of a memory-impaired older person (George 1986). The Duke project, the Family Survival Project, and Mace and Rabins (1984) noted that placement in an institution and death of the patient with dementia are consistently the most frequent reasons for families to terminate respite (George et al. 1987; Petty 1981; Petty and Wolf 1982–85).

Where deterrence of placement is a program objective, eligibility based on risk of institutionalization may be the reason for late involvement in respite services (Montgomery 1986). The lack of available residential care and nursing home beds for people with dementia would also affect the timing of placement, as might, conversely, the availability of community services. Rather than establishing program policies that require deterrence of facility admission as an outcome, the placement of persons with dementing illness in facilities should be an optional outcome (i.e., an option that mutually benefits the caregiver and the patient). Respite care cannot possibly preclude the need for more intensive care in the late stages of dementing illness, in the event of severe or acute illness of the caregiver, or in other circumstances calling for more formal intervention. However, its role in keeping individuals at home should be evaluated separately from the issue of institutional utilization.

Maintenance of the Caregiver's Health

Most respite programs would point to improving the caregiver's health as a respite program benefit. No studies have been done to specifically determine the long-term impact of respite or related services on caregiver health. Duke University evaluated the impact of its respite project on caregiver well-being. The caregivers' perceived their feelings of relief as a positive result (George 1986). However, the well-intentioned goal of preserving the caregiver's health and well-being is frequently debated. As one family member (whose brain-impaired husband is deceased) has asked often, "In providing these services, are we possibly just helping caregivers to suffer longer?" Potential exploitation of caregivers by service providers also deserves closer examination. Questions raised concern caregivers who abuse prescription drugs (for themselves or for the patient), those who are physically smaller than the patient, and those caregivers and patients confronted with violence (U.S. Congress 1987). There is, coincidentally, a rise in programs to prevent abuse of elders. The two topics are related in that no study has been made of the possible negative experiences of caregivers and patients.

Preservation of the Family's Financial Resources

For those families who pay for respite, cash resources are preserved. The average annual nursing home cost is $22,265.16 [National Center for Health Statistics (Strahan) 1987]. However, no specific studies of these cost comparisons are known to exist. Costs of respite programs vary. Most are low cost: Duke University provided a maximal subsidy of $32 per week (George 1986); some day respite centers cost only $6 a day. California regional resource centers and their client families each spend an average of only $200 to $300 per month (Family Survival Project 1986–88). Most families say that they want more service (George 1986), and many supplement agency-provided respite with additional service (Family Survival Project 1986–88).

Stretching Agency Resources

There is no doubt that provision of a respite (i.e., temporary) service will stretch agency dollars further than will twenty-four-hour care programs if the costs of the program are capped. Program start-up and initial administrative costs seem to be burdensome initially and ebb over time (George 1986). Also, components of a respite program can be shared: one agency can train workers while another matches workers with family clients. In fact, many providers cite interagency involvement in the community as necessary for a respite program to succeed (Dickman and Warren 1981; Lidoff 1985; U.S. Congress 1987).

Cost-Containment

The issue of cost-containment arises in all public debates about long-term care. It is possible to contain costs of respite care services: one publicly funded program (California) has successfully capped respite for caregivers of brain-impaired persons by allowing a dollar amount or level of service per family per month or year. Some centers, however, have long waiting lists for respite services, and funding to meet this need fully has not been forthcoming (Family Survival Project 1986–88; Petty 1981; Petty and Wolf 1982–85). Also, the OTA reported in 1987 that provision of respite care may postpone the placement of persons who are ultimately sicker when admitted to nursing homes or hospitals. This would contribute to higher costs at that stage (U.S. Congress 1987). Montgomery (1986) pointed to the need to study cost benefits of respite programs in terms of their relationship to institutional care, the length of time that services are provided, and the indirect costs incurred by the family recipients.

Perceived Relief

Nevertheless, the one completed long-term study (twenty-eight months) of respite (conducted at the Duke University Center for the Study of Aging and Human Development) showed that respite is the most desired but least available service. Caregivers surveyed indicated that the *perceived relief as a result of respite was the greatest advantage.* Steady relationships with respite workers is also a documented benefit (George 1986). Other programs and studies report similar findings through observation, anecdotes, or client satisfaction surveys (Petty 1981; Petty and Wolf 1982–85; Family Survival Project 1986–88; Lidoff 1985; Harder et al. 1986).

The desirable goals of respite programs are multiple and include:

- alleviation of caregiver stress;
- a "break" in routine;
- time for family members to be apart;
- time to run errands and attend to personal or family business;
- the availability of someone else (the respite worker) with whom to share caregiving problems and knowledge; and
- the availability of someone or a program on which to call in emergencies.

More difficult to measure but still significant goals are:

- to delay or prevent institutional placement when desirable for both the family and the person with dementia;
- to protect the caregiver's health; and
- to preserve the family's financial resources.

Types of Respite Care and Programs

A wealth of options present themselves to service providers in developing respite programs. Services and methods of service delivery can be designed to fit almost any need. Services can be paid or unpaid (voluntary); offered in the home or out; available in day care centers, nursing facilities, residential care homes, or foster homes; and provided on an emergency or ongoing basis. Most importantly, respite can be a combination of all of these. Methods used to administer and provide respite programs may take many forms: subsidies, vouchers, service credits, cooperatives, brokerages, registries, and, in some states, Medicaid. The Office of Technology Assessment and the Brookdale Foundation have examined various models of respite settings (e.g., university-sponsored and community grassroots programs) in more depth (U.S. Congress 1987; Schwartz and Dobrof 1987).

In-Home

In-home respite care is the most common type of program because caregivers seem to prefer it, at least initially, and most communities have home care services of some kind (George 1986; U.S. Congress 1987). A wide variety of in-home options are available. The caregiver can hire an aide through a home health agency or registry, volunteer companions may be available through local service agencies or church-sponsored groups, or families can trade or barter sitting time. Many home health agencies offer a respite aide or service category. A wide range of costs for in-home respite is found from minimum wage to a set rate of $100.00 or more overnight (twenty-four hours). Home health aides in California cost between $8.00 and $12.00 per hour. A New York program costs $35 per hour for a licensed professional nurse with special training (Schwartz and Dobrof 1987). Such expensive professionals are not often used for respite.

The keys to success of respite at home include the comfort felt by the family and patient with the aide, the aide's level of knowledge and skill in caring for a person with dementia, the caregiver's ability to use free time out of the home, and an affordable cost. Involvement of a family-aide matching service is, therefore, desirable.

At home services fail when the caregiver or patient does not trust the aide (or any "stranger" in the house), when the caregiver does not leave or become occupied away from the patient, or when the aide is asked to clean house, run errands, or serve as a personal maid rather than as a trained professional who is present to care for and spend time with the patient. Many in-home respite providers have noted the inability of some families to accept an outsider in the home. Some providers arrange for reluctant caregivers to meet other respite recipients to hear firsthand success stories (Lidoff 1985; Eastman and Kane 1986). Other problems with in-home respite are associated with the respite aide or agency. Aides may not show up, may not "fit in" with the family (i.e., differences in age, religion, culture), or may not be trained to deal with the patient's behavior or supervision needs.

Most families surveyed by in-home respite programs, however, find them to be beneficial, particularly because the person with dementia remains in and near familiar environments. Planners urge involvement of all participants—family members, attendants, the home care agency, and, if appropriate, the fiscal agent—in the planning and monitoring of home care services (Lidoff 1985; Petty 1985; U.S. Department of Health and Human Services 1985; Eastman and Kane 1986; George 1986; Schwartz and Dobrof 1987).

Out-of-Home

Day Care Centers

The most common and fastest growing form of out-of-home respite involves adult day care centers or programs where the caregiver arranges to leave the person with dementia at the center for a specified period. Until awareness of the needs of those with dementing illness increased in the 1980s, adult day care centers did not, in most cases, serve severely cognitively impaired adults. The two types of day care centers, day health and social day care, were intended originally to serve adults with medical and rehabilitation needs or high levels of social functioning. Formal adult day care programs integrate social, recreational, rehabilitative, medical, and nutrition services (Harder et al. 1986). Mace and Rabins (1984) reported that, by 1983, 45 percent of nearly 1,000 day care centers surveyed indicated that they served clients with dementia. Center operators reported that demand by family members was the main factor in a center's decision to accept these cognitively impaired clients.

The same survey also found that many adult day care programs were not operating at capacity (Mace and Rabins 1984), which means that perhaps space could be found for new respite care clients. To meet the special needs of persons with dementing illness, however, day care programs must be modified. Providers must be able to deal with disorientation, agitation and restlessness, wandering, withdrawal, and a longer period of adjustment. Ideally, centers could also handle incontinence, combativeness, and immobility. Mace and Rabins listed the most successful activities for persons with dementia at day care centers surveyed to be sing-alongs, physical exercise, walks, reminiscence groups, visits from children, active games, outings, listening to music, reality orientation, and visits from pets. Help with grooming and naps were also mentioned. By contrast, activities offered to cognitively well clients included shopping trips, poetry groups, self-governance, reading the newspaper, and current events discussion.

One of the first day care programs in the United States to accept persons with dementia was the Harbor Area Adult Day Care Center (Costa Mesa, California), which follows a social day care model (U.S. Congress 1987). This center shaped an already existing program to adapt to the needs of these patients. Two other types of out-of-home day care programs have emerged to serve specifically persons with dementia or similar disorders: Alzheimer's day care centers and out-of-home day respite programs. Although essentially alike—both provide a day care setting—these two program models differ in the extent and method of the service provided. Alzheimer's day care centers such as the Atlanta Community Services Program and the Alzheimer's Family Center (San Diego, California) were established to provide adult day care daily to people with dementing illness. (Both programs also arrange at-home care.) Respite for the family is one of several program goals, along with a primary goal of care, activity, and stimulation for the patient (Glenner and Moses 1986; U.S. Congress 1987).

Day respite programs provide activities for and supervision of the patient, but the primary goal is respite. The centers may be open only one or two days or half-days a week, staffed by volunteers and family members, and located in church halls, community centers, extra hospital space, or any other large available space. Centers can be inexpensive to run and offer sources of pride to the participants, families and volunteers alike. Early models of respite day centers were formed at Diablo Respite Center (Walnut Creek, California), where families paid $6 per day at a church center, and the Alzheimer's Respite Center (Santa Rosa, California), where services cost even less. Some day care centers combine their existing programs with specialized respite care. The space used by an Adult Day Health Center (ADHC) in a hospital can serve as an Alzheimer's respite center during hours when the ADHC is usually closed.

One of the most extensive day care programs for people with Alzheimer's disease is sponsored by the Brookdale Foundation (New York City) (Schwartz and Dobrof 1987). By 1988, fifteen respite program sites provided social and recreational activities for patients. In 1987, the foundation reported the cost of implementing one four-hour day care session for an individual to be $385.00. The cost per session for an individual ranged from $32 to $77, with the higher cost in programs with a smaller number of participants. The foundation works with collaborating agencies and sites and can establish a new program in six to nine months. Sites are located at churches and synagogues, senior centers, community Ys, and congregate housing facilities throughout New York City.

Co-sponsorship by community groups; involvement in service planning by the families of persons with dementia; a central, safe, and accessible location; transportation; low cost; and well-trained staff and volunteers lead to successful day care programs. However, day care does not work for everyone, particularly if a center's goals are seen as being too diverse. Another drawback has been the somewhat haphazard development of adult day care programs and the resultant lack of formal regulations in some centers (Harder et al. 1986). Also, many day care centers limit participation to mildly or moderately impaired dementia patients, those who are continent, and those who can be transported by the family or at the family's expense. It can be different, however; the San Diego Alzheimer's Family Center is one that continues to accept clients who are near death, although partially ambulatory.

A benefit of day care can be improvement in the quality of life for the individual with dementia who might otherwise sit at home in front of a television all day. In a survey of day care centers, Mace and Rabins (1984) examined changes in behavior related to the status of clients' dementing illness and changes in social behavior. Centers were inconsistent in reporting improvements in memory and walking; about as many centers said clients stayed the same or gradually declined. Greater consistency was noted for changes in social behavior; high numbers of day care centers reported that clients with dementia had developed a friendship, liked or expected to be at the center, paced or wandered less, became upset or agitated less often, and had learned where the bathroom was. However, centers were more likely to observe improvements after the client had been attending for some time.

Other researchers found that all studies of adult day care (not specifically for people with dementia) that examined client morale or satisfaction found the attitudes of day care clients to be more positive than those of clients in control groups or other care settings (Harder et al. 1986). The Brookdale Foundation Respite Program found that participants with Alzheimer's disease usually returned home in good spirits and that caregivers enjoyed seeing their relatives enjoying themselves in center activities (Schwartz and Dobrof 1987).

Short-Term Stays

Short-term stays away from home can be set up in nursing homes, residential care homes, hospitals, and the homes of other individuals as a form of foster care. This type of respite is sometimes available without formal program structure, particularly in rural areas. For instance, in a small town in Idaho, a hospital and nursing home share one two-story facility. Individuals with more intensive medical needs can be moved easily from the "acute" floor to the "nursing" floor. In the case of confused, frail patients, the hospital may allow them to stay in the same hospital room at night while participating during the day in the nursing home's activities. Individuals are also admitted into the nursing facility for short stays while the caregiver takes a break. The hospital does not have a name for this service; it's a service that simply makes sense in a sparsely populated mountain community.

One of the earliest inpatient respite programs for older people— including those with dementia—is at the Palo Alto Veterans Administration facility in Menlo Park, California. Stays begin with a trial visit, and patients can stay for several weeks at a time, returning home as is feasible (Ellis 1986a). They may stay during the week and go home on weekends. The facility collaborates with other community service agencies that provide help to the family when the patient is home. Recently, the Palo Alto facility opened an Alzheimer's Respite Center. Participants are eligible for ninety days of inpatient care annually and must stay a minimum of two weeks at a time. An assessment is conducted during the initial stay.

Weekend respite also utilizes short-term placements, although it can also be provided at home with twenty-four-hour aides or companions. In facilities, the caregiver arranges for the person with dementia to stay overnight in any available bed or in a bed previously reserved specifically for respite (Lidoff 1985; Dickman and Warren 1981). According to the Brookdale Foundation, facility stays are most helpful when the person with Alzheimer's disease has additional health problems and in helping families to prepare when they know that long-term placement is imminent (Schwartz and Dobrof 1987).

When using facilities for respite, many of the same debates occur that emerge over the use of special units for persons with dementing illness. No matter which side of the debate over segregated versus integrated units families or providers are on, they will have significant concerns about out-of-home respite options. Costs of facility-based programs may be a barrier to many families (Rabbitt 1986). If the placement is in an acute care hospital, staffing levels must be sufficient for care and supervision of dementia patients. These beds can be expensive if the hospital needs to fill empty acute beds. It is also generally easy to walk in and out of hospitals (Ellis 1986a). The same concerns exist for residential care and foster homes. If the facility or home does not normally serve persons with dementia, it may not have staff and physical features conducive to safety for the confused and agitated individual. State and local licensing issues are important in establishing facility-based respite care.

A project that tested the concept of foster care for elderly patients found it to be less costly than nursing home care. The Community Care Program begun by the Johns Hopkins University Department of Social Work found that patients in foster care maintained or improved activities of daily living and mental status scores, had higher life satisfaction, got out more, and participated more in social and recreational activities than did nursing home clients (Oktay and Volland 1987). Other programs that have tested inpatient respite are the Respite Care for Frail Elderly Project (Albany, New York) and Columbia Lutheran Nursing Home (Seattle, Washington) (The Foundation for Long-Term Care 1983).

Funding Methods

Methods for delivering and funding respite are also varied and include subsidies, volunteer programs, cooperatives, and center-based systems.

Subsidized Respite Services

Services are provided via vouchers, grants-in-aid, or other direct payment or credit. Sources of the subsidy can be funds from federal, state, or private foundation grants; waiver projects utilizing Medicaid- and federal Medicare-reimbursed home care, day care, and inpatient services; and pilot studies by the insurance industry and private agencies. Either the caregiver buys respite service or a provider arranges the service and handles the fiscal management.

In practice, with the exception of the State of New York, government is not funding large quantities of respite care. Because the care provided to the patient is often defined as "personal care," Medicare does not reimburse for respite. (The newly enacted Catastrophic Care Act may change this.) Medicaid allows for such care through its waiver projects (which permit states to "waive" certain requirements). In 1985, twenty-four Medicaid waiver projects provided respite care. Medicaid also pays for out-of-home day care (Rabbitt 1986; U.S. Congress 1987; Kemper et al. 1987).

California's regional resource centers for caregivers of brain-impaired adults offer the most extensive example of "brokered" respite services (California Health and Welfare Agency 1987; Family Survival Project 1988). Modeled after the Family Survival Project's San Francisco Bay Area program, eleven resource centers are slated for development. State-funded subsidies in the form of vouchers for respite, usually about $400 per month, are available to families. Families contribute to the cost on an ability-to-pay basis, but income is not an eligibility restriction. Assessments of the caregiver are to be conducted before the service begins and at six-month intervals. The service to the patient is arranged through home health agencies, day care centers, and other agencies under contract to the regional resource center. Some centers permit families to hire aides directly. To avoid duplication with other public agencies, the centers do not serve anyone who can receive the same service from another government program such as Medicaid or county social services. The 485 caregivers served in 1987 paid an average of $237.00 per month to receive thirty-seven hours of assistance monthly. The cost to the state-funded centers, excluding administrative costs, was $221.00 per month per family. Respite service participants cannot be terminated after an arbitrary length of time in the program. This conforms with earlier findings of the Family Survival Project and other programs that the demand for respite is not met after a few service hours but tends to increase over time (Petty 1981; Petty and Wolf 1982–85; Lidoff 1985; U.S. Department of Health and Human Services 1985; George 1986). Other services provided by the centers include information and referrals; "family consultations," which help families and caregivers plan for all of their needs from the onset of symptoms or illness through and even after the death of the patient; legal and financial consultations with private attorneys; support groups; training; and, in some sites, neuropsychological or diagnostic consultations. (The regional resource centers are a different program than California's recently initiated Alzheimer's

Day Resource Centers, which are day care programs for people with Alzheimer's that are administered by the state department of aging. Most Day Resource Centers are operated by already-existing adult day care programs. A third state-sponsored program funds Alzheimer's Diagnostic and Treatment Centers located in major medical facilities.)

A respite program of the Metropolitan Commission on Aging (Syracuse, New York) compared results when special funds enabled the project to provide respite to participants who were eligible and not eligible for Medicaid (Rabbitt 1986). Further study of funding sources for respite might reveal other ideas for models as some programs have been successful in paying for program costs with fees for service alone (Schwartz and Dobrof 1987).

There is potential for further public and private funding of respite through proposed long-term care insurance and programs. However, policy questions pertaining to eligibility, service provision, quality assurance, and payment will intensify when and if universal long-term care service is available. Will government programs and insurance companies require that service be provided through licensed entities or workers? How will small programs cope with payment reimbursement, training and reporting requirements, and liability insurance issues? Will payers allow well clients (i.e., caregivers) to be recipients of a subsidized national service? These and many other questions must be addressed by those who promote the inclusion of respite in the long-term care continuum.

Volunteer and Cooperative Respite Services

In-home respite, day center, day and night sitting, inpatient respite, and group or foster home respite and respite retreats are now provided by trained volunteers, families, and friends. A project conducts or arranges for appropriate training of volunteers and maintains a registry of trained volunteers. Families may accrue credits toward future service, pay for service, or simply trade. People in the field of developmental disabilities have vast experience in developing and managing such programs (Dickman and Warren 1981; Lindsay/Ferguson Associates 1984). Similar programs for other populations (frail aged people, people with disabilities) are beginning to proliferate, but the adequacy of volunteer respite for persons with dementia is in question, and the questions differ among in-home, day care, and facility-based programs. Issues include liability; willingness of volunteers to care for adults with problem behaviors or who need intensive supervision; scheduling difficulties; additional resources needed by agencies or groups for recruiting, training, and maintaining an adequate and regular pool of volunteers; unavailability of volunteers for extended periods; and families' unwillingness to accept unpaid workers in their homes. Emotional attachment to the program and the client can be both a benefit and a drawback. Programs must also take great care that volunteers understand confidentiality standards (Danaher et al. 1986).

Center-Based Services

In center-based services, a day care center or other agency provides and manages all aspects of respite care provision. The Alzheimer's Family Center in San Diego and similar programs in Atlanta and Virginia are models (Glenner and Moses 1986; U.S. Congress 1987).

What Makes Respite Work

Respite services work best when the family (and, if possible, the patient) works with the service provider to structure the care plan (Petty 1985; Schwartz and Dobrof 1987). Provision of a full and flexible range of options is also best (Petty 1985; Rabbitt 1986). Before a program is set up, the ages and traditional values of both the disabled person and the caregiver (and others in the home) should be considered, as should the home environment and the relationship between the patient and the caregivers. The patient's functional level and behavioral status should be assessed in conjunction with the caregiver's health status and needs for relief. In day care programs, the number of participants is important. The Brookdale Foundation thinks that ten to twelve participants is best (Schwartz and Dobrof 1987). The size of a program, however, should depend on the level of functioning of the attendees: those who are aggressive should be with a smaller number of participants (i.e., five).

Any amount of respite seems to work for those who accept it as an option. Ten hours a week of home care, one day a week in a day care center, an occasional weekend, two weeks in a foster home—all achieve some degree of relief and help to postpone or avoid institutional placement and family breakdown (Petty 1985). Alzheimer's Association surveys found that a half-day or six hours per week was most often needed (U.S. Congress 1987). Respite during the day seems to be requested by families of dementia patients more than at night or on weekends (U.S. Congress 1987; Eastman and Kane 1986). Duke University's respite project, however, discovered that caregivers of memory-impaired patients want respite to be available at night and on weekends (George 1986). A New York study found that hours of respite should not be limited because families of developmentally disabled persons are tempted to "save up" their hours for an emergency (Dickman and Warren 1981). The Family Survival Project now urges families to use respite only as needed initially, rather than on a rigid schedule, to allow the service to be phased in and begin to match life-styles.

In cases where the patient or caregiver faces a deteriorating situation, usually because of failing health, respite must be seen as a temporary solution. It is not a substitute for the family but for a much needed community-based and coordinated long-term care program. In fact, research must address the concern that respite programs might exploit families and continue stress and burden longer than is healthy. Another assumption often made by service providers is that skilled medical personnel (doctors and nurses) are needed for assessment or the provision of respite. The Family Survival Project (FSP) (San Francisco Bay Area) and the Allentown Community Center (Buffalo) both learned in the first year of their programs that skilled personnel were not critical. The FSP discovered that none of its family clients utilized the services of a professional more skilled than a home health aide or "practical nurse" (Petty 1981). Allentown reduced its nurse assessor to half-time (Rabbitt 1986).

As many community resources as possible should be utilized in designing and providing a respite service. What works in a respite program will depend on what supports it in the community. Support services include volunteer programs, day care centers, nursing homes, companion programs, transportation, housekeeping and home meals programs, counseling, information and referral services, senior centers, and recreation programs (Petty 1981; Petty and Wolf 1982–85; Lidoff 1985; Schwartz and Dobrof 1987).

Training of families and caregivers has been found to be critical for respite to succeed. Two areas benefit from training: home care techniques, so as to increase the caregiver's ability to provide patient care while reducing the caregiver's own stress, and steps for hiring and supervising home aides and attendants who would be employed directly by the family. Training of family members in physical patient care, behavioral problem management (particularly for persons with dementing illness or mental disability), financial management, and stress reduction all enhance the potential for the success of respite (Petty 1981; Petty and Wolf 1982–85).

Training of paid workers is essential, beginning with an overview of such basics as normal and abnormal aging processes. Several programs now train part-time respite aides. The senior Respite Care Program (Portland, Oregon) conducts training and has published an extensive manual that includes sections on cognitive impairment and Alzheimer's and Parkinson's diseases (Cleland 1984). A program of the National Council of Catholic Women has trained several thousand volunteers to be companions to elderly persons. In at least one community (San Francisco), the program is linked with Catholic Social Services to provide a registry (Eastman and Kane 1986). The Somerville-Cambridge Elder Services Respite Program, selected by the National Council on the Aging as the model for its innovative program series, trains and places respite companions (Lidoff 1985). Training resources may be a major advantage for joint ventures with research and educational institutes (Schwartz and Dobrof 1987). All personnel of a program who come in contact with patients and their caregivers (receptionists, drivers, and secretaries, for example) should receive at least an orientation (Mace and Rabins 1984).

Finally, there can be no doubt that a respite program's principal benefit can be the sense of control that a family feels when decision making, free time, and new roles are gained or regained by a family or caregiver. Participation in payment for these services also seems to contribute to success.

In the Duke respite project, George et al. (1987) examined the length of time that caregivers use respite and the reason for dropping out of the program (which primarily was institutional placement or the death of the memory-impaired adult). Participants stayed in Duke's respite project an average of 8.9 months [range, one to twenty-eight months (which was the length of the project)]. The researchers concluded that there were substantial individual differences in response to the program. Patient symptoms and illness characteristics seemed unrelated to the caregiver's length of service use and the reason for terminating service. Sex of the caregiver and that person's relationship to the patient, however, were found to be important predictors of both length in the program and reasons for termination:

male caregivers used the service longer and were more likely to terminate services because the patient died. Female caregivers were more likely to terminate because they institutionalized the patient. Spouses used respite service longer than did adult children and tended to use the service until the death of the patient. Adult children were more likely to place the patient.

The role of social support was also examined. Family support tended to be more important than support from friends. The perception of support by caregivers related more strongly to outcomes than did an objective measure of the actual support received. The Duke researchers also concluded that employed caregivers were at high risk for institutionalizing their relatives.

George et al. determined that predictors associated with longer use of respite care by caregivers included more hours per week spent in caregiving, the perception that social support from the family was inadequate, lower income, the perception that economic resources were inadequate, a spouse (rather than adult child) as the caregiver, fewer hours per week of recreational activity, dissatisfaction with recreation, less negative affect, and male caregivers. Predictors that were not significant included length of time of caregiving, support from friends, use of other community services, caregiver stress symptoms, use of psychotropic drugs, alcohol consumption, self-rated health, age, race, and employment status.

Limitations of Respite/When It Doesn't Work

All situations will not be served by respite care. Many family members do not seem to give up their care role easily, even when twenty-four-hour care extends over ten or twenty years. For some caregivers, the concept of respite is simply unknown and, once the new term is explained, they seek the service readily. Others fear that one small vacation will disrupt their ability to continue as they did before. Some fear that, once the patient is out of the home for even a short period, the door to permanent institutional placement will be opened. Some caregivers experience guilt when faced with the possibility of getting away and leaving their loved one behind. For home care services, having strangers in the home presents problems to some families. In addition to the anxiety anyone might feel over an outsider's presence in the home, caregivers fear the disruption of routine. Some persons with dementia refuse to be left with a stranger. Caregivers are sometimes reluctant to do what respite care requires of them: leave the home. Visits beforehand by the respite provider might alleviate anxieties. Many patients (and even their caregivers) are too ill or disabled to be cared for at home, and respite will help only in a short-term, limited way. The intake and assessment process should be viewed as a time of mutual information exchange. Many programs now mandate that home visits be made first to give and receive accurate information (Ellis 1986b; California Health and Welfare Agency 1987; Schwartz and Dobrof 1987).

In some cases, respite should not be considered at all. If the patient is violent or much larger physically, if the caregiver is very frail or in declining health, if physical or mental abuse of the patient or of another person in the home is evident, or if substance abuse is occurring, a professional or other adviser to the family should help seek other options. Also, a family may have a history of discord or be too disorganized to realize the benefits of respite services (Lidoff 1985; George 1986; U.S. Congress 1987; Schwartz and Dobrof 1987). Some programs, notably the Family Survival Project and the Allentown Community Center, discovered that the level of care needed by a person with dementia may be too intense for the level of care available from respite aides. In these cases, placement in a longer-term care facility should be explored with the family or other responsible relative or friend (Petty 1981; Petty and Wolf 1982; Rabbitt 1986). Occasionally, respite workers discover reasons for discontinuing or at least temporarily interrupting respite. This is one reason why involvement of a monitoring agency is important. Monitoring is also essential to spot potential abuse or neglect by respite aides.

Special difficulties confront respite providers and potential clients in rural areas. If demand is sporadic, regular workers may not be available when needed, and formal services are spaced far apart or are nonexistent (Lidoff 1985; Family Survival Project 1986–88). Several National Council of Catholic Women projects found it easier to locate willing volunteers in rural areas, however. Although demand for respite may be greater in urban areas, the potential volunteer pool is smaller because of a larger paid work force (Eastman and Kane 1986).

Respite is not intended to be a hospice program for the terminally ill. By virtue of the involvement of respite agencies and aides with a family, the needs of the dying patient and the family must be anticipated and incorporated into a program's care plans. Also, programs for the frail elderly and disabled have found a need for brief respite.

When offered to caregivers of dementia patients, however, brief respite does not seem to be utilized. One reason may be the time needed for these families and patients to adapt to intermittent assistance (Petty 1981; Petty and Wolf 1982–85; Rabbitt 1986).

In addition to start-up costs, respite providers confront other problems. The need for liability insurance poses problems for providers, particularly day care centers and volunteer programs, if such insurance is expensive or not readily available. Legal advisers differ in opinion about an agency's responsibility and liability in sponsoring respite services in the home. Some agencies cannot find and keep enough trained workers. Overall, however, agencies and aides report benefits from offering respite (George 1986). Outreach is particularly needed in services for dementia because many caregivers are socially isolated and community professionals may not be sufficiently aware of the need for and availability of respite care (Schwartz and Dobrof 1987).

Minority Group and Cultural Programs

A frequent and seemingly well-deserved criticism of providers of service to people with dementia and their families is the lack of programs targeted to members of minority groups. Few respite programs are targeted to patients who are black, Spanish-speaking, Asian, or in some other way identified as needing special programming because of their ethnic or cultural background. Even fewer respite programs are established solely for minority clients with a dementing illness. Many programs acknowledge the gaps in services for minority groups and are employing professionals and volunteers who are members of minority populations or speak languages other than English. Some adult day care centers are located in areas of particular ethnic groups. Training and outreach programs are also implemented to reach other agencies or professionals who could serve or refer minority clients.

In the following, three innovative programs that serve minority clients are described. The search for these programs, however, uncovered large gaps in services to minority members with dementia and their families. One service provider in an Asian community said identifying dementia clients is a basic problem; another provider mentioned the need for training about dementia to enhance the experience of the bilingual staff of his geriatric program.

- *Time Off Promotes Strength (T.O.P.S.)*, a program of the Benjamin Rose Institute, is a three-pronged respite program targeted to low income black caregivers of people with Alzheimer's disease or related disorders in Cleveland and some adjacent suburbs. In the first year of the program, 70 percent of the clients were black and half had monthly incomes lower than $1,200. Funded primarily by a grant from the Ohio Department of Aging under the Hobsen Act, T.O.P.S. provides in-home care, day care at a skilled nursing facility, and short-term overnight stays at the same facility. The day care program provides intermediate and skilled levels of care. Thirty hours per month of respite and family-caregiver choice in services received are goals (G. Deimling, pers. com. 1988).

- In Chicago, the *Elderly Support Project* reaches black clients via a home-based caregiver support program and twelve adult day care centers. The program has a behavioral management and training component to deal with difficult behaviors. Although not originally focused solely on dementing illness, more of these clients are now participating (depression and stroke patients are also included). The project is part of the University of Chicago School of Social Services Administration. It also teaches participants to link with community services and to establish or reestablish personal relationships (E. M. Pinkston, pers. com. 1988; Pinkston and Linsk 1984).

- *Altamed Health Services* in East Los Angeles, probably the largest service program in the country serving the Hispanic community, has recently received a state respite care demonstration grant. The project offers a registry of in-home and out-of-home respite care and, in most cases, matches a service with each client. Additionally, Altamed's Adult Day Health Care Center has made provisions for intermittent participation for respite purposes. The agency, which serves a twelve-square mile area, also works with long-term care providers to make respite beds available in board and care homes and skilled nursing facilities. Other California-funded long-term care case management services (Linkages and Multipurpose Senior Service Program) are also located at Altamed. More than 5 percent of Altamed's clients are believed to have dementia, and staff members believe that the number of such clients is increasing. No fees are charged for respite service (P. Ayala, pers. com. 1988).

People with dementia due to acquired immune deficiency syndrome (AIDS) are an emerging subgroup of those with dementing illness. Ultimately, AIDS dementia patients will benefit from the experience gained by providers of specialized respite programs and other services for people with Alzheimer's and similar disorders. Even in San Francisco, however, which currently has the nation's richest service community for people with AIDS, few services exist to meet the dementia-specific needs of patients and caregivers (K. Kelly, pers. com. 1988). It is generally held that persons with AIDS dementia need assistance sooner and have a shorter life expectancy than persons with other dementing illness. Patients are also younger and may have less stable environments than do persons with Alzheimer's or multi-infarct dementia. These assumptions point to a need for programs that can provide earlier intervention and respite over a shorter duration.

In developing programming for persons with varied ethnic and cultural backgrounds, the Brookdale Foundation offers a model worthy of replication. It uses one of the hallmarks of Alzheimer's disease to enhance its day care programs. The tendency of people with a dementing illness to retain long-term memory means that they may remember long-ago spoken languages, songs, and traditions. The foundation developed ethnically related programming such as musical programs, meals of ethnic foods, periods for sharing of "brief glimpses" of participants' reminiscences, and observances of holiday traditions (Schwartz and Dobrof 1987). This mixing of program options with the special characteristics of persons with dementia and those who love them most eloquently defines the possibilities of respite care.

References

California Health and Welfare Agency. Department of Mental Health. 1987. *Regional Resource Centers for Families and Caregivers of Brain-impaired Adults operations manual: Policies and procedures pursuant to the implementation of Chapter 1658.* Sacramento.

Cleland, M. 1984. *Caring that makes a difference: Senior respite care program training program.* Portland, OR: Education and Family Support Services, Good Samaritan Hospital and Medical Center.

Danaher, D., J. Dixon-Bemis, and S. H. Pedersen. 1986. Staffing respite programs: The merits of paid and volunteer staff. In *Developing respite services for the elderly,* ed. R. J. V. Montgomery and J. Prothero, 78–90. Seattle: University of Washington Press.

Dickman, I. R., and R. D. Warren. 1981. *For this respite much thanks: Concepts, guidelines and issues in the development of community respite care services.* New York: United Cerebral Palsy Association, Inc.

Eastman, P., and A. Kane. 1986. *Respite: Helping caregivers keep elderly relatives at home. Guidelines for a program whose time is now.* Washington, DC: National Council of Catholic Women.

Ellis, V. 1986a. Respite in an institution. In *Developing respite services for the elderly,* ed. R. J. V. Montgomery and J. Prothero, 61–68. Seattle: University of Washington Press.

Ellis, V. 1986b. Introducing patients and families to respite. In *Developing respite services for the elderly,* ed. R. J. V. Montgomery and J. Prothero, 69–77. Seattle: University of Washington Press.

Enright, R. B., Jr., and L. Friss. 1987. *Employed caregivers of brain-impaired adults: An assessment of the dual role.* San Francisco: Family Survival Project.

Family Survival Project. 1986–1988. *Annual reports of programs under Chapter 1658 of 1984 for brain-impaired adults and their families.* San Francisco: Family Survival Project.

The Foundation for Long-Term Care. 1983. *Respite care for the frail elderly: A summary report on institutional respite research and operations manual.* Albany, NY: The Foundation for Long-Term Care.

George, L. K. 1986. Respite care: Evaluating a strategy for easing caregiver burden. *Center Reports on Advances in Research* 10 (2). Durham, NC: Center for the Study of Aging and Human Development.

George, L. K., L. P. Gwyther, E. L. Ballard, G. G. Fillenbaum, and E. B. Palmore. 1987. *Respite care use: Predicting length of use and reasons for dropout.* Durham, NC: Center for the Study of Aging and Human Development.

Glenner, J., and D. V. Moses. 1986. *Sharing the caring: Alzheimer's respite aide training manual.* San Diego, CA: Alzheimer's Family Center, Inc.

Harder, P., J. C. Gornick, and M. R. Burt. 1986. Adult day care: Substitute or supplement? *Milbank Quarterly* 64 (3): 414–41.

Illinois Department of Public Health. Office of Health Services. Division of Chronic Diseases. 1986. *Illinois Alzheimer's disease program: Acts, rules and regulations.* Springfield, IL.

Kemper, P., R. Applebaum, and M. Harrigan. 1987. Community care demonstrations: What have we learned? *Health Care Financing Review* 8 (4).

Lidoff, L. 1985. Respite Companion Program model. *Program Innovations in Aging, Volume VII.* Washington, DC: The National Council on the Aging, Inc.

Lindsay/Ferguson Associates. 1984. *The Respite Care Co-op Program.* Kalamazoo, MI: Lindsay/Ferguson Associates.

Mace, N. L., and P. V. Rabins. 1984. *A survey of day care for the demented adult in the United States.* Washington, DC: The National Council on the Aging Inc.

Montgomery, R. J. V. 1986. Researching respite. In *Developing Respite Services for the Elderly,* ed. R. J. V. Montgomery and J. Prothero, 18–32. Seattle: University of Washington Press.

National Center for Health Statistics. G. Strahan. 1987. Nursing home characteristics: Preliminary data from the 1985 National Nursing Home Survey. *Advance Data from Vital and Health Statistics,* No. 131, DHHS Pub. No. (PHS) 87–1250. Hyattsville, MD: Public Health Service.

Oktay, J. S., and P. Volland. 1987. Foster home care for the frail elderly as an alternative to nursing home care: An experimental evaluation. *American Journal of Public Health* 77: 1505–10.

Older Women's League. 1983. *Model legislation for respite care services.* Washington, DC: Older Women's League.

Ory, M. G., T. F. Williams, M. Emr, et al. 1984. *Families, informal supports and Alzheimer's disease: Current research and future agendas.* Working document by the Work Group of Families, Informal Supports, and Alzheimer's Disease, Department of Health and Human Services Task Force on Alzheimer's Disease. Washington, DC.

Pacific Northwest Long-Term Care Center. 1982. *Respite care options for the frail elderly.* Seattle: Pacific Northwest Long-Term Care Center.

Petty, D. 1981. *Annual report of a state pilot project to assist families of brain-damaged family members.* Report for Years 1980–81. San Francisco: Family Survival Project.

Petty, D. 1985. *Family Survival Project: A joint community/state response to an unserved population.* San Francisco: Family Survival Project.

Petty, D., and L. Friss. 1987. A balancing act of working and caregiving. *Business and Health* (October) 22–26.

Petty, D., and A. Wolf. 1982–1985. *Annual report of a state pilot project to assist families of brain-damaged family members.* Reports for Years 1981–82, 1982–83, 1983–84, and 1984–85. San Francisco: Family Survival Project.

Pinkston, E. M., and N. L. Linsk. 1984. *Care of the elderly: A family approach.* New York: Pergamon Press.

Rabbitt, W. J. 1986. The New York Respite Demonstration Program. In *Developing respite services for the elderly,* ed. R. J. V. Montgomery and J. Prothero, 33–49. Seattle: University of Washington Press.

The Robert Wood Johnson Foundation. 1987. *Dementia Care and Respite Services Program: Application guidelines.* Princeton, NJ: The Robert Wood Johnson Foundation.

Schwartz, S. L., and R. Dobrof. 1987. *How to start a respite service for people with Alzheimer's and their families: A guide for community-based organizations,* ed. T. Quinn and J. Crabtree. New York: The Brookdale Foundation and The Brookdale Center on Aging of Hunter College.

Stone, R. 1985. *Recent developments in respite care services for the caregivers of impaired elderly.* San Francisco: Aging Health Policy Center (now Institute for Health and Aging), University of California at San Francisco.

U.S. Congress. Office of Technology Assessment. 1987. *Losing a million minds: Confronting the tragedy of Alzheimer's disease and other dementias.* OTA-BA-

323. Washington, DC: U.S. Government Printing Office. April.

U.S. Department of Health and Human Services. 1981. Respite and crisis care. *Human services bibliography series.* Rockville, MD: Project SHARE.

U.S. Department of Health and Human Services. 1985. *How-to manual on providing respite care for family caregivers.* Rockville, MD: Project SHARE.

Suggested Readings

Ballard, E., and L. P. Gwyther. 1988. *Training in-home respite workers to serve memory impaired older persons.* Durham, NC: Duke Family Support Program, Center for the Study of Aging and Human Development.

Gwyther, L. P., and E. Ballard. 1988. *In-home respite care: A strategy for easing caregiver burden.* Durham, NC: Duke Family Support Program, Center for the Study of Aging and Human Development.

Montgomery, R. J. V., and J. Prothero. 1986. *Developing respite services for the elderly.* Seattle: University of Washington Press.

Panella, J. 1987. *Day care for patients with Alzheimer's disease and related disorders.* New York: Demos Publishers.

Addresses for Publications

Alzheimer's Family Center, Inc. 3686 Fourth Avenue, San Diego, CA 92103

Center for the Study of Aging and Human Development, Duke University Medical Center, Durham, NC 27710

Duke Family Support Program, Center for the Study of Aging and Human Development, Box 3600, Duke University Medical Center, Durham, NC 27710

Education and Family Support Services, Good Samaritan Hospital and Medical Center, 1015 NW 22nd Avenue, Portland, OR 92710

Family Survival Project, 425 Bush Street, San Francisco, CA 94108

Foundation for Long-Term Care, 194 Washington Avenue, Albany, NY 12210

Lindsay/Ferguson Associates, 2324 West Main Street, Kalamazoo, MI 49007

National Council of Catholic Women, 1312 Massachusetts Avenue, NW, Washington, DC 20005

The National Council on the Aging, Inc., 600 Maryland Avenue, SW, West Wing 100, Washington, DC 20024

Older Women's League, 1325 G Street, NW, Lower Level B, Washington, DC 20005

Pacific Northwest Long-Term Care Center, 3935 University Way, NE, JM20, University of Washington, Seattle, WA 98195

Project SHARE, Post Office Box 2309, Rockville, MD 20852

United Cerebral Palsy Association, Inc., 66 East 34th Street, New York, NY 10016

The Wheeler Clinic, Inc., 91 Northwest Drive, Plainville, CT 06062

11

Planning for the Future: Legal and Financial Considerations

DAVID F. CHAVKIN

The onset of dementia has significant implications for the affected individual and for family members. Other chapters discuss the options available to meet the care needs of the relative with dementia. They also focus on the efforts that can be undertaken to strengthen and support the rest of the family. Although these concerns will necessarily dominate a family's attention, there are three specters that may haunt the family as it plans for the future. These three specters are guardianship, probate, and impoverishment.

As the relative with dementia loses the ability to make informed personal and financial decisions, families must often confront the possibility of guardianship over the relative's person and property. Similarly, as the relative with dementia moves into the final stages of the disease, families must consider the nature of that relative's estate and the implications for other family members when the person with dementia dies. Finally, because of the enormous costs of prolonged care for a person with dementia, there is the real possibility that the relative's spouse, children, and others may be impoverished as the disease runs its course.

Although these specters are all too real for many families, there are ways to lessen or avoid their impact. The key is to develop and implement a coherent financial and legal plan as soon as possible.

This chapter reviews some of the considerations that must be addressed and identifies some of the approaches that can be used in developing such a plan. It is not designed to turn the health or social services professional into a lawyer, estate planner, or financial consultant. In many ways, the health or social services professional plays a far more significant role. Other demands on the family may seem far more important and urgent. It is the role of the professional to persuade the family that the time and energy spent on financial and legal planning will be rewarded over the next few years. It is also the role of the professional to help the family find the strength and energy to pursue this effort.

Delay, Denial, and Ineptitude

Just as the families often deny the existence of the symptoms of dementia in a family member and delay taking that relative to a qualified health professional for a diagnostic work-up, so delay and denial may also affect financial and legal planning. Families do not like to think about death or disability and therefore often put off consideration of such issues as powers of attorney and estate planning.

Unfortunately, for most families, the sooner that these issues are addressed, the better off they will be. It is critical for professionals to encourage families to consider legal and financial planning as they begin to address the other emerging issues in their lives. The role of the health or social service professional in this area is to assist and encourage the family in seeking these resources.

The professional may also need to play a role in guiding the family through an obstacle course of misinformation and ineptitude. For example, many families are told that all of their assets will be taken if they apply for Medicaid benefits or that spouses must support husbands or wives. Other families seeking admission to a nursing home are told that they must agree to pay private rates for a period or that their relative will be discharged if Medicaid eligibility is sought. In other instances, a physician may refuse to honor a valid living will.

Ineptitude on the part of the legal or financial professionals may pose even greater risks. All too often, the general practitioner or financial consultant may design a plan for a client with dementia without considering the special impact of the disease on the future needs of the client and family. The outcome may be ineligibility of the client for public benefits and resulting impoverishment of the family.

Almost by default, the health or human service professional will be the one to try to link the family with legal or financial professionals. In this role, word-of-mouth will often be the best tool for identifying both the best and the worst resources available. In more and more communities, qualified professionals already will be working with local Alzheimer's Association chapters or through programs funded under the Older Americans Act. In other areas, however, health or social service professionals will have to do their own investigations.

Moral Norms

Most professionals would not presume to direct a family to institutionalize a relative or to maintain that relative at home. Instead, they would provide the family with all of the information necessary to identify all options clearly. Once a particular option was chosen by the family, the professional would then attempt to assist the family in identifying resources to support that decision.

In the area of financial and legal planning, however, some professionals presume to impose their moral norms on the families with whom they work. For example, some professionals regard estate planning to avoid impoverishment as distasteful. Although the failure to plan may leave a spouse to support a child on less than $4000 a year, such professionals view planning with the Medicaid program's eligibility requirements in mind as immoral.

This chapter takes a very different approach from that perspective. The philosophy of this chapter is that all lawful alternatives should be discussed with the family and person with dementia. An informed choice can then be made among those alternatives.

Identifying the Client

A family seeking assistance may include the person with dementia, that person's child or children, daughters-in-law and sons-in-law, grandchildren, and siblings of that person. Some or all of these individuals may have priorities that conflict with or complement the priorities of other family members.

The health professional may have a difficult time in sorting through these conflicting directions and competing demands. The starting place for nearly all professionals will be at the applicable ethical code of professional responsibility.

Regardless of the source of reimbursement, most such codes require the professional to advocate on behalf of the person with dementia. If the client is able to make an informed judgment, this means advocating the position expressed by the patient or client. Too often the person with dementia is viewed as having lost any legal capacity. That is often not the case.

Even if the person with dementia has significant limitations at some times, because of the variable nature of the disease the individual may still be able to make informed decisions at other times. The professional will necessarily have to seek out the individual at these times (e.g., early mornings) to involve the dementia patient in the planning process to the maximal extent possible.

Even if the person with dementia no longer has the capacity to make an informed decision, that person should not be excluded from the decision-making process. Capacity is ordinarily not an all or nothing proposition. Persons with dementia may still be able to indicate their desires. In addition, persons with dementia may have made oral statements or writings at an earlier stage that indicated their wishes for the future. These will help guide the professional in sorting through competing concerns.

The actual process for the professional will depend on the state involved and the specific discipline of the worker. In some circumstances, the professional may be asked to undertake "substituted judgment" on behalf of the patient. This means that the professional will assume the place of the patient while reaching a decision. In other circumstances, the professional may be asked to act "in the best interests" of the patient. These two formulations may lead to somewhat different results in specific cases.

In undertaking this process, it is also important for the health professional to recognize that family members are not adversaries. It is only in the most infrequent situations that family members place their own interests above those of the patient. In fact, in the vast majority of circumstances, family members subjugate their interests to those of the patient. Most family members simply do not meet the stereotype of placing their parents in nursing homes and stealing their assets. Moreover, in most cases, family members will play a vital role in providing the health professional with the necessary information for identifying the wishes of the client.

Conflicting Considerations

No one plan can serve all needs of all families. Families differ in terms of relationships among family members, and this will influence the options appropriate for that family. The extent and forms of income and resources may also differ significantly. This again will dictate different approaches.

Families must also recognize that the importance of certain values to the family may conflict with other considerations. For example, the desire by parents to maintain full control over their resources may interfere with attempts to avoid probate and to maximize eligibility for government programs that will help avoid impoverishment. Therefore, where possible, I identify countervailing considerations inherent in different approaches.

Guardianship

The Nature of Guardianship

Guardianship (or conservatorship as it is known in some jurisdictions) is a judicial proceeding that permits one person to act in the place of another. It requires a judicial finding that the person over whom the guardianship is sought is not able to make informed decisions because of a disability. This disability can result from one of the forms of dementia.

Guardianship can be ordered over the disabled individual's person and/or property. A guardianship over the property permits the guardian to control the disabled person's income and assets. A guardianship over the person permits the guardian to make other decisions in place of the disabled person.

An individual may be sufficiently disabled to be unable to manage property and affairs effectively, thereby justifying a guardianship over the property. However, that same person may still be able to make appropriate decisions about health care, food, clothing, and shelter. In such a case, only a guardianship over the property would be appropriate.

Guardianship can be either limited or general, depending on the jurisdiction involved. In a jurisdiction with a limited guardianship law, the guardian is permitted to make only the types of decisions specified by the judge in the order granting guardianship. In a general guardianship jurisdiction, the guardian will have a wide variety of powers authorized by state law.

The Problems with Guardianship

Although guardianship is sometimes necessary to meet the needs of a disabled person, it can present major problems for a family. First, it can be expensive because of the need to hire an attorney and be represented through a court hearing. Second, although attempts can be made to lessen this effect, a guardianship proceeding is often viewed as an action against the disabled relative by family members. This may exact a significant emotional toll on the disabled person and the relatives. Third, guardianship takes time. Months may elapse between the filing of the guardianship petition and the issuance of a final order. Fourth, there is an ongoing administrative burden imposed on the family. If a guardianship of the property is ordered, most jurisdictions require the guardian to file periodic reports with the court accounting for the disabled person's estate. In many situations, these problems can be avoided through advance planning and the use of other devices.

Powers of Attorney

To the extent that management of the disabled person's estate is the primary issue, a power of attorney may address all of the family's needs. A power of attorney is a legal document authorizing a person or persons to act on behalf of that individual.

The power of attorney must be executed at a time when the individual is competent. However, this does not mean that the individual must always be able to make informed decisions. It is sufficient if the individual granting the power of attorney is lucid when the document is executed.

The scope of a power of attorney varies somewhat depending on the jurisdiction in which the family resides. In most jurisdictions, a power of attorney can authorize an individual to make decisions only over financial issues. In other jurisdictions, the power of attorney can also authorize an individual to make decisions over medical issues.

The utility of a power of attorney also varies somewhat depending on the jurisdiction. In some jurisdictions, a power of attorney becomes invalid once the individual granting the power of attorney no longer has the ability to revoke it. In such states, the power of attorney becomes useless at the very time that it will be most needed.

However, most jurisdictions have now authorized a "durable" power of attorney. A "durable" power of attorney is one that survives the disability of the person who executed it. Such a power of attorney contains explicit language indicating that the power of attorney is to stay in effect even if the individual loses the ability to revoke it because of physical or mental disabilities.

If a durable power of attorney has been granted to a spouse or children, there is seldom any need for guardianship of the property. The power of attorney will instead authorize those individuals to take necessary actions enumerated in the power of attorney with regard to the property of the person executing the power of attorney.

Powers of attorney are inexpensive to obtain and do not even require the services of an attorney. They can be executed with a minimum of legal formality and with a minimum expenditure of time and resources. The key, however, is that they must be executed sufficiently early so that the grantor will still understand the consequences of the action.

The negative aspects of a power of attorney are a direct result of its relative informality. Because there is no ongoing court supervision, there is a greater potential for abuse than with guardianships. Powers of attorney are therefore most appropriate when trust is fully warranted.

Substitute Consent

One of the most common reasons for seeking guardianship of the person is the need for consent to a medical procedure. Where an individual is unable to give informed consent to a medical procedure, a guardian of the person may be appointed to give that consent.

Because of the time and expense involved in this process, a number of states have developed a different procedure for obtaining consent to medical procedures. This procedure involves the designation by state law of a list of relatives who can give consent to a medical procedure in the place of a disabled individual. This list ordinarily extends, in decreasing order of priority, from the spouse of the disabled individual to the adult grandchildren.

Living Wills

Another of the problems that frequently gives rise to the need for a guardian of the person is the situation where an individual cannot give informed consent to the nonimposition or to the removal of resuscitators or other heroic measures. In such instances, a health care provider will frequently be unwilling to allow an individual to die without such measures for fear of later liability.

A number of states have attempted to address this problem through legislative recognition of living wills. A living will is a document voluntarily executed by an individual when competent that directs health care providers not to utilize life-sustaining procedures that will only artificially extend the dying process. Generally, a living will authorizes only the administration of medication, the provision of food and water, and the performance of any medical procedure that is necessary to provide comfort or care or to alleviate pain.

Ordinarily, state statutes require that the individual executing the living will satisfy certain formal requirements, such as the inclusion of witnesses. However, once the living will meets these requirements, health care providers are generally required to implement it and can be held liable if they do not. Similarly, they are immunized from liability for following the living will.

For those individuals who believe in the concept of "death with dignity," the living will provides a tool for requiring others to honor that belief. A living will can also free family members from difficult decisions and can avoid the need for a medical guardianship proceeding.

Probate

Another of the specters to avoid is the need for probate. Probate is the process whereby an individual's estate is divided among persons designated by the decedent to receive specified shares of the estate or, in the absence of such designation, among persons designated by state law. A person designates heirs through a will. A person who dies without a will is commonly referred to as dying intestate.

The problems with the probate process are similar to those with guardianship. Probate ordinarily requires the assistance of an attorney. It is frequently very costly as a result. It also often drags on for years.

Although the available approaches to avoiding probate go far beyond the scope of this chapter, there are certain methods that can be reviewed. The approach used will take on special importance when the specter of impoverishment is discussed.

Joint Tenancy

One of the easiest ways to avoid probate is to place property in joint tenancy with right of survivorship. When real or personal property is held in such a joint tenancy, the death of one joint tenant places the entire property in the ownership of the other joint tenant or tenants. Generally, only a copy of the death certificate for the deceased joint tenant is required to modify the title to the property.

A similar result is achieved in some jurisdictions through a device called tenancy by the entirety. This is really a special type of joint tenancy with right of survivorship that is used when the property is owned by a husband and wife. In other jurisdictions, this is simply included as a type of joint tenancy with right of survivorship.

These two approaches are not for everybody. If an individual does not have confidence in the other party, joint tenancy should be avoided because either joint tenant can gain access to the entire property. Similarly, a property placed in joint tenancy by a parent with a child can be reached by the creditors of that child. Despite these disadvantages, between most husbands and wives and between most parents and children joint tenancy may provide a simple and cost-effective way to transfer property while avoiding probate.

Trusts

A trust is a legal arrangement whereby one person holds specified property for the benefit of another person. The person administering the property is ordinarily called the trustee. The person for whose benefit the property is being held is ordinarily called the beneficiary. The person who establishes the trust is referred to as the settlor, grantor, or donor.

Trusts can be created in two ways. A trust that is created while the grantor is alive is called an inter vivos or living trust. A trust that is created upon the death of the grantor is called a testamentary trust.

One purpose of a trust is to set aside certain assets for the care of a disabled person. The trustee can then authorize expenditures from the trust income or principal to meet the living expenses and service needs of the disabled beneficiary.

Another purpose of a trust is to set aside certain assets that will be available to a beneficiary when alive, but that will pass upon the death of the beneficiary to the settlor, to the settlor's estate, or to specified other persons. In this way, a trust instrument can be another device for avoiding probate.

One common use of trusts has been limited by Congress. Discretionary or restricted trusts are types of trusts in which use of the trust principal and income is controlled by the trust instrument. In a discretionary trust, for example, the trust principal and income are spent at the sole discretion of the trustee for the benefit of the beneficiary.

Such discretionary or restricted trusts are generally exempt from consideration by the various states in assessing charges for state-funded services. Such trusts were also traditionally exempt from consideration in determining an applicant's Medicaid eligibility. Because of changes in federal law, however, some discretionary trusts (referred to as Medicaid-qualifying trusts) are no longer exempt from consideration. Other approaches must therefore be utilized to preserve assets and maximize Medicaid eligibility.

Effect on Financial Entitlements

Many lawyers engage in estate planning for families. Unfortunately, not all such lawyers are equally skilled in this service. This is especially true where eligibility for a government entitlement program may be at issue. This problem is discussed further in the next section, but one example may highlight the problem.

Frequently, when a husband and wife are still alive, a lawyer may advise them to place everything in joint tenancy. This approach ensures that either spouse can gain access to the bank accounts and other marital property. In addition, on the death of one spouse, the title to the property will be automatically vested in the other.

Although this approach may achieve basic estate planning goals, it may ensure that the family will be impoverished if one spouse requires long term nursing home care. In such a situation, the institutionalized spouse will be ineligible for Medicaid until nearly all of the assets have been used for the costs of care. Only at that time will Medicaid eligibility be available to the institutionalized spouse. Unfortunately, by that time the noninstitutionalized spouse will have no assets on which to live. That outcome can be avoided with some effective advance planning.

Impoverishment

Impoverishment of a family including a member with dementia usually occurs for three reasons. First, dementia may prevent a wage earner from continuing in employment. The family may thereby lose a salary that is needed to meet the costs of shelter, food, and clothing for the family. Second, dementia may prevent a family member from performing such noncompensated services as the care of children in the home. In this case, the family will be forced to incur costs to meet these needs. Third, the costs of caring for a family member with dementia are significant. In the absence of third-party coverage for these costs, nearly all lower and middle class families will become impoverished if these services are needed over an extended period.

Again, advance planning and immediate action will be critical if impoverishment is to be avoided. In addition, several of the potential solutions require a high level of persistence on the part of the family. Although this may be difficult in light of the other demands on the family, the potential financial and other benefits are substantial.

Income Support Programs

There are a number of income support programs that may be available to replace lost earnings of a disabled wage earner. The specific programs available to the family depend on the circumstances of the wage earner and the jurisdiction in which the family resides.

Disability Insurance

The first type of income support that may be available is a private short- or long-term disability insurance policy. These policies are most often available on a group basis through an employer, but may also be purchased on an individual basis.

A short-term disability policy is designed to provide income support for a short period (generally not more than one year) after the person becomes disabled. This is designed to fill in the gap before Social Security or other benefits can begin. The payment level is usually a fixed percentage of the individual's earned income when she or he became disabled.

A long-term disability policy is designed to provide income support over a prolonged period after a waiting period. The waiting period may be thirty, sixty, or ninety days or some other period specified in the policy. This kind of policy is designed to provide long-term income support to the family regardless of the availability of such other benefits as Social Security.

Disability insurance policies are usually very inexpensive and represent a good investment for many working families. Although advance planning is preferable, some policies, especially those offered on a group basis, may have a very short exclusionary period for preexisting conditions. Thus, a family may still be able to buy some income protection even after the onset of the symptoms of dementia.

Social Security Benefits

Another program that can assist a family in these circumstances is the Social Security program. Although commonly thought of as a single program, Social Security actually has several parts. These parts are reflected in the initials OASDHI.

The OA part of *OASDHI* is the program of income support for former workers and certain dependents who are at least sixty-two years of age ("old age"). This is the part of the program frequently referred to as Social Security retirement benefits. If the disabled person is at least sixty-two years of age and is not receiving Social Security benefits already, an application should be immediately filed.

The S part of OASDHI is the program of income support for the survivors of deceased workers. Although this will be of no assistance while the disabled former wage earner is alive, it may provide needed benefits for the family later, especially if there are still young children in the home.

The HI part of OASDHI is the program of health insurance or Medicare benefits. This will be discussed in a later section.

The D part of OASDHI is the program of income support for disabled workers. To be eligible, wage earners must have become disabled when they had worked at least twenty of the previous forty calendar quarters. The wage earner must also be no longer able to engage in any substantial gainful activity by reason of a medically determinable physical or mental impairment that will result in death or that has lasted or will last for at least twelve months.

The Social Security disability program presents several problems for applicants with dementia. First, because of the requirement that the impairment be "medically determinable" and the fact that many diagnoses of dementia are made by exclusion, it may be difficult for the applicant to demonstrate that the impairment exists. This is especially true with such forms of dementia as Alzheimer's disease.

Second, because the functioning levels of many persons with dementia fluctuate widely, especially in the early stages of the disease, applicants may not be able to demonstrate disability at a time when they still meet the twenty/forty requirement of connection to the labor force. This is especially true where the applicant may be examined by a consultative medical examiner for only thirty minutes. That examiner may observe none of the problems that family members must confront on a daily basis.

Third, applicants with dementia must deal with the same problems as those faced by applicants with other disabilities. Too many persons are denied on initial application and give up in the process. Only through persistence and the exercise of appeal rights can the odds be shifted in favor of the applicant. Again, the lesson is to not give up too easily.

After an initial denial, an applicant can request a reconsideration. This is a paper review by an individual not involved in the previous determination. Additional medical and social documentation can be submitted at this stage.

If an applicant is denied on reconsideration, a hearing before an administrative law judge can be requested. This is ordinarily an applicant's best chance to overturn a denial. Chances of winning are increased if the applicant is assisted at the hearing by a lawyer or paralegal. Nearly half of the hearings are decided in favor of the beneficiary.

An individual who is denied at the hearing stage may request review by the Appeals Council. Judicial review is also available in the federal courts.

Welfare Programs

In addition to the Social Security program, which is a social insurance program, there are a number of welfare programs that may be of assistance. The common element of these welfare programs is that they are all programs subject to "means tests." Only persons with insufficient means will be assisted. By contrast, the Social Security program generally pays benefits regardless of the financial means of the beneficiary.

The major welfare program available to people with dementia is the Supplemental Security Income (SSI) program. The SSI program provides financial assistance to low-income aged, blind, and disabled persons throughout the United States. It is administered by the Social Security Administration. Aged persons must be at least sixty-five years of age; disabled persons must meet Social Security disability criteria.

There are two major differences between the SSI and the OASDHI programs. No work history is required to qualify for SSI, unlike OASDHI. Strict income and resource criteria are applied under SSI, which are inapplicable under OASDHI.

The benefit levels under the SSI program vary somewhat depending on the state or territory involved. Most states provide most recipients with only the federal benefit. However, some states supplement the federal benefit with an additional state-funded benefit.

Another welfare program that can provide needed income support is aid to families with dependent children (AFDC or ADC). Although dementia ordinarily affects persons later in life, a family including children under the age of eighteen may be aided under the AFDC program. The AFDC program is administered by the various states and territories ordinarily through local or county departments of social services or welfare. Federal funding is available to meet part of the costs of assistance in those states meeting federal criteria.

The third major welfare program available to assist people with dementia is the general assistance (or home relief or general public assistance) program. The general assistance program is funded solely with state and/or local appropriations. Eligibility criteria are extremely restrictive, and grant levels are very limited. However, for those families that cannot meet SSI or AFDC eligibility standards, general assistance may be the only program available.

Health Insurance Programs

The costs of health services required to care for a person with dementia can bankrupt most families. These costs can be avoided somewhat through third-party coverage. The problem for many families is that their third-party insurance coverage is usually not up to the task ahead. Most health insurance programs do not cover the very services required by an individual with dementia. Even covered services may be subjected to extensive cost-sharing. (For a discussion of Veteran's Administration benefits, see Chapters 12 and 15.)

Private Health Insurance

Most Americans have at least some health insurance coverage. Many of these policies are group policies paid for at least in part by employers. Other policies are purchased by individual families. These policies differ widely in terms of services covered and reimbursement available.

One of the first things that a family should do is to assess the coverage that will be available under their policies. These policies will ordinarily be of significant value to persons who need reimbursement for diagnostic services, for medications, and for acute care. However, most families are surprised to discover that nursing home services required by people with dementia are not covered. Other services that are commonly excluded are personal care services, respite care services, and adult day care services. At the same time, such services as inpatient hospital care, which are not of major importance for people with dementia, are fully covered.

Another factor that can impoverish a family is the extent of reimbursement available under the policies. Most policies require three types of cost-sharing. A deductible excludes coverage until a specified level of medical bills is incurred (e.g., hospital coverage after the first day of hospitalization). A co-insurance requirement limits insurance coverage to only a specified percentage of the costs of care (e.g., 80 percent of all covered physician services). A copayment requires a policy holder to pay a specified amount for each type of service received (e.g., $1 per prescribed drug).

Efforts are under way throughout the insurance industry to explore new policies that can address the long-term care needs of people with dementia. At present, however, these policies are very costly and do not provide enough coverage to meet the needs of most families. Private health insurance therefore remains a resource that is not particularly relevant to the long-term care needs of people with dementia.

Medicare

The Medicare program is a social insurance program linked to Social Security eligibility. Medicare coverage is automatically provided to people at least sixty-five years of age who receive Social Security old age benefits. Medicare coverage is also available for people who have been receiving Social Security disability benefits for at least twenty-four consecutive months.

Medicare coverage includes two parts—Parts A and B. Part A (known as the Hospital Insurance Program) covers hospital, nursing home, and home health care. Part B (known as the Supplementary Medical Insurance Program) covers physician and related outpatient services.

As a result of the Medicare Catastrophic Coverage Act, unlimited hospital days and increased skilled nursing home days are available under Part A. Also as a result of the Act, a cap has been placed on the amount of Part B expenses that must be paid by beneficiaries and the scope of Part B services has been expanded to cover certain costs of prescription drugs. Eighty hours of respite care per year has also been added as a Part B benefit. To finance these expansions, a new supplemental premium has been imposed on most persons eligible for Medicare Part A. This supplemental premium is computed on a sliding scale based on federal income tax liability.

Although nursing home care is a covered service under the Medicare program, the limitations on this coverage render it useless for most beneficiaries with dementia. The Medicare program excludes all custodial care from coverage. Most nursing home care required by a person with dementia is characterized as custodial by the Medicare program, so little coverage is actually authorized.

However, those persons with dementia who require skilled nursing care are entitled to Medicare coverage. In addition, persons with dementia and other conditions may qualify for skilled care on the basis of other conditions. The key, as with other OASDHI benefits, is to pursue appeal rights through at least the hearing stage.

Similar problems arise with regard to home health and physical therapy services. These services may be needed to help maintain an individual at home. However, these services will generally only maintain the functioning level of a person with dementia or may retard deterioration in these skills. Because they will not "cure" the person with dementia, coverage is often denied on the ground that the service is not active care and treatment.

A different problem arises with physician services. Physician services are reimbursed under Medicare at 80 percent of the physician's approved fee. This fee is ordinarily substantially below the level actually charged by the physician. As a result, a Medicare beneficiary must ordinarily pay not only 20 percent of the approved fee, but also the difference between the approved fee and the actual physician charge. The only exception is when the physician agrees to accept the Medicare-allowable fee as payment in full. This is known as accepting assignment. Only a small percentage of all beneficiaries are able to find physicians willing to treat them on this basis.

Although the Medicare program is extremely important for many older and disabled Americans, the limitations under the program reduce its importance for most persons with dementia. Unfortunately, many families believe that the Medicare program will protect them from financial catastrophe. The actual experiences of many families demonstrate the necessity of not relying on Medicare.

Medicaid

The Medicaid program is a social welfare program linked to eligibility under the SSI and AFDC programs. It has become the most important third party payment source for long-term care of people with dementia.

Everyone eligible for AFDC benefits automatically receives Medicaid coverage. In most states, everyone receiving SSI benefits also receives Medicaid coverage. However, a separate application is sometimes required.

In addition to recipients of cash welfare benefits, many states extend eligibility to other groups. Although eligibility varies widely from state to state, two optional groups are commonly aided. The first of these is the nursing home cap population. The second is the medically needy.

Under the nursing home cap option, a state can provide Medicaid for individuals who have too much income to qualify for SSI benefits, but who live in a nursing home. In such cases, the state can use a higher income standard, called the nursing home cap, to determine eligibility. An individual with income under that cap who is otherwise eligible for SSI can then qualify for Medicaid coverage. After limited set-asides for a spouse and children living at home, the individual must pay over all of his or her income to the nursing home, other than a small personal needs allowance. The State then pays for the remaining costs of care in the nursing home.

The medically needy option is presently used by more than half the states. However, not all states cover aged and disabled persons under the medically needy programs. In a state with a comprehensive medically needy program, all individuals who would be eligible for SSI benefits but for excess income can qualify for Medicaid coverage if they incur sufficient medical expenses. Any income in excess of the state-established medically needy income level, after allowable income disregards, becomes the applicant's spend-down liability. Once the applicant has incurred sufficient medical expenses to meet that liability, Medicaid coverage will be available to pay for additional medical bills incurred during the eligibility period for services covered under the state plan.

Although the nursing home cap and medically needy options are important financial resources for people with dementia and their families, there are numerous factors that limit their impact. Some of these factors can be avoided by careful planning; other factors are inherent in the scope of the programs.

First, the financial eligibility standards for Medicaid are extremely restrictive in most states. In many states an individual cannot have more than approximately $2,000 in nonexempt assets. The major exempt asset is a home occupied by the applicant, a spouse, or a dependent child. In some states, an individual cannot have more than approximately $100 in income per month.

Second, although the Medicaid program generally treats a nursing home resident as separate from other family members, serious problems can arise if the noninstitutionalized spouse or children do not have their own sources of income. Under current Medicaid law, a noninstitutionalized spouse with no other sources of income will be allocated one-half of the couple's total assets up to $12,000. States, at their option, can allocate increased amounts as long as the noninstitutionalized spouse is not left with more than $60,000 in nonexempt assets. Income may also be allocated from the institutionalized spouse to the noninstitutionalized spouse as long as the total monthly income of the noninstitutionalized spouse does not exceed $1,500 per month.

Both of these asset and income limitations may be superseded by court orders for support of the at-home spouse. However, most individuals are reluctant to sue their institutionalized spouses for support, and the amounts mandated by the federal law will ordinarily be inadequate to maintain current standards of living.

Third, there is a strong bias under the Medicaid program toward institutionalization of an individual with dementia. Services required to maintain an individual in the community (such as respite care, adult day care, and personal care) are optional services not covered in many states. In addition, the separation of the income and assets of an institutionalized spouse and a noninstitutionalized spouse (beginning with the first day of the first full month of institutionalization) does not apply if the spouses are living together.

However, despite all of these limitations, Medicaid is more and more frequently the payment source of final resort for a family. Approximately two-thirds of the residents of nursing homes nationwide receive Medicaid reimbursement for at least part of their costs of care. The percentage of residents who will receive Medicaid reimbursement for at least part of their stay in a nursing home is even higher because of the speed at which even substantial estates can be exhausted by the high costs of nursing home care. The key then is planning around the availability of Medicaid reimbursement so as to preserve sufficient income for the nondisabled spouse and children, if any.

The major complicating factor in this process is the Medicaid transfer of assets prohibition. Ordinarily, it is excess resources, not income, that make a family ineligible. A family with relatively high income can be eligible for Medicaid if it has sufficient medical expenses. By contrast, a family with extremely limited resources may be ineligible because of the low resource limits.

To prevent applicants from transferring assets to other family members for less than fair consideration for the purpose of establishing Medicaid eligibility, Medicaid law penalizes all transfers of nonexempt assets within thirty months of applying for assistance. Transfers of exempt assets, however, are not prohibited. This includes a transfer of the applicant's home to the spouse, a child under 21, or a blind or disabled adult child. Transfers more than thirty months before applying for assistance are also not penalized. This time limit becomes a key element of any planning.

Another common problem arises when spouses living in the community are informed that they must support their institutionalized spouses receiving Medicaid reimbursement. Policies in this area vary greatly from state to state, but spousal responsibility is not enforced in most jurisdictions. Because this issue is in flux nationally, spouses should be advised to seek competent legal representation before such actions as divorce are undertaken.

Social Service Programs

In addition to the income support and health insurance programs discussed, there are also several social service programs available to help meet the needs of people with dementia and their families. These programs are also generally "means-tested," but have eligibility criteria that are more liberal than the social welfare programs. Thus, a family may be ineligible for SSI or Medicaid benefits, but may still be able to qualify for some assistance.

The Social Services Block Grant is a federal law that provides grants to states to provide services pursuant to an approved state plan. Although many social services state plans have tended to focus on families with children or on the mentally alert disabled and elderly, more and more plans cover some needed services for persons with dementia. These services may include attendant care, homemaker chore services, respite care, adult day care, and similar services essential to maintaining a disabled family member in the community. The program is generally administered by a state welfare or social services agency through local or county departments.

The Older Americans Act also provides federal funding to states for social services. Whereas the Social Services Block Grant is primarily directed at low-income persons, the Older Americans Act provides assistance to persons over the age of sixty. Again, however, some income and resource criteria must generally be met to qualify for services. The program is ordinarily administered through a state office on aging and area agencies on aging.

As with the Social Services Block Grant, many state plans have tended to exclude people with dementia. However, more and more services are now being provided for families including people with dementia. These services may include respite care, minor home modifications, nutritional services, and day care. In addition, legal services to the elderly are funded under the Act. These specialized legal services programs can be a major source of assistance for families in undertaking the planning described in this chapter.

The Legal Services Corporation Act is also an important source of legal assistance. The Act provides funding for state, county, and local programs to serve low-income residents. These programs may be known as legal aid societies or legal services programs. In general, they are extremely proficient at providing representation with regard to financial entitlements and similar issues.

Putting It All Together

The next step is to put all of these considerations into place in a coherent financial and legal plan for the family. The following discussion describes how such a plan might be developed.

Drawing the Family Tree

The first step in the process is to get a clear picture of the family members and their individual situations. Age, health status, marital status, and sources of income are critical factors if an effective plan is to be developed. In which children do the parents have confidence? Which children might have special needs that should be addressed? These questions must be asked and answered.

Identifying Income and Assets

The next step is to identify all sources of income available to the individual with dementia and the family. Special issues, such as the effect of death on a payment source, must also be investigated. For example, certain pensions provide for continued payments to the spouse of the deceased worker for a specified period and at a specified level.

A similar review must be made of all assets. Here the focus is not merely on the amount of the asset and its form, but also on the title or ownership of the asset and any limitations or penalties that may be incurred if the asset is transferred.

Working It Through

With these factors in mind, we can see how a coherent legal and financial plan might be developed.

John and Mary have two daughters, Amy and Sue. John is in generally good health and is seventy-one years old. Mary has Alzheimer's disease and is sixty-seven years old. Mary is living at home, but her needs have increased to such an extent over the past year that John is not certain that he can continue to care for her at home.

John and Mary own the house in which they are living. It is worth approximately $80,000 with a $10,000 mortgage still outstanding. Title to the house is in both names. They also own stocks, bonds, and certificates of deposit worth approximately $60,000. These stocks, bonds, and certificates of deposit are also in joint ownership.

John receives Social Security retirement benefits of $550 per month. Mary receives Social Security retirement benefits of $300 per month. John also receives a small pension of $210 per month.

Amy lives in the same city as John and Mary. She is married with one child. Amy has a close relationship with John and Mary. Sue lives in another state. She has a history of emotional problems that interfere with her ability to work and manage her affairs. She is single and receives Social Security disability benefits. She occasionally comes home for holidays but has little other contact with her parents.

Because it seems that Mary will need nursing home care in the near future, the primary question is how to establish Medicaid eligibility for Mary. Although Mary's income is low enough to make her financially eligible, the resources to which she has access would make her ineligible.

In considering resources, the house is not a problem. As long as John continues to live there, the house is an exempt asset for purposes of Medicaid eligibility. We should, however, consider as part of the estate plan what will happen to the house when John dies. This will be especially important if John should predecease Mary because we do not want title to the house to vest in Mary while she is in the nursing home. Because at that point it would not be occupied by her, by her spouse, or by a dependent child, it would not be exempt and would make her ineligible.

The immediate problem is the liquid assets. Most states limit eligibility to people with nonexempt resources of less than $2,000, so Mary is significantly over the limit. As the need for nursing home care is relatively imminent, transferring the assets to her husband may not be the best approach; this would result in her ineligibility for at least thirty months (and potentially longer in some states).

The first step might be to take $10,000 of the cash assets and pay off the remaining mortgage on the house. Because John and Mary do not have high incomes, the tax deductibility of the mortgage interest is probably not important. Moreover, most of the payments by this time are principal rather than interest. In this way, we can convert a nonexempt asset into an exempt asset without wasting any of it.

The next step could be to split the remaining assets ($60,000 minus $10,000) down the middle. Instead of each spouse being a joint owner of all of the stocks, bonds, and certificates, each spouse would own one-half of the liquid assets. Eligibility for Medicaid would then not be affected.

If this approach is used, Mary would have approximately $25,000 ($50,000/2) in assets in her name. (If the state in which John and Mary live permits the noninstitutionalized spouse to receive even more assets, more than half of the assets may be transferred to John, the noninstitutionalized spouse.) She would use these assets to pay for her costs of care until her assets fell below $2,000. At that point, she would convert from private-pay status in the nursing home to Medicaid reimbursement. This will probably occur in less than twelve months based on average nursing home costs.

Another approach would be immediately to transfer all of the assets into John's name. This approach recognizes that John's income is probably not going to be sufficient to support him in the community without interest and dividends from the liquid assets. This approach would probably require John and Mary to forego Medicaid eligibility for thirty months. During this period, John would have to utilize adult day care, personal care, respite care, and similar services to meet Mary's needs at home. Whether John would come out better under this approach would necessarily depend on some projection of Mary's condition and likely needs over the next few years.

Whatever assets are placed in John's name should be arranged to avoid probate. If he has sufficient confidence in Amy, he could simply give the liquid assets to her with the understanding that he would utilize them while he is alive. A more formal approach would be to place the liquid assets in joint tenancy with Amy with right of survivorship. Again, there would have to be some understanding that one-half of the assets would be used to support Sue after John's death.

John could utilize a more formal approach. He could place half of the assets in joint tenancy with Amy and the other half in an inter vivos trust. John would continue to have access to the trust funds while he is alive. This is known as a life estate. On his death, the remaining principal in the trust would be used to support Sue in the form of a discretionary trust with Amy as trustee.

With regard to the house, steps should also be taken to deal with it while John is alive. By transferring it to John while he is residing in the house, the transfer is an exempt transfer under Medicaid law. Once transferred, John can later transfer title to the house to Amy or can make some other arrangement.

A second approach for the house would be a transfer to Sue. Because Sue receives Social Security disability benefits, she qualifies as a disabled adult child. The house could even be placed in a spend-thrift trust for Sue's benefit (perhaps with Amy as trustee) without having any impact on Medicaid eligibility.

A third approach would be for John to sell the house to Amy. Amy and her husband might be able to use the tax advantages (deductibility of depreciation, interest, taxes, and maintenance costs) of the house, which they would then rent back at fair market value to John. John would finance the purchase at commercially reasonable terms to Amy and her husband. John's will might also provide that any remaining balance on the loan would be forgiven upon his death.

All of these transfers would be expedited by having John and Mary sign durable powers of attorney. These powers of attorney could permit John and Amy to act on behalf of Mary and Amy to act on behalf of John. If these durable powers of attorney were not already in existence, the attorney working with John and Mary would attempt to have them executed at a time when Mary was lucid and appreciated the nature of the document.

Conclusion

This example gives some sense of the factors that would be considered and the approaches that could be utilized in planning for a family that includes a member with dementia. The role of service providers in this process would be to assist the family in recognizing the need for timely and effective action and to assist the family in linking up with legal and other assistance to develop and implement a coherent plan.

Probably the most important role that service providers can play, however, is to give the family a sense that all is not hopeless. As dark as things may look and as difficult as the years ahead may be, there are steps that can be taken to make the situation better. The key is finding the strength and energy to take those steps.

III THE COMMUNITY

12

Formal Long-Term Care Services and Settings

KATIE MASLOW, M.S.W.

Long-term care for people with dementia necessarily involves supervision, personal care, and assistance with activities of daily living. Family and friends provide this care informally for most people with dementia, but some patients have no family or friends who are able and willing to provide care. Many other patients require formal or paid services beyond the care that family and friends can give.

In addition to supervision and personal care, a variety of medical, social, rehabilitative, legal, and financial services may be needed (see Table 12.1). Most of these services can be provided in any of a number of settings—the patient's home, community agencies such as adult day care centers, or residential settings such as nursing homes and board and care facilities. Because of the lengthy course of most diseases that cause dementia, patients generally require care for a prolonged period. Because many such diseases are progressive, each patient may require different kinds of care at different stages of the illness to correspond to changes in level of functioning.

Formal long-term care services for people with dementia are provided primarily by the public and private agencies that serve elderly people. The services are funded in part by federal, state, and local government, in part by out-of-pocket payments by patients and their families, and in part by charitable contributions.

We have no comprehensive long-term care policy in this country, and the services that are available for all kinds of patients vary greatly from state to state and in different jurisdictions of the same state. Overlapping services and gaps in services are common, and there is often no reliable source of information about what services are avail-

TABLE 12.1   Care Services for People with Dementia

Physician services: Diagnosis and ongoing medical care, including prescribing
   medications and treatment intercurrent illness

Patient assessment: Evaluation of the individual's physical, mental, and
   emotional status; behavior; and social supports

Skilled nursing: Medically oriented care provided by a licensed nurse, including
   monitoring acute and unstable medical conditions; assessing care needs;
   supervising medications, tube and intravenous feeding, and personal care
   services; and treating bed sores and other conditions

Physical therapy: Rehabilitative treatment provided by a physical therapist

Occupational therapy: Treatment to improve functional abilities; provided by an
   occupational therapist

Speech therapy: Treatment to improve or restore speech; provided by a speech
   therapist

Personal care: Assistance with basic self-care activities such as bathing, dressing,
   getting out of bed, eating, and using the bathroom

Home health aide services: Assistance with health-related tasks, such as
   medications, exercises, and personal care

Homemaker services: Household services, such as cooking, cleaning, laundry, and
   shopping, and escort service to accompany patients to medical appointments
   and elsewhere

Chore services: Household repairs, yard work, and errands

Supervision: Monitoring an individual's whereabouts to ensure safety

Paid companion/sitter: An individual who comes to the home to provide
   supervision, personal care, and socialization during the absence of the
   primary caregiver

Congregate meals: Meals provided in a group setting for people who may benefit
   both from the nutritionally sound meal and from social, educational, and
   recreational services provided at the setting

Home-delivered meals: Meals delivered to the home for individuals who are
   unable to shop or cook for themselves.

Telephone reassurance: Regular telephone calls to individuals who are isolated and
   often homebound

Personal emergency response systems: Telephone-based systems to alert others that
   an individual who is alone is experiencing an emergency and needs
   assistance

Transportation: Transporting people to medical appointments, community
   facilities, and elsewhere

Recreational services: Physical exercise, art and music therapy, parties,
   celebrations, and other social and recreational activities

Mental health services: Psychosocial assessment and individual and group
   counseling to address psychological and emotional problems of patients and
   families

Adult day care: A program of medical and social services, including socialization,
   activities, and supervision, provided in an outpatient setting

TABLE 12.1 (continued)

Dental services: Care of the teeth and diagnosis and treatment of dental problems

Legal services: Assistance with legal matters, such as advance directives, guardianship, power of attorney, and transfer of assets

Protective services: Social and law enforcement services to prevent, eliminate, or remedy the effects of physical and emotional abuse or neglect

Case management: Client assessment, identification and coordination of community resources, and follow-up monitoring of client adjustment and service provision

Information and referral: Provision of written or verbal information about community agencies, services, and funding sources

Hospice services: Medical, nursing, and social services to provide support and alleviate suffering for dying persons and their families

Respite care: Short-term, in- or outpatient services intended to provide temporary relief for the primary caregiver; respite care can include personal care, supervision, and many of the other services listed above

Source: U.S. Congress Office of Technology Assessment 1987.

able in a community (U.S. Congress, Office of Technology Assessment 1987). Thus, what is sometimes referred to as "the long-term care system" is, in most communities, not a system at all but rather a patchwork of services with many holes in it (Cohen et al. 1983).

Some long-term care facilities and agencies have developed special services for persons with dementia and, in some communities, public or private agencies and individual health care or social service providers offer specialized counseling and referral services to help families and others locate appropriate long-term care services for dementia patients. In general, however, specialized services are not available. Although such services will probably increase in coming years, it is unlikely that they will serve more than a fraction of all persons with dementia.

As a result, most dementia patients and their families face all of the same problems as other elderly and physically or mentally impaired persons who need long-term care: lack of needed services in many communities; lack of information about available services; lack of coordination among long-term care agencies; poor quality of care provided by some agencies; and inadequate third-party funding for needed services.

In addition, some pervasive characteristics of existing services are particularly inappropriate for dementia patients.

- Existing services generally focus on medical and skilled nursing care needs as opposed to the personal care and social service needs that are more common among dementia patients.
- Existing services focus almost exclusively on discrete physical care needs as opposed to the ongoing supervision that is often needed by people with dementia.
- Existing services are primarily intended to address specific needs of the patient as opposed to supporting the family or others who are caring for the patient.
- Mental health services for patients or their families are seldom available.

These characteristics of long-term care services reflect the focus and intent of the federal programs that fund long-term care. They not only hamper the efforts of families and other to locate and arrange services for persons with dementia but also obstruct efforts of health care and social service providers to develop and maintain appropriate services for these patients.

Federal Programs That Fund Long-Term Care

About eighty federal programs provide or pay for some long-term care services, either directly or indirectly, but six programs—Medicare, Medicaid, Supplemental Security Income (SSI), the Social Services Block Grant, Title III of the Older Americans Act, and Veterans Administration Programs—are the main sources of support. Medicare, Medicaid, SSI, the Social Service Block Grant, and Title III of the Older Americans Act are discussed in Chapter 11.

The Veterans Administration (VA) provides long-term care for eligible veterans in 116 VA nursing homes, in sixteen large domiciliary care facilities, in state veterans' homes across the country, and under contract in community nursing homes and board and care facilities. As of 1985, home care services were provided at forty-nine of the 172 VA Medical Centers, and adult day care was provided at nine medical centers (Mather and Abel 1986). Respite care is provided at twelve centers (VA 1984).

Federal programs pay for a large portion of long-term care services, and federal regulations that govern these programs play a significant role in defining and structuring long-term care services overall. Some programs, such as the Social Services Block Grant, leave decisions about who is eligible and what services are covered primarily to the states, but Medicare, Medicaid, and the VA all have federally mandated eligibility, coverage, and payment requirements. In addition, each has requirements for the facilities and agencies that are certified to provide covered services. Thus, program regulations determine not only who is eligible, what services are covered, and how much is paid for them, but also who can provide them.

In addition to federal programs, state and local government programs and private health care and social service agencies provide some services for people with dementia. Medicare and Medicaid also fund waiver programs and demonstration projects. In some communities, these programs provide services that are not otherwise covered and may be especially appropriate for dementia patients—for example, respite care. In the fall of 1986, Congress authorized more than $40 million for new Medicare and Medicaid demonstration projects for persons with dementia. However, waiver programs and demonstration projects can serve only a small proportion of all people with dementia. For the others—the great majority—the lack of appropriate services can usually be traced to eligibility, coverage, or payment policies of the major federal programs that fund long-term care.

Some knowledge of the federal programs that fund long-term care and their limitations is essential for health care and social service professionals who treat dementia patients or advise families about their care. Without this knowledge, professionals can convey inaccurate information and raise false expectations about available services, thus increasing the frustration of family members already stressed by caregiving responsibilities.

Settings and Services

Little reliable information is available about the number of persons with dementia in most settings or the number who receive specific services, such as respite care in any setting. Although the importance of cognitive deficits and dementia in determining the long-term care needs of individuals is well recognized by many health care and social service providers, most large-scale surveys of the elderly and long-term care populations have not collected information about cognitive status or the prevalence of dementia. An exception is the Epidemiological Catchment Area (ECA) Survey, a study of community-dwelling people of all ages conducted in five cities. A cognitive assessment instrument, the Mini-Mental State Exam (MMSE) (Folstein et al. 1975) was used in the survey, and at the Baltimore site respondents with suspected dementia were evaluated by a psychiatrist and a neurologist. The resulting data described the prevalence and causes of cognitive impairment and dementia in the community, some characteristics of dementia patients, and their use of health care services.

In other large-scale surveys of elderly and long-term care populations, patient diagnosis has been obtained. However, a diagnosis of dementia or lack of such a diagnosis is often unreliable outside of specialized diagnostic and treatment centers. Measures of cognitive ability that could be used to verify diagnosis and to establish the severity of dementia frequently have not been obtained. As a result, information about the number of persons with dementia in each setting and about their characteristics and care needs often must be derived from small-scale studies that may not be representative and from retrospective analysis of data from research not intended for this purpose.

Nursing Homes

Nursing homes are health care facilities that provide skilled nursing care, personal care, and twenty-four-hour supervision. They are now the most frequently used residential setting for persons with dementia. Although Medicare, Medicaid, and VA regulations emphasize the nursing aspects of nursing home care, for persons with dementia (and perhaps many other long-term care patients) the most important aspects of nursing home care are the availability of personal care and twenty-four-hour supervision.

Nursing homes serve a heterogeneous population that includes terminally ill patients who have been discharged from hospitals because they do not need acute care or, increasingly, because their length of stay or cost of care has exceeded the average length of stay or cost of care for their diagnostic category (DRG) under the Medicare prospective payment system; individuals admitted from a hospital for recuperation and rehabilitation after a hip fracture, surgery, or other treatment; and individuals who are medically stable but functionally impaired due to a variety of chronic physical, cognitive, and psychiatric conditions. Some of the latter group are deinstitutionalized state mental hospital patients or chronically mentally ill people who would

have been admitted to state mental hospitals before the deinstitutionalization movement.

In this context, it is difficult to determine how many nursing
home residents have dementia. Residents who do not have dementia
may be, or seem to be, cognitively impaired because of depression,
speech and hearing impairments, mental retardation, or the effects
of acute or chronic diseases or medications used to treat them. Mental
status tests and cognitive assessment instruments have not been routinely used in most nursing homes, and the diagnosis in the resident's
medical chart may not be correct—especially if the patient was admitted some years ago and the chart diagnoses have not been updated.

Data from several recent studies indicate that 40 to 60 percent of
nursing home residents have dementia (Texas Department of Health
1985; Foley 1986; Rhode Island Legislative Commission 1984) and that
the proportion may be as high as 75 percent in some facilities (Rovner
et al. 1986). The 1985 National Nursing Home Survey found that 63
percent of elderly nursing home residents were disoriented or memory
impaired to the extent that they needed assistance with personal care.
Forty-seven percent were reported to have senile dementia or chronic
organic brain syndrome (U.S. Department of Health and Human Services 1987).

Many nursing home employees and others believe that dementia
patients are more difficult to care for and require more staff time than
other patients. One study (Rovner et al. 1986) found that many nursing
home residents with dementia also have psychiatric disorders (including delusions, hallucinations, and depression) and behavioral
problems (such as restlessness, agitation, and wandering).

Retrospective analysis of data on New York State nursing home
residents showed that those with dementia were, on average, more
impaired than other residents in activities of daily living (eating, bathing, dressing, toileting, bowel and bladder control, and personal hygiene). They were also more likely than other residents to have behavioral problems (wandering, verbal abuse, physical aggression, and
regressive or inappropriate behavior). On average, residents with
dementia required about 6 percent more staff time than other residents
(Foley 1986). Thus, as many nursing home employees and others have
suggested, persons with dementia tend to be "heavy care" patients.

The New York State data were collected in nursing homes that
for the most part did not have special units or special programs for
persons with dementia. There are some indications that dementia

patients may be less difficult to care for in facilities where the physical environment and daily routine are adapted to their needs and the staff is trained to care for them.

Nursing homes vary greatly in the quality of care that they provide for all residents. Recent reports document very poor care in some facilities (U.S. Senate 1986; Institute of Medicine 1986). Even in "good" nursing homes, some aspects of the care provided may be inadequate or inappropriate for persons with dementia. Space is often insufficient for physical exercise, and regular exercise is not promoted. Noise and activity associated with housekeeping, shift changes, and other routine occurrences may agitate these residents. Staff members are frequently not aware of behavior management techniques that might lessen agitation and reduce behavioral problems, and medications that might lessen agitation are sometimes not used appropriately. Finally, the common practice of rotating staff from one unit to another can be a problem for persons with dementia, who may be able to remember a staff member they see every day but cannot remember over longer periods and may become agitated when repeatedly confronted with staff members whom they do not recognize.

Despite these problems, some persons with dementia adjust well to nursing home placement. For some, this may be because expectations for their behavior and functioning are lower in the nursing home than at home. If the primary caregiver at home has been frustrated, angry, or upset by caregiving responsibilities, the person with dementia may experience less disapproval and criticism in the nursing home. In the extreme, if there has been physical abuse or neglect at home, the nursing home is likely to be an improvement.

For caregivers, placing the person with dementia in a nursing home can result in guilt or relief or a combination of both. Widespread negative social attitudes about placing one's relative in a nursing home—attitudes that are shared by some doctors, nurses, social workers, and others—can intensify the guilt that families feel in this situation. There is no evidence that cognitive and functional impairments associated with dementia progress faster in patients cared for in nursing homes than in those cared for at home. Many experts agree that institutionalization is necessary for many persons with dementia at some time in the course of their disease. In this context, health care and social service professionals should be aware of and help families recognize the positive as well as negative aspects of nursing home placement.

Even when a decision is made to seek nursing home placement, finding a nursing home bed and paying for it are very difficult in many communities. Nursing home beds are often readily available to people who can pay privately for care, but the cost—$20,000 to $30,000 a year or more in most areas of the country—is prohibitive for most individuals and families, especially when care is needed for prolonged periods, as it may be for persons with dementia.

Medicare seldom covers the cost of nursing home care for dementia patients for reasons that are discussed in Chapter 11. The Medicare Catastrophic Coverage Act of 1988 increased the maximum number of days of nursing home care that Medicare can cover from 100 to 150 and decreased the required patient copayment from $67.50 a day for the 21st to 100th days to $25.50 a day for the first eight days. Neither of these changes resolves the problems that limit the availability of Medicare coverage for nursing home care for persons with dementia, however.

VA nursing home care is available for veterans with service-connected disabilities, but veterans without service-connected disabilities—the great majority—are eligible for only six months of nursing home care. Medicaid eligibility varies in different states, but financial eligibility requirements must be met. Until recently, if there was a spouse, he or she had to live on a very small amount of money in the community if Medicaid was going to pay for the patient in the nursing home (see Chapter 11). The Medicare Catastrophic Coverage Act allows states to raise the level of income and assets that the spouse can retain while the patient is in the nursing home.

Even when payment is available, some nursing homes are reluctant to admit persons with dementia, whom they perceive as "heavy care." In states where Medicaid reimbursement is very low, they may be reluctant to admit individuals who are likely to stay long enough to deplete their private funds and become eligible for Medicaid. Finally, limitations on nursing home bed supply in many states restrict access for all kinds of patients.

Board and Care Facilities

Many health care and social service professionals are less familiar with board and care facilities than nursing homes. Board and care facilities are nonmedical, residential care settings that provide room and board and some degree of supervision. Some also provide personal care. They differ from nursing homes in that nursing care is generally not provided. They differ from rooming houses and other room and board situations in that supervision and assistance with some activities are provided.

Beyond this general definition, however, the category "board and care facilities" is diffuse and, to a great extent, theoretical. Board and care facilities vary greatly in size, staffing, organization, activities, and atmosphere. They include small adult foster homes that may take in one or two persons, personal care or group homes that may serve five to ten residents, retirement homes and homes for the aged that may serve 100 or more residents, and large domiciliary care facilities that care for several hundred residents. Small board and care facilities may be run somewhat informally by a single individual or couple, whereas larger facilities have a larger, more formally organized staff. Some board and care facilities—usually smaller ones—are "homelike," whereas others—often the larger ones—are more "institutional." Yet smaller facilities do not necessarily provide better care.

There is no information about the number of persons with dementia in board and care facilities. Research on these facilities has generally categorized residents as aged, mentally ill, or mentally retarded. One large-scale study found, for example, that of 230,000 residents about whom any information was available, 45 percent were elderly, 37 percent were mentally ill, and 15 percent were mentally retarded (Reichstein and Bergofsky 1980). Other studies have shown that about one-third of elderly and mentally ill residents of board and care facilities were disoriented or forgetful (Sherwood and Gruenberg 1978; Dittmar and Smith 1983). It is not known how many of these individuals have dementia.

Little is known about the care provided in board and care facilities. One study of small facilities in Pennsylvania found that the majority provided laundry, shopping, cleaning, transportation, and assistance with medications and handling money. One-third or less provided assistance with bathing and dressing (Sherwood and Morris 1983).

Board and care facilities that provide twenty-four-hour supervision may be a particularly appropriate setting for some persons with dementia. The best board and care facilities encourage self-care to the extent of the resident's capability, promote resident involvement in some housekeeping tasks, and foster positive relationships between residents and staff and among residents.

Unfortunately, quality of care varies greatly in board and care facilities. Although some provide good or adequate care, physical abuse, neglect, and exploitation have also been reported. Persons with dementia are particularly unlikely to be able to resist abuse and exploitation or to inform others about it.

All states license some types of board and care facilities. However, licensing regulations may address only physical plant and fire and life safety code requirements, rather than quality of care. Few states inspect board and care facilities regularly, and some types of board and care facilities are not licensed or regulated at all in most states. Thus, there is no uniform or reliable quality assurance mechanism. For families and health care and social service providers, this means that any board and care facility should be carefully inspected before placing persons with dementia, and ongoing supervision of their care is necessary.

Access to board and care for all kinds of people is limited by a lack of information about the facilities—especially small ones—in many communities. Access may be further limited for dementia patients because some facilities do not accept persons with behavioral problems or incontinence (Gutkin and Morris 1981).

Access may also be limited by cost. Although in general, board and care costs significantly less than nursing home care, it may still cost more than the individual or family can pay. Neither Medicare nor Medicaid pays for board and care, but many states provide a supplement to the federal SSI benefit (or other state funding) for residents of some types of board and care facilities.

Variations in funding among states and great differences in the number and types of board and care facilities in different states and localities mean that no general statements can be made about the availability of this mode of care for dementia patients. The potential positive features of board and care facilities for these patients suggest, however, that health care and social service professionals should familiarize themselves with local board and care facilities and potential sources of funding for them.

Home Care

Many of the services listed in Table 12.1 can be provided in the home. Perhaps the most important of these for persons with dementia are supervision, paid companion, and personal care—all services that provide respite for the primary caregiver. It is widely believed that such services lessen the burden of care for families and other informal caregivers and consequently support their efforts to keep persons with dementia at home. Many other home care services, including skilled nursing, physical therapy, occupational therapy, home-delivered meals, and transportation, can also be helpful, depending on the needs of the patient and the primary caregiver.

Although some persons with dementia receive home care services through home health care agencies, many families hire maids or sitters to provide supervision and personal care for persons with dementia (George 1984). This is primarily because of the high cost of services provided by home health care agencies. As one woman told the Kansas Alzheimer's and Related Diseases Task Force (Kansas 1986): "I was told that I might be able to get someone in for an hour a day—that might be long enough to bathe and dress my husband. When I asked how much, I was told it would cost $40.00 an hour from the minute they left the office until they returned."

Medicare is the largest public payer for home care services, but Medicare coverage of home care services is limited to skilled nursing care; physical therapy, speech therapy, and occupational therapy; medical social services; medical supplies and equipment, but not medications; and home health aide services. Medicare home care services must be prescribed by a physician and supplied by a home health care agency that has been certified to participate in the program, of which there were about 5,000 in 1985 (*Health Care Financing Review* 1985).

Home health aide services, which can include personal care such as bathing, dressing, and feeding, are probably the most useful Medicare-covered home care services for persons with dementia. However, home health aide services are covered only if the individual also meets Medicare's strict eligibility requirements for skilled nursing care, physical therapy, or speech therapy—a condition that many persons with dementia do not meet. Moreover, home health aide services are covered only when they are provided on an intermittent and part-time basis. Thus, ongoing personal care is seldom covered by Medicare. Supervision and paid companion services—both very important for persons with dementia—are not covered, although home health aides usually serve these purposes when they are in the home.

Medicaid covers skilled nursing care, home health aide services, and, in some states, personal care. Under the 2176 waiver program, some states also provide homemaker and respite care and other home care services. However, the financial eligibility criteria for Medicaid (i.e., limits on income and assets) are so restrictive in most states that most individuals are not eligible.

Respite care, which is intended to relieve families of caregiving responsibilities temporarily, is a particularly appropriate service for persons with dementia. However, the provision of respite care is problematic within the context of Medicare, Medicaid, and VA program regulations for two reasons. First, home care services covered by these programs are intended to meet specific health-related needs of the patient, whereas respite care can involve any services that relieve the primary caregiver of caregiving responsibilities. Second, eligibility for home care services covered by these programs is based on the needs of the patient, while respite care is also responsive to the needs of the family. These problems can be circumvented in waiver programs and demonstration projects, but eligibility and coverage rules will have to be changed considerably to allow respite care as a part of regular benefits. The Medicare Catastrophic Coverage Act of 1988 authorized Medicare coverage for eighty hours of respite care per year for individuals who meet certain requirements. The regulations to implement this new benefit had not been published at the time of this writing, however.

In some localities, Social Services Block Grant funds and funds available through Title III of the Older Americans Act are used to provide respite care and other home care services that are not covered by Medicare or Medicaid or pay for services for people who are not eligible for Medicaid because they have income or assets above allowable limits. However, Social Services Block Grant and Title III funds are insufficient to meet the need for services in most communities.

In summary, although a large proportion of home care is publicly funded, the services most often needed for persons with dementia are not covered by some programs and are not adequately funded by others. Because such services are costly, especially when they are needed for prolonged periods, they may be essentially unavailable to patients and families who are unable to pay privately for them.

In addition to the high cost and the lack of adequate public funding for home care services, the worker's expertise in working with people with dementia, family expectations, and cultural differences create problems (see Chapter 10).

Another problem may be the general lack of quality assurance mechanisms for home care. A recent report of the American Bar As-

sociation's Commission on Legal Problems of the Elderly points out
that:

> In-home location of services makes their actual delivery essentially
> invisible, and, therefore, largely beyond the reach of public or pro-
> fessional scrutiny . . . . On the one hand, home care services bring
> enhanced opportunities for elderly to live longer and indepen-
> dently in their communities. Yet they also bring enhanced risks of
> poor care, unreliable services and outright neglect, abuse, and ex-
> ploitation. Anecdotal reports leave little doubt that all these prob-
> lems exist but to what degree is not known (U.S. Congress, Select
> Committee on Aging 1986).

These concerns are particularly relevant for persons with dementia,
who may be unable to report poor care or abuse to the primary caregiver.

One question that has received almost no attention in public
discussion about home care services is whether it is advisable to provide such services for persons with dementia who are living alone
and, if so, under what circumstances. Yet this question is faced daily
by hospital discharge planning units and home health care agencies
that must decide whether a given patient can manage safely at home
with only a few hours a day of personal care and supervision, intermittent visits of a nurse, and perhaps home-delivered meals.

Twenty-four-hour care is almost never available through publicly
funded programs and is too expensive for most people to pay for
themselves. Thus, the following paradox occurs repeatedly in communities across the country: persons with dementia who live alone
are provided with an aide to bathe and perhaps prepare a meal for
them or help with shopping and housekeeping *because they are too
confused to care for themselves,* and then they are left alone for the
remainder of the day and night and often for the whole weekend
because twenty-four-hour care is not available.

This paradox arises because the conceptual model of home care
services that underlies most public programs that fund home care is
based on the needs of physically impaired people. At present, the
eligibility and coverage regulations of these programs are stretched
to meet some needs of cognitively impaired people, but they cannot
encompass the needs of very confused people who live alone.

Thus far, there have been no reports of hospital discharge planning units or public or private case management or home care agencies

being sued for failure to ensure the safety of persons with dementia who are discharged home or maintained at home alone with part-time home care services. Such suits seem likely, however, in view of the relatively frequent cases brought against social service agencies for placing children in unsafe home situations.

Greater understanding among health care and social service professionals about what home care services are actually available in a given community and greater consideration of the needs of dementia patients who live alone could lessen liability risks and, more importantly, decrease instances of patients being sent home with inadequate supervision and assistance.

Adult Day Care

Adult day care can include a variety of medical, social, recreational, and mental health services. Many adult day care centers serve only one or primarily one group of people, for example, physically impaired people; retarded and developmentally disabled people; mentally ill people, particularly those who have been discharged from a mental hospital; or the frail elderly. Persons with dementia are most likely to be cared for in adult day care centers that serve the frail elderly, but client groups in different centers overlap, and some persons with dementia are cared for in centers that serve each type of client.

Some adult day care centers have been established specifically for persons with dementia. Other centers have admission policies that restrict access by persons with dementia, for example, policies that deny admission to people who are disruptive, combative, too confused, or in need of constant supervision (Behren 1986; Mace and Rabins 1984).

During the past fifteen years, the number of adult day care centers in this country has increased from less than ten to more than 1,200 (Behren 1986). Yet many communities do not have an adult day care center, especially communities in rural areas.

Unlike nursing homes and home health care agencies, adult day care centers have developed largely without federal or state regulation. As a result, they differ greatly in staffing, mode of operation, and services provided (Behren 1985).

The Alzheimer's Association and many health care and social services professionals are enthusiastic about the role of adult day care in the treatment of persons with dementia. Although there is no research to demonstrate that adult day care postpones the need for nursing home placement, many people believe that it does. Anecdotal evidence and some research indicates that very severely physically and cognitively impaired people can be effectively cared for in adult day care centers (Rathbone-McCuan and Elliott 1976–77), but other studies indicate that adult day care centers serve a different group of clients than do nursing homes (Harder et al. 1983).

Referrals to adult day care should not be automatic. One important factor is whether the dementia patient has a family member or friend who can provide care when the patient is not at the day care center. In addition, although adult day care is helpful for some and perhaps most persons with dementia, other such persons may not benefit. Some patients cannot adjust to a new environment or to certain aspects of an adult day care program. Moreover, for some families, the difficulty of getting an uncooperative patient dressed and out to the day care center outweighs the benefits of being temporarily relieved of caregiving responsibilities. In these cases, home care or residential care may be more appropriate.

The average cost of adult day care is $27 to $31 a day in late 1985 and 1986, although some programs cost considerably more (Behren 1986; Ransom and Kelly 1985). Some state Medicaid programs cover adult day care, and some states (twenty-nine in 1984) use Social Services Block Grant funds to pay for it (U.S. Senate 1985). Other state and local funds and United Way and other charitable contributions also support adult day care in some communities. Yet client fees are the primary source of funding. Paying for such care is difficult or impossible for many clients and families, especially if the client attends frequently—which many adult day care providers believe is important if the confused client is to adjust to the new environment and program.

State Mental Hospitals

Thirty years ago, before the deinstitutionalization movement, state mental hospitals were the primary residential care setting for people with dementia. Now most people with dementia who need residential care are in nursing homes, and there is no information about how many such people are in state mental hospitals. The 1980 census counted 51,000 elderly people in all mental hospitals (Lerman 1985), but it is not known how many of these people have dementia.

Persons with dementia who are in state mental hospitals now may have behavioral problems that cannot be handled by a nursing home. Alternatively, they may have been admitted to the state hospital with a psychiatric condition some years previously and may have developed a dementing disorder while in the hospital.

On the one hand, state mental hospitals have been criticized for providing only custodial care and in some cases for providing very poor care. On the other hand, anecdotal evidence suggests that some dementia patients receive excellent care in state mental hospitals (Massachusetts Governor's Task Force 1985). In general, for patients who wander, more space is available in mental hospitals than in nursing homes. Staff members are trained to expect and manage behavioral problems and may have a greater knowledge of the use of medications to control agitation than is available in nursing homes.

Access to care in state mental hospitals is limited in many jurisdictions by a general requirement that patients must be considered a danger to themselves or others to be kept in the hospital without their consent. In addition, many states support aggressive discharge planning programs in state mental hospitals, partly because it is believed that patients of all kinds are better off in the community and partly because the public cost of care in a state mental hospital is generally higher than the public cost of nursing home care. Medicaid covers the cost of care in a state mental hospital for persons who are financially eligible and over age sixty-five but not for persons who are under age sixty-five. This is an important consideration for anyone who is evaluating service options for younger dementia patients.

Thus, for a variety of reasons, care in a state mental hospital may not be an option for persons with dementia. However, the Rhode Island Legislative Commission on Dementias Related to Aging (1984) proposed the development of a special care unit for persons with dementia in one state mental hospital, and some other state mental hospitals already have "psychogeriatric units" that care for such persons. Health care and social service professionals should familiarize themselves with any special services for dementia patients that may be available in a local state mental hospital, the admission criteria, and the cost to families of care in this setting.

Outpatient Mental Health Care

Dementia is an organic condition, not a mental illness per se, but some of the emotional and behavioral problems often associated with it may be best understood and treated by mental health specialists. Families of dementia patients may need short-term counseling to deal with the difficult caregiving situations that they face, equally difficult decisions about placement, and the conflict that may develop among family members about caregiving responsibilities and decisions about placement. In addition, health care and social service providers who work with dementia patients can benefit from consultation with a mental health specialist to increase their understanding of patient behavior and to learn techniques to lessen agitation and disruptive or inappropriate patient behaviors. Caregivers may also learn methods of coping with the stress associated with caring for these patients.

For all of these reasons, involvement of mental health specialists in the care of dementia patients is appropriate in many cases, yet many mental health specialists are not experienced in treating these patients or counseling their families. Thus, health care and social service professionals who make such referrals should be knowledge-able about the qualifications of the mental health specialists to whom they refer the patients.

Community mental health centers (CMHCs) provide a variety of mental health services, primarily on an outpatient basis, although some also provide short-term inpatient treatment. Some do not pro-vide any services for persons with dementia. The results of one survey (Light et al. 1985) indicate, however, that CMHCs that provide special services for elderly people often also provide services for persons with dementia and their families. These agencies are also likely to offer mental health services in satellite sites, such as senior centers, nursing homes, and other residential facilities where persons with dementia are seen and cared for. Thus, in some jurisdictions, the CMHC may be a valuable resource for persons with dementia, their families, and the long-term care facilities and agencies that serve them.

Outpatient mental health services are also provided by mental health specialists in private practice, including psychiatrists, clinical psychologists, psychiatric social workers, and psychiatric nurses. It is not known how often mental health specialists in private practice treat persons with dementia or their families, however.

Apparently, very few persons with dementia see mental health specialists. Data from the ECA survey in Baltimore indicate that no respondent who was over 65 and cognitively impaired had seen a mental health specialist during the preceding six months (German et al. 1985). The reason for this may be a reluctance on the part of some mental health specialists to treat persons with dementia and their families, resistance on the part of some families to seeking help from a mental health specialist, the cost of the treatment, lack of third-party reimbursement, or a combination of these.

Locating and Arranging Formal Long-Term Care Services for Persons with Dementia

Most discussion about long-term care services for persons with dementia has focused on which settings and services are most appropriate for them. There has been less discussion of how families and others can locate and arrange the needed services, assuming that they are available. Yet lack of information about available services is clearly a problem, as anyone can testify who has been quoted in the newspaper or other public media as having information about services for persons with dementia, only to be inundated with calls from families who are desperately looking for such services.

One problem in locating services for persons with dementia is that appropriate services may be provided in any of four systems: the medical or physical care system, which includes nursing homes and home health care agencies; the mental health system, which includes state mental hospitals and CMHCs; the aging services system, which includes Area Agencies on Aging, senior centers, and programs funded through the Older Americans Act; or the social service system, which includes local social service and welfare agencies, protective service agencies, and services funded by the Social Services Block Grant. Each of these systems also includes many private agencies, and each has administratively separate funding sources, at least for funds originating at the federal level.

Some communities have developed effective methods for coordinating two or more of these systems, but most have not. Thus, individual service providers in one system may not be aware of services provided in other systems. The mental health system seems to be particularly isolated from the other three in many communities. For persons with dementia and their families, who may need services from any of the systems, the lack of coordination among them is a major problem.

Another problem in locating long-term care services for persons with dementia is that some agencies may say that they have special services when they do not. The experience of the Massachusetts Governor's Committee on Alzheimer's Disease (1985) is instructive in this regard: "At the beginning of our examination of available community

THE COMMUNITY

services, one member was assigned the task of calling facilities on a random list and asking if they had specialized services for Alzheimer's patients. Without exception, the caller was told that such specialized services existed. When questioned more specifically, most facilities failed to demonstrate any special capability to assist the Alzheimer's client."

Even if facilities and agencies that have services for persons with dementia can be located, there are no standards for evaluating them. This lack of standards reflects the lack of agreement among experts about what constitutes good care for these patients and the lack of research comparing alternate forms of care for them.

A related problem in this relatively new area is that many self-proclaimed "experts" actually know very little about dementia or the care of persons with dementia. Families that are desperate for help and health care and social service providers looking for better ways to care for these patients are easy targets for such "experts."

In a few communities, there are agencies specifically set up to help families and others locate and arrange services for persons with dementia. One example is the Family Survival Project in San Francisco. In other communities, the local Alzheimer's Association chapter may be a valuable source of information. However, many local Alzheimer's Association chapters have no paid staff, and it is sometimes difficult to locate the person in the chapter who knows the most about community services. Some chapters have formal information and referral programs. For example, the Chicago chapter has an 800 telephone number for questions about services in Illinois.

Local Area Agencies on Aging (AAAs) may also be helpful in some communities. Since 1984, the federal Administration on Aging has funded a program to train AAA staff about Alzheimer's disease and to develop support groups for families of these patients. Not all of the more than 600 AAAs nationwide participate in this program, but many do, and they may be able to direct families and others to appropriate services.

Finally, individual health care and social service providers who care for persons with dementia often know about other long-term services for these persons in their communities. For example, staff of an adult day care center that serves persons with dementia may have considerable knowledge about the availability and quality of care provided for such persons by local nursing homes, board and care facilities, and home care agencies.

Arranging long-term care services for persons with dementia is, in some respects, more difficult than arranging services for other kinds of patients. Individuals are often unaware of their condition and care needs and may refuse needed services. In addition, they are usually unable to evaluate different care options or to participate in important decisions, such as nursing home admission or the sale of a home. Thus, family members or others must make these decisions, often without knowing what the individual would have wanted. Finally, because appropriate services for these individuals are not available in many communities, families have held back from seeking formal services until the situation is desperate. As a result, decisions about long-term care services are often made in an atmosphere of crisis.

This chapter has emphasized the federal programs that fund long-term care. Because persons with dementia often require long-term care services for prolonged periods, they are likely to exhaust their own resources and to need publicly funded services. Understanding the eligibility and coverage regulations of the federal programs that pay for long-term care and of the state and local programs that supplement them is, therefore, essential in arranging services for these patients.

Also essential for this purpose is an awareness of the family's feelings and attitudes about the person with dementia, the person's care needs, and the service options. These feelings and attitudes are part of the patient/family reality and must be taken into account in assessing long-term care needs and arranging appropriate services. Decisions about long-term care tend to evoke strong feelings—sadness, loss, anger, and guilt, among others—and emotion-laden memories, for example, promises to one's spouse or parents about never putting them in a nursing home. Discussion of these feelings can often relieve tension and facilitate decision making.

A final element in arranging long-term care services for persons with dementia is a recognition that the person's needs will change over the course of most diseases that cause dementia and that decisions about long-term care should not be considered "final." This is especially true because so little is known about the usual course of most of the diseases that cause dementia.

References

Behren, R. V. 1985. Adult day care: Progress, problems, and promise. *Perspective on Aging* 14 (6): 5–39.

Behren, R. V. 1986. *Adult day care in America: Preliminary report of the results of the National Institute of Adult Daycare/National Council on Aging Survey, 1985–86.* Washington, DC: National Council on Aging. July.

Cohen, D., J. Hegarty, and C. Eisdorfer. 1983. The physician's desk directory of social resources: A physician's reference guide to social and community services for the aged. *Journal of the American Geriatrics Society* 31 (6): 338–41.

Congressional Research Service. 1987. *Financing and delivery of long-term care services for the elderly.* 87-143-EPW. Washington, DC: Library of Congress. February 24.

Dittmar, N. D., and G. P. Smith. 1983. *Evaluation of board and care homes: Summary of survey procedures and findings.* Denver, CO: Denver Research Institute, University of Denver. February 22.

Doty, P., K. Liu, and J. Weiner. 1985. An overview of long-term care. *Health Care Financing Review* 6 (3): 69–78.

Foley, W. J. 1986. *Dementia among nursing home patients: Defining the condition, characteristics of the demented, and dementia on the RUG-II Classification System.* Contract report. Washington, DC: U.S. Congress, Office of Technology Assessment.

Folstein, M. F., S. E. Folstein, and P. R. McHugh. 1975. Mini-Mental State: A practical method for grading the cognitive state of patients for the clinician. *Journal of Psychiatric Research.* 12:189–98.

George, L. K. 1984. *The dynamics of caregiver burden.* Washington, DC: American Association of Retired Persons. December.

German, P. S., S. Shapiro, and E. A. Skinner. 1985. Mental health of the elderly: Use of health and mental health services. *Journal of the American Geriatrics Society* 33:246–52.

Gutkin, C. E., and S. A. Morris. 1981. A description of facility and program characteristics in nine domiciliary care programs. In *Domiciliary care clients and the facilities in which they reside,* ed. S. Sherwood, V. Mor, and C. E. Gutkin, V-1–V-7. Boston: Hebrew Rehabilitation Center for the Aged.

Harder, W. P., J. C. Gornick, and M. R. Burt. 1983. Adult day care: Supplement or substitute. Washington, DC: The Urban Institute.

Health Care Financing Review. 1985. Health facilities participating in Health Care Financing Administration programs, 1985. *Health Care Financing Review* 6 (4): 143.

Institute of Medicine. 1986. *Improving the quality of care in nursing homes.* Washington, DC: National Academy Press.

Kansas Alzheimer's and Related Diseases Task Force. 1986. *Final report to the Kansas Department on Aging.* Topeka, KS: Kansas Alzheimer's and Related Diseases Task Force.

Lerman, P. 1985. Deinstitutionalization and welfare policies in the welfare state in America: Trends and prospects. *American Academy of Political and Social Science Annals—1985* 479:132–55.

Light, E., B. Lebowitz, and F. Bailey. 1985. CHMCs and elderly services: An analysis of direct and indirect services and services delivery sites. *Community Mental Health Journal* 22 (4): 294–302.

Mace, N. L., and P. V. Rabins. 1984. *A survey of day care for the demented adult in the United States.* Washington, DC: National Council on the Aging.

Massachusetts Governor's Task Force on Alzheimer's Disease. 1985. *Final report.* Boston: The Commonwealth of Massachusetts.

Mather, J. H., and R. W. Abel. 1986. Medical care of veterans: A brief history. *Journal of the American Geriatrics Society* 34 (10): 757–60.

Ransom, B., and W. Kelly. 1985. Rising to the challenge. *Perspective on Aging* 14 (6): 13–14.

Rathbone-McCuan, E., and M. Elliott. 1976–77. Geriatric day care in theory and practice. *Social Work in Health Care* 2 (2): 153–77.

Reichstein, K. J., and L. Bergofsky. 1980. *Summary and report of the National Survey of State Administered Domiciliary Care Programs in the Fifty States and the District of Columbia.* Boston: Horizon House Institute. December.

Rhode Island Legislative Commission on Dementias Related to Aging. 1984. *Final report.* May.

Rovner, B. W., S. Kafonek, L. Filipp, M. J. Lucas, and M. F. Folstein. 1986. Prevalence of mental illness in a community nursing home. *American Journal of Psychiatry* 143:1446–49.

Samuel, F. 1984. Health Industry Manufacturers Association. Personal communication, February 14.

Sherwood, S., and L. Gruenberg. 1978. *A descriptive study of functionally eligible applicants to the Pennsylvania Domiciliary Program: Commonwealth of Pennsylvania.* Boston: Hebrew Rehabilitation Center for the Aged.

Sherwood, S., and J. N. Morris. 1983. The Pennsylvania Domiciliary Care experiment: Impact on quality of life. *American Journal of Public Health* 73:646–53.

Texas Department of Health. 1985. *Alzheimer's Disease Initiative Nursing Home Study.* Austin, TX.

U.S. Congress. Office of Technology Assessment. 1987. *Losing a million minds: Confronting the tragedy of Alzheimer's disease and other dementias.* Washington, DC: U.S. Government Printing Office. April.

U.S. Congress. Select Committee on Aging. 1986. *The black box of home care quality,* prepared by the American Bar Association, committee pub. No. 99-573. Washington, DC: U.S. Government Printing Office.

U.S. Department of Health and Human Services. 1987. *Use of nursing homes by the elderly: Preliminary data from the 1985 National Nursing Home Survey.* National Center for Health Statistics, No. 135, May 14.

U.S. Senate. Special Committee on Aging. 1985. *Developments in Aging, 1984,* Vol. 2. Washington, DC: U.S. Government Printing Office. February.

U.S. Senate. Special Committee on Aging. 1986. *Nursing home care: The unfinished agenda*, No. 99-J. Washington, DC: U.S. Government Printing Office. May.

Veterans Administration. 1984. *Caring for the older veteran.* Washington, DC: U.S. Government Printing Office. July.

Vladeck, B. C. 1980. *Unloving care: The nursing home tragedy.* New York: Basic Books.

13

Tapping an Unlimited Resource: Building Volunteer Programs for Patients and Their Families

VIRGINIA BELL, M.S.W.

Volunteerism is considered by many to be a great American tradition. In settings such as churches, schools, museums, libraries, and hospitals, volunteers play an integral role. A 1985 Gallup poll measured the breadth of volunteerism in the United States. Among its findings:

1. Almost one-half of Americans over the age of 14, or approximately 89 million people, volunteered.

2. Volunteers contributed an average of 3.5 hours per week in 1985, up from 2.6 hours measured by a previous (1980) poll.

3. Volunteers are found in all age and income groups. In 1985, 51 percent of females and 45 percent of males were volunteers. Teenagers between fourteen and seventeen had the greatest percentage of volunteers, 52 percent. Forty-four percent of persons between the ages of fifty and sixty-four volunteered; 43 percent of those between sixty-five and seventy-four also volunteered. Perhaps surprising to some, one in four over the age of seventy-five volunteered!

4. Most volunteers (80 percent) contributed time to charitable organizations.

5. The most popular form of volunteer work was assisting the elderly, the handicapped, or social welfare recipients.

6. The primary reasons for volunteering were a desire to do something to help others (52 percent), an interest in the work or activity (36 percent), or enjoyment of the volunteer activity (32 percent) (*Americans Volunteer* 1986, 4).

For organizations concerned with the elderly, there is much good news in this survey. Older people, even those over seventy-five, are active participants in the nation's volunteer pool. The elderly are also beneficiaries of the volunteer effort, with "helping an elderly neighbor," often cited as an example of informal volunteer efforts (*Americans Volunteer* 1986, 15).

Despite this good news, I have often been told by organizations working with patients with dementia and their families that volunteers remain difficult to attract, particularly in direct service areas such as respite care. This chapter discusses strategies for building such programs based on my experience directing a dementia-specific day care program, the Helping Hand.

The primary focus of the chapter will be on involving volunteers in direct service programs such as in-home and day care dementia-specific respite programs. However, the principles discussed should benefit program planners seeking volunteers in other settings such as staffing help-lines, building counseling and referral programs, and developing support groups. For readers requiring more detailed information on the mechanics of volunteer program management, a brief bibliography at the end of the chapter offers suggested texts for further reading and gives addresses and publications of national organizations promoting volunteerism.

The Helping Hand

The Helping Hand respite program provides families with time away from their often twenty-four-hour caregiving day by offering a safe, creative environment for persons with Alzheimer's disease or related disorders (referred to as "participants" in the program). Founded in 1984 by the Lexington/Bluegrass Alzheimer's Association and the Sanders-Brown Center on Aging at the University of Kentucky, Helping Hand currently operates five days a week and is staffed almost entirely with volunteers. Professional staff work part-time and offer supervision to volunteers. The program is based on an activities model; in a relaxed, friendly setting participants are offered sensitive one-to-one care and attention by the same volunteer each week.

The volunteers include both men and women from all backgrounds and professions. They range in age from 25 to 87, from young mother to great-grandmother. Almost half of the volunteers are former caregivers who bring special expertise and experience to the program. Currently, fifty-five volunteers are active in the program. Most of the volunteers give one day of care per week; others act as substitutes when needed.

Involving volunteers as staff of the Helping Hand program began as an economic necessity. Little funding was available for dementia-specific day care in 1984. The logical way to solve this problem was to recruit and educate volunteers to provide that care. At that time, much skepticism existed about the involvement of volunteers in such an effort. Questions included:

How can volunteers do what families find so difficult?
Are volunteers reliable?
Are volunteers willing to attend study sessions?
Will volunteers keep information confidential?

The Helping Hand program has demonstrated that what began as a necessity has resulted in a gold mine of expertise and love from volunteers. Volunteers can provide quality care, are reliable, will attend educational programs, and can maintain confidentiality. The following sections will describe our four years experience of recruiting, educating, effectively involving, and nurturing volunteers.

Recruiting Volunteers

Before beginning a recruitment effort, it is necessary to have a clearly defined job description for the volunteer. In the Helping Hand, volunteers are asked to relate one-to-one with the program participant. In addition, the volunteers become a valuable part of a team effort to provide friendship, information, and support to the family caregiver. Volunteers assist in the design of individual and group activities. The volunteers also provide role models of dementia-specific respite care for students and professionals and assist in the ongoing decision making and evaluation of the program.

To fulfill these responsibilities, the Helping Hand seeks individuals who can value all human beings, regardless of their disabilities. As Mary Howell (1984) wrote, the Alzheimer's patient should be viewed as "fully a person." Translating this belief into action requires patience, calmness, flexibility, a sense of humor, and a determination to seek ways to fill the huge deficit left by the dementing illness. Volunteers must be able to contribute to a safe, secure, joyful milieu; it is critical that volunteers be able to put aside their own disappointments or anxieties for a given period and project a positive outlook.

A first step to developing potential contacts for volunteer recruitment is to network with organizations that promote and support volunteerism. These public and private groups can be valuable sources of technical assistance and training and are often willing to help directly with volunteer recruitment.

Federal, state, and local governments are very involved in encouraging volunteerism. Nationally, ACTION is the federal agency charged with coordinating domestic volunteer efforts. Its purpose is to encourage volunteerism and to demonstrate the effectiveness of volunteerism in meeting social problems. ACTION sponsors many major programs, but of greatest interest to persons developing programs for patients with dementia is the Retired Senior Volunteer Program (RSVP) because this program actually recruits and places volunteers over 60 in a variety of programs. There are over 750 RSVP programs in the United States.

Also, on the national level several private, nonprofit groups are dedicated to promoting volunteerism and assisting individual program managers. VOLUNTEER—The National Center offers technical assistance and support to volunteer programs. The Association of Volunteer Administration is a professional organization for individuals serving in the field of volunteer management.

State and local governments also have made efforts to support volunteerism. In early 1988, more than thirty-five states had offices of volunteerism. These offices are often willing to assist in the development of volunteer programs, sponsor training programs and conferences, and help with grantsmanship. At the local level, governments sometimes offer support through the office of the mayor.

Community-based groups (sometimes chapters of national organizations) involved in volunteerism are too numerous to mention. Groups with a particular interest in programs for older persons include the nonprofit Volunteer Centers (sometimes called Voluntary Action Centers) that exist in many communities to encourage volunteerism. These Volunteer Centers, part of an informal national network of such centers, are particularly helpful to groups planning new programs because they maintain comprehensive listings of local volunteer resources.

Other community groups helpful to volunteer programs include the American Association of Retired Persons, the National Association for Retired Federal Employees (NARFE), Red Cross chapters, and Junior League organizations. In addition, private business and industry, "newcomer's clubs," churches, synagogues, high schools, colleges and universities, and various clubs and organizations have volunteer programs.

Although the mentioned resources can prove invaluable to volunteer programs for Alzheimer's patients and their families, the only national organization with local chapters specifically devoted to serving this population is the Alzheimer's Association. By working with a local Alzheimer's Association chapter, program planners can tap a rich source of volunteers and ensure coordination of services.

Once a program planner has contacted national, state, and local groups for information and support, recruitment efforts can begin. As a result of networking with other groups promoting volunteerism, the planner should have an extensive listing of sources for volunteers. When the Helping Hand staff developed this initial list, staff began making approaches to specific organizations, asking for names of potential volunteers. These individuals were then contacted one by one and asked if they could help. This individualized approach is particularly important in the area of Alzheimer's disease because dementing illnesses are still largely misunderstood by the community and caring for persons with Alzheimer's disease is an unfamiliar experience to many potential volunteers.

Also at this time, the Helping Hand began a media campaign to make people aware of volunteer opportunities. Advertising volunteer opportunities in newspapers, radio, television, and posters brought visibility and credibility to the program and planted seeds of interest. However, persons interested in giving time as volunteers do not readily respond to a mass appeal for help. These appeals compete with many other messages and make it easy for one to feel that the need for help is being addressed to someone else (Wilson 1976).

The Helping Hand has had great success in attracting volunteers from area Alzheimer's support groups. Former family caregivers have actively participated in volunteer work. These volunteers, who have finished the long journey of caring, know how much it means to have someone to help. They may also feel that they have expertise from their caregiving experience that would be valuable to share with others. One former caregiver said, "I felt that I was giving care in the dark. Now that I am more knowledgeable about the disease and the care needed, I am able to share this by helping others."

Among its volunteers, the program also counts family members whose loved ones are being cared for in other cities. Persons who are miles away from the caregiving of a family member may respond to a volunteer task near home. "Someone is helping with my mother and since I can't be there I would like to give care to someone here" is an often-expressed sentiment.

As the community has become more familiar with Helping Hand, volunteers have become easier to recruit. The program has received strong support from several organizations, including Junior League, the Kiwanis Club, NARFE, and the RSVP program.

The very best contacts for volunteers are from enthusiastic volunteers already on the job. The Helping Hand encourages volunteers to be involved in the recruitment process. They often know someone who would be "perfect" to love and care for a person with a memory disorder.

Once potential volunteers are identified, they are invited to observe the program from beginning to end. It is always made clear that the invitation has "no strings attached." This visit allows them to observe the spirit of the program and helps them, and the staff, determine whether they will feel comfortable working with a person with dementia. After they have reflected on their visit to the program, a staff member arranges a time to discuss the program, offer information, and answer questions. If still interested, the person is invited to attend the next scheduled training session.

Training Volunteers

Rigorous training for volunteers is a critical component of any program serving persons with dementing illness. To receive expert help in designing its training program, Helping Hand staff turned to the Alzheimer's Disease Research Center at the University of Kentucky, one of twelve such centers funded by the National Institute on Aging. These centers, other colleges and universities, Alzheimer's Association chapters, private physicians, nurses, social workers, physical therapists, and others can provide assistance in developing and leading training programs.

Volunteers in the Helping Hand receive sixteen hours of training covering the following major areas: changes in normal aging, Alzheimer's disease and related disorders, families under stress, relating and communicating with a demented person, and assisting with motor abilities and handling emergencies. The first four-hour training program covers the biology of aging and offers an overview of Alzheimer's disease and other dementing illnesses. A critical concept conveyed in this section is that confusion and memory loss are not a normal part of aging. The training stresses that individuals suffering memory loss or confusion *at any age* should receive a complete medical evaluation.

Resources used in this segment include copies of *The 36-Hour Day* (Mace and Rabins 1981) given to each volunteer and copies of literature about Alzheimer's produced by the Alzheimer's Association. Continuing educational efforts included the distribution of current articles and quarterly updates at volunteer meetings.

The second segment of training for Helping Hand volunteers is four hours on the impact of dementing illnesses on families. Because the volunteer will inevitably spend time with the caregiver, understanding the impact of dementia on the family is vital. The most effective teaching tool is to ask several caregivers to come to the session to "tell their stories." No one better knows the stress of caregiving than one who has experienced the physical, emotional, and financial stress of dementing disease. In addition to the caregiver interviews, the training program has involved social workers, psychologists, and other professionals to discuss how families are affected by diseases causing dementia.

A number of resources are used in this segment. *The Hidden Victims of Alzheimer's Disease: Families under Pressure* (Zarit et al. 1985) focuses on the impact of dementing illness on families. The Alzheimer's Association has several publications aimed at teenagers and young children that can be helpful. A 1986 video made by the Alzheimer's Association, "Caring: Families Coping with Alzheimer's Disease," is an effective introduction because it follows three different families and their approaches to caregiving. Also, reprints of selected academic articles on caregivers are offered.

The third four-hour training segment covers relating to and communicating with persons with memory disorders. When a person with dementia can no longer respond to the usual flow of conversation or participate in day-to-day activities, it is easy to converse inappropriately or ignore the person entirely. Being sensitive to the participant's level of functioning and learning to communicate and relate within that framework is often the key to improved self-esteem. To underestimate a person's functional level can be as frustrating as to overestimate his abilities.

Role playing is the technique that has proved most effective in this third segment of training. Role playing is an excellent way for volunteers to begin to understand the feelings of anxiety, frustration, depression, and anger that often accompany a memory disorder. Role playing at different levels of dementia can be very helpful in teaching volunteers to assess the functional level of each participant.

The following is a sample of role playing used in training programs. Two persons are chosen to participate. Mr. A is talking to his friend with Alzheimer's disease but is unaware of how one should communicate with a person with a memory loss. Mr. B plays the role of a person who cannot recall recent events and names of persons, places, or things. The dialogue begins with:

Mr. A: Hello, how are you today?

Mr. B: (smiles and responds) Great!

Mr. A: What brings you here?

Mr. B: (looks away, shifts from one foot to another, and finally answers) Not really.

Mr. A: (not knowing what to say next but feeling that he must say something) Hear that you've had a trip recently. Where did you go?

Mr. B: (wrings his hands and looks for someone to help him with an answer)

Mr. A: (embarrassed, begins to guess) Did you head south?

Mr. B: (walks away from an impossible situation)

Because Mr. A asks inappropriate questions, Mr. B becomes anxious and frustrated.

When the same situation is presented after Mr. A has attended a study session on communicating with a person with dementia, the results are much more positive:

Mr. A: Hello, how are you today?

Mr. B: (smiles and responds) Great.

Mr. A: So glad to see you, *Tom.*

Mr. B: Yes. (smiles)

Mr. A: How's your wife, *Mary*?

Mr. B: (points in his wife's direction) Over there. (seems pleased to be identifying his wife)

Mr. A: I understand that you and Mary have just had a trip to the *beach.*

Mr. B: (pleased) Yes.

Mr. A: Bet that was fun. I love the *ocean.*

Mr. B: Yes and those big things come rolling in.

Mr. A now has knowledge about Mr. B's family and background, provides verbal cues, and shows greater sensitivity to Mr. B's memory problem.

Another important part of this section on communication is the explanation of the Helping Hand's use of biographical information on each participant. Before admission to the program, families help staff and volunteers create brief "life stories" that include the persons, places, events, and things that may help persons with dementia recall positive aspects of their lives. During the training, the life story is introduced and volunteers are taught to use the biographical facts to give verbal and nonverbal cues that may help the demented person find pleasant moments of recall. For example, Mr. A's knowledge of Mr. B's life story in the second role playing episode greatly improved their ability to relate and communicate.

Because volunteers work so closely with participants on a weekly basis, training stresses that volunteers will come to know very well the individuals with whom they work. Through the participant's life story and day-to-day companionship, volunteers can recognize life-long patterns of behavior and be able to anticipate and often avoid problem behavior. Building on the information learned about the effect of Alzheimer's disease on the patient, the training stresses those activities and areas of interest appropriate given functional limitations. Thus, knowledge about communication and the weekly, ongoing relationship that volunteers form with participants allow volunteers to develop skill and confidence when working with participants who have dementia.

Behaviors difficult to manage can occur despite all efforts, however. Role playing again is used to demonstrate improved methods of handling such behaviors. Two resources helpful on the subject of difficult behavior include *Care of Alzheimer's Patients: A Manual for Nursing Home Staff* (Gwyther 1985) and *The 36-Hour Day* (Mace and Rabins 1981).

The final four hours consist of lectures and demonstrations by a nurse and physical therapist. Simple rules of lifting, moving, standing, and walking a person with dementia are covered, as are handling emergencies such as choking, fire, and medical problems. Ample time is provided for volunteers to practice all techniques presented. Comments are often made that this training has proved useful in settings other than the respite program.

Although training program content may vary from program to

program, I recommend that volunteers be exposed to a vigorous training program and an ongoing learning process. Before making a definite commitment, the volunteer should be encouraged to work in a
program several weeks after training. Trained and committed volunteers will have greater skills and more confidence in their work.
They are likely to stay involved longer, and training is certain to
improve the quality of the program.

Effectively Utilizing Volunteers

No matter how good a recruitment program or how extensive
the training, the key factor for success in developing a volunteer
program is the quality of the experience for volunteers. Because volunteer programs serving patients with dementia and their families
are fairly recent, there are few models for volunteer program planners
to follow on what tasks volunteers can perform. The following volunteer sketches look at four roles assumed by volunteers in the Helping Hand program: volunteer as caregiver, volunteer as family friend,
volunteer as group leader, and volunteer as teacher/role model.

Joan—Volunteer as Caregiver

Joan had cared for her mother with Alzheimer's disease. When
her mother died, Joan wanted to offer some help to another family
by using the skills she had gained helping her mother.

As a Helping Hand volunteer, Joan shared each Wednesday afternoon with Frank, a former executive director of a large government
agency. When he had started in the Helping Hand program, he had
still been able to describe his feelings about his illness, once saying
of his problem, "It's like your head is a big knob turned to off." The
disease progressed, and after three years he spoke in a jumble of
seemingly meaningless words. Although his communication skills
were severely impaired, when he arrived for the program he often
greeted Joan by saying, "That's the one." Frank may not have known
Joan's name or exactly who she was, but down deep he seemed to
know that Joan was his friend who cared for him every week.

Joan became Frank's memory. She knew the names of his family,
his dogs, his favorite vacation spots, his love of jazz music, and much
more. She was like a barometer reading his emotional needs; she
could almost always predict what would bring him joy and what
would be stressful for him. Testing every six months showed that he

was experiencing a steady cognitive decline, but Joan learned to be more resourceful in adapting the environment of the program to meet Frank's needs and to help him maintain his dignity. The week before Frank died, he and Joan danced to the music of Benny Goodman.

Comment

Volunteer programs often fail because volunteers feel that the work they are doing is not important. In the Helping Hand program, volunteers become primary caregivers one afternoon per week. This sense of responsibility motivates volunteers in a number of ways. They develop a strong relationship with the person for whom they care. The volunteers know that their work does make a difference; participants often seem appreciative and value the attention of the volunteers.

Mark—Volunteer as Family Friend

Mark is a retired minister and has been active in the Helping Hand since it began. Today he carefully helped Laura with her coat and hat and watched for her car to arrive. Instead, her caregiver son-in-law, John, appeared in the hallway. "Could I see you for a few minutes, Mark?" he said with a sense of urgency in his voice. Mark placed Laura's hand in the hand of another volunteer and quietly went down the hall for a few private moments with John.

"We're concerned about Mom. Did you notice a big difference in her behavior today?" John was obviously worried. Mark was quick to answer affirmatively. Certainly he had noticed a gradual decline over the past two years, but today Laura was more restless than usual and seemed to be in pain. Together they agreed that she should see her doctor. The medical examination revealed a bladder infection that was causing her to be very uncomfortable.

During his time as a volunteer working regularly with Laura, Mark had developed a close relationship with Laura's children. Mark regularly meets the family when they drop off and pick up Laura. The conversations often help Mark to learn more about Laura's past. Once he learned that she had enjoyed crocheting. The conversation resulted in Laura bringing an example of her work, a crocheted bedspread, to show. Laura smiled as she recognized something her hands had created. Time with Mark also allows the family to talk with someone who knows Laura and understands the difficulty of caring for her. "You won't believe what Mom did today!" is a common opening.

Comment

Although the volunteer's primary role is to serve the program participant, volunteers interact with the family as well. One caregiver recently wrote, "The volunteers are my best friends. They care about me in the same loving way that they care for my loved one." Volunteers are part of a team effort to help both participant and caregiver.

Mary—Volunteer as Group Leader

Mary is a retired elementary school teacher and is adept at involving every participant and volunteer in the topic of the day. "You're right, Sid, that is an old-fashioned apple-peeler," Mary commented as she moved from table to table to discuss other articles related to apples. There was a miniature apple basket, a picture of a cider press, a jar of apple jelly, and many varieties of apples. Volunteers also brought in sayings and songs about apples. There was a time to talk about favorite recipes and to touch and taste the apples. On this day, Mary had given much thought to the participants and their backgrounds and present abilities and had worked to design ways of involving even the most demented participants.

Previously, Mary had helped plan other topics for the program and had had the opportunity to decide which subjects she would like to discuss with the group. Mary is also a part of the weekly and quarterly program evaluation. She enjoys reviewing past activities and interests to determine the most successful approaches.

Comment

On a rotating basis, volunteers in the Helping Hand lead the program's class. The activities are often based on special interests of the volunteers (e.g., volunteers sometimes bring in shells, antique toys, or other items that they have collected). At first it was planned to develop four or five classes as perfectly as possible by using all five senses to stimulate and challenge participants. It soon became obvious that volunteers were not challenged by repetitive topics and participants noticed the enthusiasm of volunteers when new topics were discussed. Thus the format was changed to discussion of a different topic each week.

The results have been strongly positive. Volunteers who have experience in public speaking or teaching enjoy using these skills. Yet other volunteers who may not have strong confidence in their speaking ability are still encouraged to share their interests with the group. Being sensitive to the needs of patients with dementia is more important than producing a "perfect" presentation.

Sarah — Volunteer as Teacher

Sarah has volunteered in the program for two years. As a retired nurse and exercise enthusiast, she enjoys leading the weekly exercise and dance program. Sarah regularly suggests new activities to keep participants physically active. From experience with participants and their life stories, she knows which participants enjoy dancing and their favorite type of music. Sarah recently said, "I'm amazed at the joy and happiness that music can create for both participants and volunteers."

Present that day were two nursing students from a nearby university and an observer from a local nursing home. Before and after the program, Sarah talked with these visitors about her volunteer work and the activities that day. Sarah spoke with great confidence about the kind of activities appropriate for persons with memory loss. In addition, she answered questions about Alzheimer's disease, the importance of respite care for families, and how the program functions.

Comment

Volunteers often speak to community groups and visiting students and professionals. In effect, volunteers become role models for persons caring for individuals with dementia. If volunteers can succeed, our staff often says, there is no excuse for professionals in other settings not to strive to improve their skills and raise their commitment to serving persons with dementing illness. One volunteer urged the staff at the nursing home caring for his wife to visit the Helping Hand. As a direct result of that visit, the nursing home reassessed their approach to patients with dementia and developed more creative activities for their residents.

Retaining Volunteers

The best way to maintain continued volunteer involvement is by offering a meaningful experience. The Helping Hand has succeeded in part because of its high expectations for volunteers. Volunteers assume many roles including caregiver, family friend, group leader, and teacher. The joyful milieu created in the program allows volunteers to get to know participants and each other. Many friendships have been formed.

Another important aspect of retaining volunteers is strong lines of communication between volunteers and staff. In our program, scheduling for absences is done one month in advance, but volunteers know that if they need time off for an unexpected event they can talk to staff and a substitute will be called. Volunteers are involved in the decision-making and evaluation process and are kept up-to-date on program news. Also, volunteers are encouraged to share concerns or problems with staff immediately.

The Helping Hand has avoided volunteer burnout in part because of its volunteer sabbaticals. Volunteers who have worked over two years in the program are encouraged to take a three-month break. They then return to the program with renewed enthusiasm and new experiences to share with the group.

Formal activities to recognize the volunteers' contributions are also important. The Helping Hand sponsors occasional social events and luncheons. Volunteers are often nominated for the local newspaper's "Volunteer of the Week" and other local and state awards.

Conclusion

The Helping Hand program, a dementia-specific day care program, has involved volunteers successfully for over four years. Initially, many believed that the volunteer model could not work. Comments at the time included, "Be sure to have the volunteers take self-defense lessons to protect them from the participants," and "Volunteer burnout will be high—the program should primarily utilize paid aides and have volunteers help out."

It is clear that these critics were wrong. Nineteen of the first twenty volunteers are still active. Families who utilize the program and professionals who visit have agreed that the quality of care is high.

For programs helping persons with dementia, volunteers can be an unlimited resource that allows one-to-one care, a ratio impossible to achieve with paid staff. Volunteer programs are not free, however. They require significant staff time and ongoing support, but the rewards can be great!

References

Americans volunteer, 1985. 1986. Washington, DC: Independent Sector.

Howell, M. 1984. Caretakers' views on responsibilities for the care of the demented elderly. *Journal of the American Geriatrics Society* 32: (9): 657–60.

Wilson, M. 1976. *The effective management of volunteer programs.* Boulder, CO: Volunteer Management Associates.

Suggested Reading

Building Volunteer Programs

Flanagan, J. 1984. *The successful volunteer organization.* Chicago: Contemporary Books, Inc.

Naylor, H. 1973. *Volunteers today: Finding, training, and working with them.* Dryden, NY: Dryden Associates.

Vizza, C., K. Allen, and S. Keller. 1986. *A new competitive edge: Volunteers from the work place.* Arlington, VA: VOLUNTEER, The National Center.

Wilson, M. 1976. *The effective management of volunteer programs.* Boulder, CO: Volunteer Management Associates.

Wilson, M. 1981. *Survival skills for managers.* Boulder, CO: Volunteer Management Associates.

Wilson, M. 1983. *How to mobilize church volunteers.* Boulder, CO: Volunteer Management Associates.

Alzheimer's Training Sessions

Gwyther, L. 1985. *Care of Alzheimer's patients: A manual for nursing home staff.* Washington, DC: American Health Care Association and Alzheimer's Disease and Related Disorders Association.

Mace, N., and P. Rabins. 1981. *The 36-hour day: A family guide to caring for persons with Alzheimer's disease, related dementing illness, and memory loss in later life.* Baltimore: Johns Hopkins University Press.

Quinn, T., and J. Crabtree, eds. 1987. *How to start a respite service for people with Alzheimer's and their families.* New York: Brookdale Foundation.

Zarit, S., N. Orr, and J. Zarit. 1985. *The hidden victims of Alzheimer's disease: Families under pressure.* New York: New York University Press.

Zgola, J. 1987. *Doing things: A guide to programing activities for persons with Alzheimer's disease and related disorders.* Baltimore: Johns Hopkins University Press.

Addresses and Publications of National Organizations Promoting Volunteerism

ACTION Public Affairs, 806 Connecticut Avenue, NW, Washington, DC 20525. Quarterly publication: *ACTION Update.*

Association for Volunteer Administration, Post Office Box 4584, Boulder, CO
80306. Quarterly publication: *Journal of Volunteer Administration.*
VOLUNTEER: The National Center, 1111 North 19th Street, Suite 500, Arlington, VA 22209. Quarterly publication: *Voluntary Action Leadership.*

14

Residential Care for Persons with Dementia
DOROTHY H. COONS

The health care system is faced with the over-whelming question of how to provide appropriate and humane care for those who are currently afflicted with Alzheimer's disease or other forms of dementia and for whom no curative treatment is known. At present, there exist two sources of care—the family and the nursing home. The role of caregiver may be long and stressful. Because the victims of dementing diseases are often very old, the family members caring for them may be themselves in late middle age or elderly. In time, families may reach a decision to place a relative in an institution because they become overwhelmed with the demands and realize that they are unable to continue to render the necessary care and attention required by the relative. The decisions for nursing home placement are frequently reached only after much agonizing and feelings of guilt. The negative images that families have of nursing homes add to the distress that they experience (Chenoweth and Spencer 1986).

Nursing homes, too, have been facing a dilemma for which they have found few answers. Neither the staff nor the nursing home system is prepared to give individualized care for this group of people. Alzheimer's disease victims remain lucid during much of their illness and, although often very disoriented, they are keenly aware of their environment and are sensitive to the behaviors of others around them. If they interpret others' behaviors as a violation of what they consider appropriate, they may quickly respond in anger and combativeness. Restless energy or agitation may also lead to incessant wandering. These characteristics can present insurmountable difficulties for the traditional nursing home staff, whose major mission is that of pro-viding continuous and sustained medical and nursing care and who must rely on unvarying schedules and routines to meet heavy daily demands.

Emerging from a number of studies (Mace 1987; Coons 1987b) is a realization of the existence of a serious gap in the continuum of care. There is a great need for settings with a social orientation that recognize the capacities and sensitivity that remain intact, at least in part, for years in many Alzheimer's victims. The establishment of special units, however, without new knowledge and new methods will result in facilities that are no more effective than those currently caring for this very special group of people (Koff 1986).

Persons in the early and middle stages of Alzheimer's disease are unique among those in need of care in old age. Some are relatively healthy from a physical point of view and are not afflicted with multiple chronic impairments and the frailties characteristic of the largest population of the elderly in nursing homes. This factor makes them aliens in our current health care system.

For most victims of the disease, their life pattern for fifty or more years has been that of the usual adult. They have had careers, families, their own homes, and, in varying degrees, have been educated and have experienced independence and success in life. Although the onset of Alzheimer's disease is slow and insidious, the victim usually recognizes early the gradual and devastating changes that are occurring and will lead only to growing dependency and eventually to a full loss of function. The pathos of the situation was vividly expressed by one Alzheimer's disease victim in his diary written, with the help of his wife, a year after his diagnosis. He wrote: "No theory of medicine can explain what is happening to me. Every few months I sense that another piece of me is missing. My life . . . my self . . . are falling apart. I can only think half thoughts now. Someday I may wake up and not think at all . . . not know who I am. Most people expect to die someday, but who ever expected to lose their self, first" (Cohen and Eisdorfer 1986). The progression of the disease affects the individual's capacity to function, and the stages of the illness have been defined principally in terms of functioning level. The identification of stages is a gross evaluation at best. The fluctuation of the impaired person's ability to function or comprehend creates many shaded areas that make the practice of categorizing persons with dementia questionable. There is also the danger that the diagnosis of the late stages of Alzheimer's disease may actually become the basis for withdrawing services from the victim. Even with severely impaired persons, there remains for many a conscious awareness of the environment and a need for social and psychological supports. Researchers have described Alzheimer's disease as having various numbers of stages from three to seven (Berg and Danziger 1984; Berger 1985; Reisberg et al. 1982). The Berger classification is used in this chapter not as absolutely distinct and separate stages but as a means of defining the range of needs in the continuum of care for persons with dementia who are not limited in performance by physical handicaps, vision or hearing losses, or delirium.

Berger (1985) used what he called a practical, understandable classification to help identify the severity of impairment as well as the specific needs of persons in each category. His system includes the following stages:

Severity Class I: can function in any surrounding, but forgetfulness is often disruptive of daily activities;

Severity Class II: can function without direction only in familiar surroundings;

Severity Class III: needs direction to function even in familiar surroundings but can respond appropriately to instruction;

Severity Class IV: needs assistance to function and cannot respond to direction alone;

Severity Class V: remains ambulatory, needs assistance to function, but cannot communicate verbally;

Severity Class VI: bedridden or confined to a chair and responds only to tactile stimuli.

Families are frequently able to care for relatives in the early stages of the disease, but one study (George 1984) found that a surprisingly large number (40 percent) of persons with Alzheimer's disease or related dementias were living at home at the time of death. For many families, however, the care becomes so stressful that the caregiver becomes ill or so exhausted that he or she can no longer provide for a relative. For those in the final stages of the illness, nursing homes are usually prepared to give the complete care needed. Alzheimer's victims in the middle Stages III and IV and, to some extent, Stage V are the ones most inadequately served by our current system. The progression of the disease varies greatly from person to person, and some may remain in the middle stages for years. Residential care settings are needed to fill the gap in the current health care system between the family that can no longer provide care at home and the traditional nursing home. Those in Stage V who are ambulatory and not in need of extensive medical and nursing care would also benefit from modified residential care that adapts staffing patterns, approaches, and the physical environment to their special needs. Such settings would give families the opportunity to make placement decisions, not out of desperation and as a last resort, but on the basis of the therapeutic benefits to their impaired family members. Table 14.1 illustrates a proposed continuum of care to accommodate the changing care needs of the person with Alzheimer's-type dementia.

This chapter describes, as a part of the continuum of care, a residential care setting especially designed for persons in the middle stages (III and IV) of Alzheimer's disease. A model called Wesley Hall was tested in a two-year demonstration project from December 1983 through December 1985. Interventions included alterations in the physical environment, extensive staff training to help staff assume new roles and relationships with residents, and the designing of a milieu that offered rich and meaningful opportunities for resident involvement. The criteria used in developing Wesley Hall are applicable to any setting seeking to provide care for dementia victims, including nursing homes, psychiatric hospitals, community hospitals, adult day care programs, respite care, and retirement homes. The cost of residential care, as implemented on Wesley Hall, was somewhat lower than the cost of nursing home care, yet residential care offered an environment better suited to those who may remain in the middle stages of Alzheimer's disease for years (Coons 1987b).

The person with a dementing disease has been described principally in terms of *loss* of cognitive abilities and functional capacities. Treatment has focused on ways to control behavior identified as symptomatic of dementia. In the Wesley Hall project, the diagnosis of dementia was considered only partially descriptive of the individual. There was emphasis also on identifying remaining capacities and abilities. The diagnosis of dementia, in the medical context, denotes brain damage that is viewed as untreatable and carries with it the prognosis of inevitable deterioration. In many instances, this can serve as the rationale for offering only custodial care.

In contrast, the therapeutic milieu for persons with dementia will *maximize* their remaining capacities and their abilities to respond and benefit from warm and supportive interactions with others. It will *deemphasize* the deficits and impairments that are characteristic of the disease. The objective is to create an accepting, enjoyable, and sup-

TABLE 14.1 Proposed continuum of care

	Family Care	Residential Care	Residential Care	Institutional Care
Location	In the home, sometimes with the help of day care and respite services	In specially designed units in nursing homes, retirement homes, or freestanding units	In specially designed units in nursing homes or freestanding units	In nursing homes or Veterans Administration facilities or community hospitals
Severity of Impairment*	Stages 1 and 2 or even until death if the family is able to provide care	Stages 3 and 4 (if there are no medical complications that require extensive nursing care)	Stage 5 (if there are no medical complications that require extensive nursing care)	Stage 6 (and Stages 3, 4, and 5 if there are medical complications that require extensive nursing care)
Type of Care	Supervision, maintenance, treatment for depression if needed, legal and financial planning, and structured supportive social activities	Total milieu responds to social and psychological needs and gives assistance with activities of daily living as needed	Total milieu responds to social and psychological needs and gives extensive assistance with activities of daily living	The milieu responds to medical, nursing, and total care needs and provides sensory and social stimulation

* Based on Berger's (1985) System for Rating Severity of Impairment.

portive milieu that will help people with progressive dementia to get pleasure from living and will serve to distract them from the constant reminders of their illness.

The following list of criteria characterizes the residential care model described here:

1. homogeneity of the resident population;
2. a small, homelike, and manageable setting with preferably no more than fifteen residents;
3. maximal resident autonomy and freedom;

4. individualization and flexibility of approaches and resident opportunities;
5. a continuity with the past and in family relationships and a continuation of normal social roles for residents;
6. a stimulating sensory and social environment;
7. staff roles and approaches that respond to the special needs of residents;
8. staff training and training methods that sensitize staff members to the special needs of persons with dementia;
9. a cohesive staff team with strong administrative support; and
10. good diagnostic and medical care.

The latter part of this chapter provides the rationale for each criterion and a discussion of its application in the Wesley Hall project.

The Development of Wesley Hall: A Residential Care Setting

The residential care setting called Wesley Hall* was designed as a two-year experimental demonstration at the Chelsea United Methodist Retirement Home located in the town of Chelsea, Michigan. The retirement home, with 159 residents, is part of a twenty-six-acre campus that also includes separate apartments for independent living and a 110-bed facility for skilled nursing care. Residents of the retirement home are expected to be capable, with a minimum of assistance, of managing basic activities of daily living.

In 1983, the home was facing a crisis typical of many such facilities throughout the country. As its resident population aged, many had become increasingly impaired and, according to estimates of the administrator, approximately 10 percent were suffering from severe memory loss. They were ambulatory and relatively healthy physically and thus were considered inappropriate candidates for the nursing area. They were no longer able to manage, however, in the large and widely separated areas of the retirement home. Some were unable to

---

* This project was highlighted in the videotape/film, *Wesley Hall: A Special Life*, produced by Inner Image Productions, Inc., and distributed by Terra Nova Films, 9484 S. Winchester Ave., Chicago, Illinois 60643. Other project staff of the Institute of Gerontology, The University of Michigan, included Anne Robinson, Director of the Wesley Hall Unit; Beth Spencer, Program Consultant; and Dr. Shelly Weaverdyck, Neuropsychological Consultant.

Note: All names of residents have been changed.

locate the central dining room; others were incontinent in their futile effort to find their hall's bathroom. As they drifted in and out of other residents' rooms, aimless in their search for places that they could not find, they became constant targets of the anger and resentment of alert residents. They soon acquired the labels of the "crazies" and the "seniles" and, with the constant verbal abuse from some of the more mentally able residents, they became increasingly agitated and fearful. Some seldom left their rooms. It was an equally difficult time for alert residents, who were disturbed both day and night by the wandering of the impaired residents.

When the home's administration approached the investigators for assistance, a decision was reached to establish a special living area that could be redesigned to accommodate the deficits and, at the same time, encourage use of the remaining skills and abilities of this vulnerable group. It was expected that there would be a constant testing and evaluation of new approaches, activities, and practices that could be used successfully with persons who were severely impaired. Staff members would be encouraged to question traditional patterns of communication and methods of working with impaired persons and to develop close, supportive relationships with residents.

The Wesley Hall project rested on the principle that both the social and physical environments can be significant factors in the care and treatment of dementia victims. A number of the therapeutic measures to be introduced in Wesley Hall required alterations in the physical environment that had the potential of conflicting with certain state codes. In anticipation of this, the institute staff met with the inspection officer of the state department of public health to explain the objectives of the project and to seek permission for the installation of a small kitchen, acceptable as a "learning resources center," and for residents to wash and dry dishes used at meals. Both of these requests were granted. The fire marshal was consulted to ensure that the new furniture and its arrangement would meet safety regulations. These are important first steps, for the process of change can be long and difficult if the alterations are viewed as violations of existing state and federal codes.

A series of meetings with the employees' union in the home before the opening of the area was especially crucial to explain why staff were taking new roles and why residents would be involved in many tasks ordinarily handled by staff in other parts of the home. The union was cooperative and supportive of the plans.

During the second year of the project, Wesley Hall had a full-time coordinator, one full-time and one half-time resident assistant (called "aides" in the retirement and nursing homes) on day and afternoon shifts, one full-time resident assistant on the midnight shift, and a part-time housekeeper to work with the eleven residents. Medications and other medical care were administered by the nursing staff from the retirement home and the nursing home. The primary physician was also medical director of the home. The staff:resident ratio was lower when Wesley Hall opened, but it was soon discovered that residents needed far more assistance with self-care activities or tasks, for example, than a small staff could provide. Even with the increase, staffing during the second year was considered to be at a minimum. The area would have benefitted from an activities person or from two full-time resident assistants on the day and afternoon shifts. A highly skilled and dynamic coordinator was seen as a critical component in the success of Wesley Hall. She worked regularly with residents in implementing many of the activities and in helping them in activities of daily living. This enabled her to model behaviors and approaches, but it also gave her direct experience with some of the problems of other staff members.

Wesley Hall was located in the home for the aged rather than the nursing home in the Chelsea complex and was designed as an intermediate level of care. This presented problems for several families, for there was no mechanism available for reimbursement for an intermediate level of care in the state of Michigan. Wesley Hall was established as a private pay area, but, with the special efforts of the home's administrator, two families were able to get supplemental support. At the time of the completion of the project in December 1985, daily costs to residents of the retirement home were $29.70; Wesley Hall residents paid $42.65 a day; and the nursing home section (intermediate and skilled) cost $60.00 a day.

Criteria for Designing a Residential Care Setting: Rationale and Application

Homogeneity of the Resident Population

Rationale

The Institute of Gerontology has long advocated the designing of treatment environments for persons of similar needs, abilities, and deficits and, through research, has documented the effectiveness of such a policy. It is essential, however, to view the grouping of persons according to capacity as an opportunity to design the physical environment, the activities, and the staff approaches in ways that are appropriate and can best accommodate the needs of special populations. Segregation alone is not sufficient; it is merely a first step in the development of the therapeutic milieu (Coons 1983).

The question of whether special units should be established for persons with dementing disease has been debated for the past several years with no consensus. The feelings are vehement on both sides of the issue (Mace 1987).

Administrators often cite the financial and logistical problems of organizing treatment according to needs. Others believe that it is reasonable to expect the alert elderly person to help an impaired roommate or neighbor on a regular basis, in spite of the fact that even staff members sometimes find such assistance stressful and difficult. Such a policy creates a distasteful situation for the alert resident, who is forced to live in close proximity with a severely impaired person who is often barely more than an acquaintance.

A frequently expressed argument for integration is that alert persons can serve as models for those who are impaired. The circumstances that led to the designing of the project described in this chapter refute that argument from two perspectives. First, it seems unrealistic to assume that cognitively impaired older persons have the capacity to use the behaviors of other persons as prototypes for their own responses. Second, alert persons who find themselves angry, frustrated, and unable to cope with their impaired neighbors would be poor behavioral models.

Homogeneity enables the designer to provide a milieu that meets the needs of each of the members of the group to the greatest extent possible. If facilities have established several units with each accommodating different levels of impairment, it becomes possible to meet the needs of residents as their conditions decline by moving them to the milieu that is most appropriate for them. A wide diversity in a group to be served leads to a design that accommodates neither the severely impaired nor the intact person. Those with severe memory loss require very specific types of supports and approaches if they are to be helped to maintain a maximal level of functioning. What is appropriate for a severely impaired group would be inappropriate and excessively protective for alert persons. On the other hand, an environment designed for well aged persons can be stressful for persons with dementia, offering them little or no protection or compensation for deficits. There is no question, however, that both the cognitively impaired and the alert elderly can benefit from environments that take into account the sensory losses that are a part of normal aging.

Application

To select a group of residents with similar needs and capacities, project staff developed the following selection criteria for Wesley Hall. Residents were:

1. ambulatory;
2. able to feed themselves using a fork or spoon with occasional help from staff to cut up meat or vegetables;
3. having problems with severe memory loss and confusion, such as being unable to locate their own rooms, the bathrooms, or the central dining room or to identify the facility or town in which they were living;
4. not in need of extensive or sustained medical care beyond that which the small number of staff in the area would be able to provide;
5. able to manage at least some self-care activities with the assistance of staff; and
6. able to follow simple instructions related to very simple tasks such as arranging cookies on a plate or pouring juice.

Wesley Hall was not a barrier-free environment, but residents could use walkers or canes. Diagnoses varied; ten of the original residents were diagnosed as having either Alzheimer's disease or multi-infarct dementia; one of the eleven residents had a diagnosis of dementia secondary to viral encephalitis.

A number of instruments designed to assess mental functioning were administered before and throughout the two-year project. On the mental status questionnaire of Kahn et al. (1960), residents scored eight, nine, or ten of ten possible errors or "don't know" answers, placing them in the range of or bordering on the severely impaired (Kane and Kane 1981). Abilities to verbalize varied considerably, ranging from several who were fairly articulate most of the time to two who had problems in forming even short simple sentences. There was much variation in capacities from day-to-day and in different situations. Most had problems with spatial orientation and in naming relatives when they visited.

When staff from the nursing, activities, dietary, and housekeeping departments of the home were asked to identify and describe persons having difficulties living in the large retirement home, they used such words as disoriented, bewildered, frightened, combative, agitated, restless, depressed, withdrawn, difficult, inappropriate in behavior, and incontinent. They adequately described the behaviors of the various residents eventually selected for Wesley Hall.

A Small, Homelike, and Manageable Setting with Preferably No More than Fifteen Residents

Rationale

Persons with dementia are overwhelmed by large, unmanageable spaces and large numbers of people with whom they must cope. Based on the experiences of Wesley Hall and those of others, a group of eight to fifteen persons in an area has the potential, if well designed, of providing a minimum of stress. More than fifteen persons may increase the frequency of aberrant behavior and make care difficult. In facilities having a large population of persons with dementia, a series of small, self-contained units with residents grouped according to their degrees of impairment can offer an opportunity to provide nonstressful environments. A small, stable group makes possible a social interchange among residents, even those who are severely impaired.

It is essential that designers look beyond the physical structure to the social consequences of their plans. A small dining room can serve, for example, as a persistent reminder that the resident is in a home, not a hospital, especially if arranged to encourage mealtime communication and congeniality (Boling et al. 1983). The creation of a homelike environment with familiar sounds, aromas, sights, and personal possessions deemphasizes the illness of residents and helps them to maintain identity. There is evidence that the presence of personal possessions increases the likelihood that staff will perceive elderly persons in a positive way and as being less decrepit than their illness would indicate (Millard and Smith 1981).

In an effort to create a homelike environment that avoids constant reminders of illness and dependency, the residential care setting deliberately omits the formal nursing station. Past trends that provided prominent nurses' stations with ready visibility of all doorways and call lights are now being questioned by geriatric nurses. The new trend is for staff members to be with residents as much as possible rather than being behind nurses' stations (Hiatt 1985). To further reduce the emphasis on illness and to encourage more friendly relationships between staff members and residents, staff members do not wear uniforms. This departure from the traditional medical model encourages more social conversations and interactions and reduces the hierarchy that often exists between staff and residents. The residential care model also discards such noxious institutional reminders as the intercom system as being inappropriate and disturbing to residents, who are often baffled and even frightened by the distorted, crackling voices that come from the speaker (Lawton 1981).

In discussing a major problem in developing warm, homelike environments, Mace stated that, unfortunately, "The emphasis of standard [is] on physical evidence of quality—shining floors and sparkling bathrooms, beds perfectly made, and everything put away. Staff are discouraged from letting patients make their own beds, even if sloppily, or talking with patients instead of tidying up. This pervasive tone of regulations, more than specific incidents, shapes patient care. This focus on the physical plant, combined with financial pressure for efficiency, has resulted in an atmosphere which more resembles a hospital than a home" (Mace, N. L., letter to the author, February 1987).

Application

The area that became Wesley Hall was located on the top (fourth) floor of one wing of the retirement home. Its long hall and lack of direct access to the out-of-doors made it far from ideal, but this space was chosen because it had two bathrooms (one for men, one for women) and was separate and unattached to other units in the retirement home. Access was by elevator or stairways, and it therefore did not serve as a thoroughfare between different areas as did most of the other sections of the home. Before renovations, it housed twelve residents in single-occupancy rooms. The rooms opened onto a long hall that also accessed the mens' and womens' bathrooms and connected two communal areas. A small area at one end of the hall became a cozy den. The lounge area at the opposite end of the hall was furnished as a small living room with dining space. The bedroom adjacent to the dining area was converted to a kitchen (or "learning resources center").

Not only was the total area sufficiently small to make it manageable and nonstressful, but each of the rooms provided a sense of intimacy and home. Residents' rooms were furnished with their own furniture and other personal possessions. Families brought in pictures and personal memorabilia to establish linkages with the past. A wooden plaque to the left of each bedroom door had a large picture of the resident and the person's name in clear, visible letters. Each door was decorated with a motif that was symbolic of the resident's earlier occupation or special interest, such as a baseball pennant, needlework, or a flower arrangement. These items not only personalized each person's room but also helped in orientation.

To accommodate sensory loss and to create a warm, inviting environment, ceilings were lowered and lighting was more than doubled. Short-napped carpeting replaced shining, dark tile in the living room, den, hallway, and a number of residents' rooms. The carpeting had specially treated fibers in both nap and backing that is used in hospitals to allow easy cleaning.

In lieu of a nursing station, staff used the small desk in the kitchen or the dining room tables for making notes or completing records. Wallpaper was used extensively to provide visual stimulation as well as to create a homelike, noninstitutional environment. Normal homelike sounds also added to the feelings of home, as the chirping of the pet parakeet and occasionally soft music from the record player created interest for both staff and residents.

Although regular meals were catered from the central kitchen, the appetizing aromas of food frequently prepared in the Wesley Hall kitchen added a homelike dimension. Residents and staff were frequently involved in baking and cooking activities, and the scents of muffins baking or simmering soup could be appreciated in all parts of the unit.

Maximal Resident Autonomy and Freedom

Rationale

A major goal in the residential care setting is to provide an environment that enables residents to maintain maximal autonomy over their own lives. This precludes the use of physical restraints and excessive drugs and assumes a flexibility in daily routines to accommodate changing moods and special needs of residents. The overuse of drugs is not only physically harmful to mentally impaired persons, but also essentially causes the dissolution of personality at a far greater rate than would be expected from the illness itself (Reichel 1983a). The use of physical restraints, including geri-chairs and bean bags, with the elderly is one of the most demeaning and infantilizing practices in use today. It is the final indignity that strips the elderly person of all autonomy. Several studies have shown that physical restraints, in addition to their negative effects on patient morale and on the attitudes of staff toward restrained persons, do not, in fact, reduce the frequency of accidents (Cape 1983; Frengley and Mion 1986). If there are occasions when restraints seem to be the only way to prevent persons from harming themselves (Bartol 1983), their use should be limited in time, prescribed for a clearly defined purpose, and reevaluated after a short period to determine their effectiveness.

In a study of agitated behaviors of nursing home residents, Cohen-Mansfield and Billig (1986) listed these reasons for the agitation as identified by professional staff: "1) frustration at loss of control, especially during ADL experiences of being changed, bathed or fed, or during forced activity against one's will, as having to get out of bed or to be dressed; 2) invasion of one's territory or personal space; 3) the behavior of other residents; 4) confusion, aggravated by lack of structure; 5) loneliness, need for attention; 6) depression; 7) past issues; 8) phase of the moon; 9) constipation; 10) deafness; and 11) restraints." The listing is remarkably perceptive, and it may identify most of the reasons for the "behavioral problems" in persons with dementia. If the causes suggested are correct, most of them could be avoided if environmental factors, including staff approaches, were changed. The challenge is to protect individuals from harm and at the same time ensure freedom of choice and movement.

A further challenge for staff members lies in the problem they face when residents refuse to do something, such as bathing, that staff view as essential. Coercion and control are considered inappropriate and nontherapeutic approaches in residential care and can quickly lead to difficult behaviors. To develop alternatives requires staff ingenuity and flexibility and an awareness of residents' moods.

Application

Wesley Hall was an unlocked unit, and residents had access to all congregate areas including the kitchen, dining room, living room, den, and bathrooms. This gave persons space to wander and areas to explore. The kitchen became a popular space where residents could always get coffee, juice, milk, or fruit. Safety timers on the stove and oven were installed to ensure that they could not be turned on if staff were not present.

Many opportunities were offered to residents throughout the project for them to share tasks with staff, such as folding towels, setting tables, preparing snacks, and making beds. Involvement was optional, but even those who chose not to participate in the actual tasks were often involved in the group's conversation and laughter. Residents had the freedom to choose when they would get up in the morning, when they would have breakfast, and when they would go to bed at night.

When residents first moved into Wesley Hall, several left the area by means of the elevator in attempts to return to their former rooms. They became lost on other floors as staff searched frantically for them. For a period, a needlepoint swatch was used as a disguise to cover the elevator button. The swatch was removed after residents became more comfortable in the area and made few efforts to leave. Doors leading to stairs were unlocked but were painted to match the surrounding walls. This served as sufficient camouflage that residents only occasionally seemed aware that they led to ways out of the area. Later in the project, when staff had become aware of individual capacities to manage, several residents left the area to pick up newspapers or to go outdoors to smoke. Most, however, were unable to leave and return without the help of staff.

Physical restraints and bedrails were never used in Wesley Hall, and only occasionally were sedatives or psychotropic drugs prescribed. Dosages were small, closely monitored, and withdrawn as soon as feasible.

The right to make decisions about how and where residents spend time is an important element in establishing their autonomy. Having this right of choice can often effect dramatic changes in behavior, as illustrated by the following description of the situations with Mr. Bartell, Mrs. Charles, and Mrs. Williams.

Mr. Bartell had become very agitated and restless while living in the large retirement home. Staff members were usually able to convince him that he should come to the dining room for breakfast, but he would return to his room immediately after eating to undress and go to bed. Staff's efforts to get him up after that met with resistance and often combativeness. This led to the retirement home staff's locking his door when he left his room, forcing him to remain in the sunroom or dayroom until after the evening meal. Other problems developed at that point. He became verbally and physically abusive to other residents, and because he could not find the bathroom he frequently urinated in inappropriate places. The policy on Wesley Hall was that no sleeping rooms in the area would be locked and that residents would have access to their rooms at all times. This, combined with a number of other interventions in Wesley Hall, proved to be effective. Mr. Bartell would get up for breakfast, occasionally go back to bed for a short nap, and then get up again to join others in the living room. He was often lured from his room by the arrival of children in the area or by the sound of activities in the kitchen or living room. He selected a comfortable chair in the living room that he considered his own, and he spent much of his time there rather than in bed, poring over his newspapers. His episodes of combativeness, although never completely eliminated, gradually diminished in frequency.

Mrs. Charles and Mrs. Williams had been agitated and restless when they first moved to Wesley Hall. They would walk constantly, sometimes together, wandering from the living room to the kitchen, to the den, and in and out of their own rooms. A rearrangement of furniture brought an unexpected solution to their restlessness. A small settee was placed in the living room giving full view of the hallway, the dining area, and the doors to the kitchen. The settee soon became theirs as they sat together watching the action and muttering about resident or staff behaviors that they considered inappropriate. Watching the behaviors of others can be a favorite and stimulating occupation for residents and can help them remain alert and aware of their surroundings.

Individualization and Flexibility of Approaches and Resident Opportunities

Rationale

Individualization as it relates to the person with dementia is often considered untenable in settings that follow the practice of treating all residents alike. The unwillingness or inability of staff to recognize unique individual characteristics and needs and the excessive standardization in the interests of institutional routine, orderliness, and predictability (among other things) shape an environment that cannot accommodate the special needs of the person in the middle stages of Alzheimer's disease (Lawton 1986). Some routines can become so ingrained and fixed that practices are seldom questioned and any suggestions for changes are met with strong resistance.

What is needed is an individual-centered approach that adjusts expectations to individual capabilities, rather than hoping that one set of norms will apply to everyone (Woods and Britton 1985). Health professionals are trained to develop care plans that are highly specific and directed toward individual needs in treating persons who are physically ill, but their training seldom prepares them to work effectively with those whose needs lie in the areas of social and psychological support (Burnside 1982).

Individualization is especially crucial, for example, in attempting to help persons who are incontinent. Hodge (1984), speaking of the complexity of dealing with incontinence in persons with dementia, stressed the need "for comprehensive behavioral analysis, taking into account all the various possibilities, both organismic and environmental which may interact to lead to the specific behavior under review." He listed the following as potential problems for persons with dementia:

1. inability to recognize need;
2. inability to find a toilet;
3. too slow to get there;
4. inability to recognize a toilet;
5. inability to undress appropriately;
6. apathy;
7. incontinence maintained by contingent staff inattention (i.e., when staff are unaware of or unresponsive to residents' needs to urinate); and
8. medical problems.

These complexities, along with variation in the frequency of individuals' needs to urinate, mean that careful planning for each individual is absolutely essential if a continence program is to be effective.

In any setting, the activities and opportunities available to residents need to be individualized to provide meaning to the residents involved and to ensure a reasonable chance for success. Settings that attempt to implement the hackneyed activities that have become identified with nursing homes meet with little success, and these experiences only reinforce the negative feelings that residents have about themselves and the frequent impressions of staff members that the person with dementia can do nothing.

Clearly related to the individualization of interpersonal relationships, opportunities, and the physical environment is the need for the milieu to be flexible and changeable to respond to the special problems residents may be facing. The fears and desolation that many persons with dementia experience, as described earlier by the diarist, accompanied by the loss of judgment and control over behaviors place them in hazardous positions in a hostile or indifferent environment. Even when residents are no longer able to express their emotions in words, their faces and actions reflect the fear, panic, and anxiety that they are feeling. Many of their behaviors must be expressions of these frightening and devastating emotions. Their inability to interpret the meaning of the events occurring around them or to adjust to changes and expectations implicit in the environment places stress on the dementia victim's already weakened abilities to cope. To the degree that the environment adjusts to and accommodates residents' needs, some of the decline in abilities may be checked.

Application

Knowledge of each resident's strengths and abilities and of the areas in which each resident needed special assistance enabled staff members at Wesley Hall to individualize planning and maximize the functioning of each person. Staff members' increasing awareness of situations that might create stress for each individual and their understanding of the signals that indicated the beginning of difficult behaviors enabled them to help residents avoid agitation, anger, and combativeness.

The development of individualized approaches was especially crucial in reducing incontinence. Four residents were incontinent before their move to Wesley Hall. Each person was examined by staff from the University's Continence Clinic to ensure that there were no problems that might need medical treatment. Immediately after they moved to the new area, staff began observations to determine how frequently each resident needed to urinate. An individualized toileting schedule was developed and tested by all the staff. On recommendation of the Continence Clinic, liquid intake was greatly increased for all residents, including the four who had been incontinent, to strengthen the signals that they needed to urinate. Except for an occasional accident, the incontinence was controlled after a few months with the scheduling and the increase in liquids.

Individualized planning was also essential in determining the extent to which each person could manage activities of daily living and the types of staff interventions needed to encourage maximal self-care (Robinson et al. 1987). Staff soon learned that all residents were able to brush their teeth or dentures if they were given special assistance. Mrs. Olsen had spatial problems and was easily distracted and confused if the countertop near the sink was strewn with articles. She was unable to locate the toothbrush or put toothpaste on the brush. The procedure followed for Mrs. Olsen was for staff to clear the countertop of all items, put toothpaste on the brush, and place it in her hand. Staff turned on the water and guided her hand to the water and then Mrs. Olsen was able to proceed. Mrs. Smith, on the other hand, was able to manage all steps except putting the toothpaste on her brush; she could locate the brush without distractions, turn on the water, dampen the brush, and proceed without instructions. These details in planning may seem excessive and time consuming, but they make the difference in whether staff increase dependency by doing steps in a task that a resident is still able to manage.

To reduce the stress of the early morning hours and to give residents the right of choice, project staff reached a decision to extend the breakfast period over several hours. The dietary department was willing to give the plan a trial period. The central kitchen sent up breakfast at the regular time, but cereal, bread, rolls, and other breakfast foods were kept on Wesley Hall for use at any time. If hot foods were sent up on the cart, staff placed part of it in a warm oven if it could be held for an hour or two. This gave a range of options and enabled residents who were early risers and those who slept late to have breakfast. Some of the residents came to breakfast in bathrobes, and then staff assisted those who needed help in dressing after the breakfast period ended.

Residents' resistance to bathing led staff to devise another flexible plan. Staff soon found that the system of bath schedules that they had followed when they worked in the nursing area not only was ineffective but also could lead to anger and chaos. A variety of approaches were tested and many were discarded, but gradually staff learned ways to help residents accept baths with a minimum of resistance. Staff members on all three shifts shared their experiences, and it became apparent that some staff persons were having success with specific residents while others were not. This enabled staff to divide the responsibility as it worked most effectively.

Staff gradually discovered the importance of presenting bath time as a social occasion. They found it helpful to sit and chat with a resident for awhile before suggesting a bath. At other times, they were successful if they suggested sharing a snack together after a bath. These approaches did not always succeed, but they were far more successful than coercion or a more direct approach and were much less stressful.

One innovative staff person had had a totally unsuccessful morning in trying to get Mr. Bartell to take a bath. She had approached him several times and then had withdrawn when he had become verbally abusive. Later she sat down with him and asked, "If you had your choice, what would you like to eat while you're taking your bath?" He replied promptly, "A dish of ice cream." She responded to this immediately, saying, "When you get into the tub, I'll come back to the kitchen and get you that dish of ice cream, and you can have it while you're taking a bath." He chuckled and said, " 'They' [meaning other staff] won't like that." The resident assistant said quickly, "We'll never tell 'them.' " This conspiracy appealed to Mr. Bartell, and the bath combined with eating the ice cream proceeded with no further problems.

Staff training had stressed that only schedules for administering medications and medical treatment needed to be adhered to. It was far more important to carry out an activity, such as bathing, with resident acceptance then to get the task done on schedule. In other words, success was to be measured by the extent to which staff could maintain a relaxed, nonstressful environment rather than by the speed and efficiency with which they could complete the day's work.

Continuity with the Past and in Family Relationships and a Continuation of Normal Social Roles for Residents

Rationale

Even though residents in a residential care setting are physically separated from their former homes and families, the setting has the potential for helping the residents to maintain a strong link with the families and a reassuring continuity with their past lives. The physical environment provides many opportunities to help the residents maintain identity. Personal furniture, pictures, and articles brought from home serve to give the resident a sense of ownership and a bond with earlier life.

In designing therapeutic environments, Institute of Gerontology research has emphasized the need for the availability of normal social roles so that residents can continue to function and be involved in activities that had meaning to them in their earlier lives. The theory supports the idea that roles prescribe the patterns of behavior that are socially acceptable for each position or function in a group or society. If, for example, the only available role is "frail, sick patient," the individual will conform to the expectations embodied in that role. If, however, a number of normal nonsick social roles, such as friend, citizen, consumer, or worker, are available and the individual is encouraged to choose freely among them, the person's behavior will be varied and far more therapeutic in its effects than when it is prescribed by the sick role. Although residents may not remember old roles and activities, they nevertheless are more likely to have residuals from the past that make the reinstitution of previous roles easier. These roles enable even the very frail to respond and to function in an environment that is nurturing and enabling (Coons 1983). With this concept in mind, the daily living in a therapeutic setting can be designed specifically to reinstate, to the extent possible, the roles of homemaker, family member, volunteer, friend, and, in some situations, worker.

The absence of meaningful roles has become the prevailing mode in many treatment settings, partly because staff members view residents as incapable and beyond involvement and partly because many state regulations preclude the implementation of activities that would offer residents opportunities to resume normal "well" roles. These regulations need to be carefully reevaluated and reinterpreted so that the individual can be protected but not deprived of the opportunities that are essential in providing a rich and active life.

The implication in the residential care model is that the residents are active participants unless they choose to be spectators. A number of special facilities for persons with dementing disease are now citing, as one of their special features, an area where staff fold towels and residents can observe the process. The assumption evidently is that the residents are incapable of being more than spectators. In the residential care setting, staff members are trained to share with residents and to break tasks down into a series of steps so that even the most impaired persons can succeed at some phase of the operation. This sharing of tasks with the staff brings about awareness and confidence among residents that are lacking if opportunities for mutual involvement are unavailable to them.

In the residential care model, families are seen as valuable resources in providing staff with information about the residents' preferences and earlier life-styles. Families and staff members frequently share in efforts to reduce stress and to give the reassurance and support needed to help residents live satisfying lives. The ambience of the residential care model provides a comfortable milieu for families as well as for residents and staff. The relaxed, homelike environment encourages visiting, and the many activities shared with families, residents, and staff reduce the stress of visits (Metzelaar and Coons 1986).

Application

Conceptualizing programming as an opportunity for residents to continue in normal social roles provides a focus to the activities and a linkage with the past. Activities based on earlier roles enable residents to participate in many of the tasks that were overlearned and were so much a part of their earlier lives. Many still retain the capacities to manage even though they are severely impaired.

In the role of homemaker, residents at Wesley Hall were involved, with the help of staff, in setting tables, washing and drying dishes, baking muffins and cookies, making homemade ice cream, and folding towels and, with the guidance of a housekeeper, they assisted in bed making, vacuuming, and dusting. The activities were genuinely a part of the life of the area and not "busy work" scheduled for set times. For example, the towels were folded by staff and residents together whenever they came from the central laundry.

In the role of volunteer, most of the residents were able to participate in carefully selected service projects. They successfully completed a variety of projects for the American Red Cross, such as folding flyers or stuffing envelopes. Another favorite service activity was making garnishes for the retirement home's central dining room. Those who were not participants in the service projects were often active observers, sharing in the excitement of the activities and in the conversation. As was mentioned previously, very deliberate efforts were made in the physical environment to provide residents with a continuity with the past in the furnishing of their rooms, in individualized door decorations, and in the display of family pictures and photograph albums.

A number of interventions jointly planned by family and staff members helped reduce agitation. Mrs. Charles, for a period of time, was convinced that her son had rejected her. She insisted that he never came to visit her, and she repeatedly asked staff to call him. In reality, he visited her at least once a week and sometimes took her for a ride or out to lunch. Within minutes after he had left, she had forgotten the visit, and she became angry when staff tried to reassure her that her son came frequently. One of the staff met with her son on his next visit to describe the situation and to suggest a plan that she thought might help Mrs. Charles. She suggested that he write a note in large letters on newsprint to say that he had visited, describing what they had done together and the good time they had had. The note was to be posted on her closet door so that his mother could see it and staff could refer to it if she became agitated. The plan was effective. Mrs. Charles could still read and she frequently pointed to it when staff were in her room and sometimes read it aloud with obvious pride.

Family potluck dinners were scheduled about every four months. These events, as well as occasional newsletters, gave staff members opportunities to keep families informed about current and future events. The dinners were festive, with small tables arranged through-out the area to enable each resident to share the dinner with relatives. The families enjoyed these opportunities to have relaxing and focused visits and to become better acquainted with the relatives of other residents. Such activities were organized to encourage family involve-ment and to strengthen and reinforce the residents' role as family members (Coons and Weaverdyck 1986).

A Stimulating Sensory and Social Environment

Rationale

Kahana (1982) hypothesized that resident morale results not from the characteristics of the environment alone or solely from the per-sonality of the resident but from the degree of fit between the needs of the individual and the ability of the milieu to gratify those needs. To accommodate the needs of a variety of persons simultaneously, an environment must offer a wide range of options and ensure the right of each individual to make choices. In the residential care setting, the stimulation lies in the visual and sensory interventions, the quality and frequency of social interactions, and the richness and abundance of opportunities for involvement.

In efforts to determine the appropriate environment for persons in the early or middle stages of dementia, implementors are exploring a variety of approaches. Stripping environments of all visual and social stimulation, a policy followed by some settings, offers an environment that gives the resident no sensory cues, no incentives, no memorabilia that provide linkages with the past, and no choices. Such impoverished settings can have strong negative impact on self-image and morale. The argument favoring such settings describes them as stress reducing, and yet boredom and sterility can be as stressful as excessive stimulation.

A rich environment, if appropriately designed and if residents have the freedom to accept or reject involvement at any time, can offer constant stimulation without stress. The interaction of the residents with their surroundings helps them remain aware and involved and has the potential for retarding deterioration and recapturing skills that were overlearned in their past lives. Well-planned programs that are satisfying and diversional and offer exercise can also greatly reduce the frequency and intensity of problem behaviors (Mace 1987).

Application

The physical environment at Wesley Hall was modified to meet many needs, one of which was to provide visual stimulation. Traditional pastel paints were discarded in favor of figured wallpaper in a number of areas. Wherever the basic colors of yellow, green, red, or blue could be tastefully incorporated, they were used to provide visual stimulation and better visibility for persons with poor eyesight. Enlarged photographs and several colorful mobiles added zest to the area and drew comments from residents from time to time (Coons et al. 1987; Coons 1987a).

The social environment provided a complexity and interest largely unavailable to residents in the large retirement home. Staff training had stressed the importance of communication between staff and residents and pointed out that any shared experience offered opportunities for verbal intervention. When staff members were helping residents in self-care activities, for example, they explained the steps involved, encouraged, reassured, complimented, and reminisced or laughed together about any funny thing that might have occurred.

The staff gradually became skillful at raising moods or reducing tension by introducing activities spontaneously. Ball tossing and sing-alongs were especially popular, and residents could join in or not as they chose. Some merely tapped a foot or clapped their hands to the singing, but even those who found it difficult to speak more than a few words could usually sing the words to old, familiar songs. Children were especially appealing, and most residents would quickly become involved in whatever activity staff might introduce when children were present. The pet parakeet or the fish in the aquarium both drew the attention of residents and, with the help of staff members, the residents kept them and the window-ledge bird feeder supplied with food.

The frequent involvement of residents in light, relaxing, and undemanding activities helped to keep them very much aware of their surroundings. It also gradually reduced the agitation, the restless wandering, and the anger that had been expressed so often by most residents during the first several months of the project.

Staff Roles and Approaches That Respond to the Special Needs of Residents

Rationale

The uniqueness of persons in the middle stages of Alzheimer's disease has been mentioned, as has their incompatibility with the practices in traditional institutional settings. The style of the residential care setting requires a revision of staff roles and approaches and a strengthening of relationships between staff members and residents. Spontaneity and innovation can provide a rich and stimulating environment for residents and for staff who are flexible and imaginative. Not all staff are comfortable in such a milieu, however; some people prefer to work in settings that are highly structured and consistent. The staff of most nursing facilities are not prepared either educationally or psychologically for the complex task of providing excellent care for the individual suffering from a dementing disease. The effectiveness and quality of the milieu in residential care relies upon staff's ability to explore and develop new and creative approaches. They also need to reach an understanding of and sensitivity to the special problems and needs of dementia victims and to develop a great amount of patience and empathy (Burnside 1979; Wells 1982; Bartol 1983).

The roles of staff in residential care are defined as "enabler" and "friend." Time is spent in helping residents to continue in activities of daily living to the extent that they are able, with staff doing no task or part of a task that residents can manage themselves. The role of aide as "caretaker" is considered inappropriate and nontherapeutic in residential care. A warm personal relationship between staff and residents is considered an essential element in the creation of a home-like environment. Because residents in the middle stages of Alzheimer's disease are often relatively well physically, they do not require that staff spend a major part of each day in nursing tasks. This frees staff members to spend time with residents in social and interactive ways.

The behaviors of persons with dementia that present some of the most formidable problems in nursing homes and for families include wandering, incontinence, agitation, and combativeness. There is always the question of how much the behaviors exhibited are a result of the disease and how much they are the result of a hostile, indifferent, or inept environment.

In the residential care model, the goal is to develop a repertoire of approaches that can reach the consciousness of individuals and enable them to thrive to the extent possible within the restrictions of their impairment. While no single approach is consistently successful, the variety provides staff with many options that can accommodate the changing moods, the alterations in the degrees of impairment, and the special and often unexpressed needs of residents. If staff become skilled in the use of the following approaches, they can avoid coercion or the aggressive methods that provoke the difficult behaviors.

DIVERSION. Diversion can be a very effective way of reducing agitation or anger and of distracting residents from whatever seems to be troubling them at the moment. When staff become sensitive to signs of distress or mood changes, they may avert an outburst or combativeness by intervening with an activity or conversation that focuses on something pleasant and appealing to the person. In this way, staff can *avoid* a difficult behavior rather than try to *manage* it after it occurs.

TOUCH. Touch from genuinely concerned and caring staff can be one of the most soothing and comforting approaches that staff can adopt. It is one sensory pathway that can reach even the most impaired individual (Wolanin and Phillips 1981). Touch at mealtime can be an effective means of encouraging severely impaired persons to eat (Eaton et al. 1986). It is important for staff to recognize that not all elderly persons like to be touched and that, at times, touch can be an invasion of privacy or personal space. Staff may therefore need to find different ways of communicating affection.

RELAXED CONVERSATION AND ACTIVE LISTENING. A very effective approach is simply a considerate, humane, and genuinely concerned response to resident needs. Easy, relaxing conversation can help residents through difficult situations, and listening to even incoherent messages can often give staff clues to the cause of agitation or anger.

The effects of relaxed conversation and personal attention by a sensitive nurse's aide are described by Cohen and Eisdorfer (1986). They tell the story of Mrs. Barnes, a nursing home resident for more than a year, who had been labeled by staff as belligerent, unpleasant, and difficult to dress and get out of bed. She frequently yelled at aides or struck them. A newly hired nurse's aide was given the responsibility of helping Mrs. Barnes. The aide began by introducing herself, chatting about the weather or news, arranging the breakfast tray, and then sitting close to Mrs. Barnes and asking how she was feeling, if she was ready to eat, or whether she wanted to freshen up. For two days, Mrs. Barnes continued to complain and yell, but on the third day she told the aide that she wanted to wash up before eating. The aide and Mrs. Barnes sat together while she ate breakfast, and then she dressed herself without assistance. When the aide prepared to leave, Mrs. Barnes reached for her hand and said slowly, "Thank you for making me feel real again."

The aide's approach with Mrs. Barnes follows no labeled therapy. She was probably treating Mrs. Barnes as she, herself, would want to be treated if the situation were reversed.

A LIGHTHEARTED APPROACH WITH HUMOR. A lighthearted approach creates a relaxed and nonstressful milieu in a residential care setting. Dementia does not suddenly end the person's capacity to enjoy life and to laugh (Mace and Rabins 1981). Staff, too, can benefit from learning to appreciate the humorous and the ludicrous to help in their own survival (Burnside 1982). Laughter helps both staff members and residents to unlock tensions. Humor can take many forms, from gentle joking, to laughing at foolish situations, to outright buffoonery. A climate of lightness and frivolity encourages residents to initiate humor themselves and enables them to laugh at and with staff. There must be a clear understanding by staff members of the difference between lighthearted humor, which can help persons relax, and ridicule or making fun of residents and their impairments, which can be destructive and cruel.

WITHDRAWING AND RETURNING LATER. The changing moods of persons with dementia and their inability at times to comprehend immediately what is being asked of them can lead to problem situations. The policies in residential care of encouraging maximal resident autonomy and of avoiding coercion require that staff members give residents time to respond and vary their approaches from one occasion to another and from person to person.

The approach becomes one of the staff member suggesting an activity, such as bathing. If the resident resists, the staff member withdraws to return later, possibly with a different way of introducing the suggestion that may be more palatable. This delay may also give residents the time needed to comprehend what is being asked of them.

ENCOURAGEMENT AND REASSURANCE. Encouragement as a suggested approach in residential care refers to staff's acknowledgement of what residents are able to manage in ways that will help them recognize their own successes. It does not imply that they should give residents false hopes or inaccurate information about their illness.

Staff's reassurance can be especially helpful when a resident seems to feel frightened, abandoned, or neglected. Praise and encouragement can help residents continue to feel good about themselves even with severe impairments if staff focus attention on their capacities rather than their deficits.

Application

Initially, staff members found it difficult to assume the role of enabler on Wesley Hall. They had become accustomed to the role of caregiver when they worked in the nursing home, and the shift from caring for persons to helping them do as much as possible for themselves meant a complete change in values, style, communication, and use of time. For a while, the staff also felt uncomfortable with the expectations that they would initiate and test out new approaches and activities and become a part of the decision-making process.

Gradually, staff members learned that these roles were exciting and rewarding, although seldom easy. They became involved with many of the decisions related to changes in the physical environment and took a major part in introducing and testing a variety of activities. Their commitment to the project was manifested in their contributions of plants, kitchen utensils, and a canary.

The variety of staff approaches developed on the Wesley Hall project led to a gradual reduction in incontinence and night wandering and a lessening of the frequency and intensity of agitation and combativeness of residents. There was also a change in the appearance of residents who, before coming to the area, had looked confused, ill, out of touch, and depressed. Gradually, the residents became more alert, well looking, and involved. This led to much speculation by staff about what specific interventions had made the difference. Special efforts were made to help residents be well-groomed. Staff worked with families to provide a variety of attractive clothing. Good hair and nail care was considered essential, as were bathing and dental care, and men were helped to shave regularly. Many of the changes, however, were more psychological. Although the residents' abilities to function declined slowly, most continued to be alert and aware of their surroundings. They smiled or laughed easily and often, and they were quick to establish eye contact with anyone approaching them.

The period after the evening meal was the most difficult for residents. A variety of interventions were tested in efforts to reduce the agitation that seemed to occur when it became dark. One of the most effective was the implementation of a variety of activities that were lighthearted and often humorous. Gradually, this evening period became the most active time of the day. Residents became quite involved, to the point that most went to bed between 9:30 and 11:00 p.m., tired, relaxed, and diverted from the problems that seemed to cause them so much distress.

Staff members need to be well supported and their efforts acknowledged if they are to maintain this flexibility and spontaneity. The unpredictability of resident responses, at times, caused staff members to become discouraged. They learned, however, to accept the fact that, although no single approach was necessarily successful every time, some approaches were consistently unsuccessful. In any case, the staff needed a variety of potentially successful alternatives from which to choose. This required imagination and a willingness to try positive, although often nontraditional, ways of helping residents through difficult situations in an effort to enable them to live with a minimum of stress.

Staff Training and Training Methods That Sensitize Staff to the Special Needs of Persons with Dementia

Rationale

Training to prepare staff in residential care settings to provide the maximum in therapeutic environments for persons with dementia requires more than the basics of good nursing care. It is helpful to include knowledge about aging as well as an overview of dementia, but staff especially need information on ways to communicate with residents and techniques that will help them to function in the role of enabler. Staff can be taught approaches so that they can help residents reduce the extent of agitation, wandering, and incontinence, and they can learn ways to create a relaxed and satisfying milieu that will help residents to enjoy life.

Training methods need to be carefully selected and designed. Lectures alone may give staff the information they need to give good physical care and to develop and maintain routines. They are not effective, however, in helping staff develop an empathy with persons with dementia, an understanding of what they must be experiencing, and a sensitivity to their psychosocial and psychological needs.

Essential training methods include: (1) information given through short lectures and handouts, (2) audiovisual aids that show effective approaches and techniques, (3) experiential exercises that help staff learn and practice new skills, (4) experiential exercises designed to help them examine their own styles and approaches, (5) opportunities and exercises that will help staff gain an understanding of and empathy for the impaired persons with whom they are working, and (6) experiential training in team building and problem solving. These training ingredients are fundamental in preparing staff for the exceedingly complex and difficult task of providing a supportive and nurturing milieu.

Application

Most of the staff for the Wesley Hall project were selected from interested persons who were already employed in the home. Interested staff members were interviewed and given an opportunity to work with a small group of cognitively impaired residents as a part of the selection process. Everyone to be involved—nursing staff, residential assistants, and housekeepers—were given a monthlong training program before the opening of the Hall. A number of new experiential training materials were developed specifically to prepare staff to work with persons with dementia.

A variety of teaching methods were used to cover the following staff training topics: (1) Dementia: An Overview; (2) Designing a Therapeutic Milieu; (3) The Impact of the Physical Environment on Residents; (4) Changing Staff Roles in a Therapeutic Milieu: Enabler and

Friend versus Caregiver; (5) The Special Technique of Task Breakdown; (6) Use of Task Breakdown in Activities of Daily Living; (7) Examining Individual Staff Approaches; (8) Developing a Repertoire of Staff Approaches; (9) Identification of Strengths and Needs of Residents; (10) Interventions: To Reduce Incontinence; (11) Interventions: To Reduce Night Wandering; (12) Interventions: To Reduce Agitation and Combativeness; (13) Interventions: To Improve the Personal Appearance of Residents; (14) Problem-solving Techniques; and (15) Team-building Techniques. Special exercises were also designed to help staff better understand their style of communication and the impact that their personal biases might have on residents. During one training session, staff members expressed concern about how they would be able to cope with Mr. Bartell, one of the men selected for the project. He was described as angry, combative, and impossible to manage. A special exercise was designed and, during the following training session, staff were asked to think of some of their experiences with Mr. Bartell and to identify what they would consider his strengths and his needs. From this perspective, staff's description was dramatically different from that of the previous session. Their comments included: "Mr. Bartell has a great sense of humor," "He was so helpful to Mrs. James the other day when she had trouble getting up from her chair," "He is very gentlemanly and polite when he isn't angry," "He loves to play 'Uno' when any of his family come to visit him," "He likes to have people pay attention to him." Staff recognized the contrast in their two evaluations—one dealing with his problem behaviors, and the other with his strengths and needs. Several staff members began visiting Mr. Bartell regularly and, even before moving to Wesley Hall, his behavior changed. His explosive outbursts were a challenge to staff, and their efforts became directed toward helping him to avoid the anger. During the project, he was one of the most popular of the selected residents.

The growth of staff insight and their greater acceptance of difficult behaviors was illustrated in a staff meeting several months after the project began. One resident assistant reported on an experience she had had several days before when she had gone to Mr. Bartell's room to suggest that it was time for him to go to the bathroom. He became furious and began screaming profanity at her. She said calmly, but firmly, "I am trying to help you, and I don't like to have you talk that way to me." She went on to say, "He stopped and looked at me in the most crestfallen way and said, 'Those are the only words I know,' and then he walked along with me with no more swearing. I felt so bad; I gave him a big hug." This story and others helped staff to recognize the powerlessness of persons with dementia and the desperation they must feel at times. In addition to the monthlong training program before Wesley Hall opened, there were training sessions throughout the two years of the project to respond to specific needs and unexpected problems or in preparation for new interventions to be tested.

Cohesive Staff Team with Strong Administrative Support

Rationale

The quality of human relationships in any setting becomes the key to defining the character of the milieu. The development of a cohesive staff team that can share information and work together to solve problems is crucial. Staff need to have opportunities to express opinions and suggest ideas and solutions, and supervisors and other administrative staff need to listen to those who are the direct caregivers. This does not mean that the administrators are abdicating their roles as leaders. It means instead that they are demonstrating their respect for direct service staff and valuing and acknowledging their insights and experiences. The staff who do the caring must also receive nurturing, and administrators need to recognize that this is an essential part of their own jobs and roles. For staff to use their own sensitivity in discerning the feelings of the residents and to be able to reach out to them in their loneliness and fear, there needs to be created a work atmosphere in which staff members feel a sense of their own self-worth and dignity and in which their morale remains high (Burnside 1982).

The style of administration is extremely critical in establishing residential care units with the philosophy described in this chapter. Administration must be willing to examine objectively existing practices, and they must be willing to question and discard those practices that inhibit the development of a therapeutic milieu that is supportive and satisfying to both residents and staff.

Application

In programs such as Wesley Hall, the demands on staff are great and unending. They cannot resort to the separation from residents and the impersonal and aloof stance that serve as protection in many traditional settings. The possibilities of burnout must, therefore, be faced, and measures must be taken to reduce stress on staff.

Rotation of staff, a practice followed in some settings, was not considered appropriate on Wesley Hall for several reasons. The special training before the opening of Wesley Hall and the ongoing sessions afterward led to staff growth and development that gave substance to the program. This would have been quickly lost if staff were to have been there for only a limited time. The practice of rotation also gives a subtle message to staff that persons with dementia are difficult to work with, the job is unrewarding, and no one can survive it for a long period. One measure taken in Wesley Hall to avert staff burnout was to use weekly staff meetings as problem-solving and training sessions and as an informal support group. This enabled staff to present specific difficulties that they were having and to develop a plan of action for the following week. The next meeting gave them an opportunity to report on the success or failure of the planned interventions. In addition to the weekly meeting, the coordinator of the project met frequently with each staff person individually in informal counseling sessions and to offer one-on-one training. These meetings demonstrated to staff that they were valued and that their special problems were of real concern to the coordinator.

Staff on all three shifts were asked to keep a daily log, not only as a means of recording information gained on the project but also as a way of sharing experiences with other staff members. The log also became an effective tool in developing a cohesive staff team. They shared their successes, their failures, and their feelings. All staff read the log and made notes in the margins from time to time. Sometimes there was only a drawing of a smiling or a sad face to show pleasure or sympathy. There were also such notes as "I had the same experience! Help!" or "That was a real success!" or "I'll get in a little early tomorrow to see if I can take off some of the pressure."

A number of social gatherings and parties away from the job also helped staff members to become better acquainted and comfortable with each other. They described these events as helping to create a team spirit and reduce the possibilities of burnout. The result of these efforts was the development of a close, cohesive team of staff members who were confident and proud of their achievements.

Good Diagnostic and Medical Care

Rationale

Good diagnostic and medical care is provided, not as an end in itself, but as a mean of helping residents maintain maximal capacity to enjoy and participate in the life of the facility. There is frequent reference to the need for careful evaluation to identify reversible dementia so that appropriate treatment may be given to restore health (Cummings and Benson 1983; Cohen and Eisdorfer 1986).

Reichel (1983b) agreed that this is one of the reasons for careful diagnosis, but he also stressed the need for ongoing diagnostic and medical treatment for persons who have been diagnosed as having senile dementia of the Alzheimer's type by a physician who will take charge of medical, social, and emotional problems. He pointed out that serious medical problems may develop that can affect the residents' health and well-being beyond the dementia. Because of the difficulties and challenges of diagnosing medical problems in persons with dementia, he suggested that it may be necessary to make referrals to specialists from time to time.

Application

The medical director of the Chelsea United Methodist Retirement Home did a diagnostic work-up on each resident, did weekly evaluations, and prescribed medical treatment. A psychiatrist who specialized in treating some of the psychiatric problems associated with dementia served as a consultant in special situations. On recommendation of the physician, several residents were admitted to a geriatric unit in a psychiatric hospital for evaluations of depression and other problems. This was followed by a 10-day observational period in the unit, during which the physician evaluated the pharmacological interventions. All residents for the project were examined by the University of Michigan Continence Clinic to rule out infections as a possible cause of incontinence.

Conclusion

Persons with Alzheimer's disease and related dementias present a very special challenge to caregivers. Even the most sensitive, creative, and imaginative staff will become discouraged when all of their efforts, at times, seem to meet with failure. Because of the shifting moods and the unpredictability of this group of impaired persons, their care is exceedingly complex and defies many of the practices that are viewed as the means by which the traditional setting survives. A relaxed, accepting approach by staff, flexibility of schedules, individualization of the social and emotional milieu, and a reinstatement of opportunities for residents to continue in normal social roles would all seem counterproductive in the setting striving for efficiency and to some who are responsible for monitoring state and federal regulations.

The memory loss, disorientation, combativeness, and wandering behavior considered characteristic of many forms of dementia tend to confound every aspect of medical and nursing care. In spite of this, there has been very little careful study and documentation of daily care techniques that could maximize the quality of life for these individuals. The studies cited on the use of physical restraints illustrate the value of carefully documented research that examines practices that have become so ingrained in our health care system that they are seldom questioned. Similar studies are needed to compare the effects of many of the traditional methods used in the care of persons with dementia with new and more humane techniques and approaches. The results may prove that it is possible for even the severely impaired to live with dignity.

Residential care offers an alternative that, with appropriate staff training and administrative support, can be adapted to any care setting attempting to provide for impaired persons an environment that is positive and responsive to their special needs. It is imperative that policymakers and health care specialists take a fresh, new look at what is possible. Dementia is devastating in itself; families and victims need models of care that ameliorate, not deepen, the devastation.

References

Bartol, M. A. 1983. Reaching the patient. *Geriatric Nursing* (July/August) 234–36.

Berg, L., and W. Danziger. 1984. Predictive features in mild senile dementia of the Alzheimer's type. *Neurology* 34 (May): 563–69.

Berger, E. Y. 1985. The institutionalization of patients with Alzheimer's disease. *Danish Medical Bulletin* 32 (1): 71–76.

Boling, T. E., D. M. Vrooman, and K. M. Sommers. 1983. *Nursing home management: A humanistic approach.* Springfield, IL: Charles C Thomas.

Burnside, I. M. 1979. Alzheimer's disease: An overview. *Journal of Gerontological Nursing* 5 (4): 14–20.

Burnside, I. M. 1982. Care of the Alzheimer's patient in an institution. *Generations* (Fall) 22–23, 50.

Cape, R. D. T. 1983. Freedom from restraint (abstract). *Gerontologist* 23 (October): 217.

Chenoweth, B., and B. Spencer. 1986. Dementia: The experience of family caregivers. *Gerontologist* 26 (3): 267–72.

Cohen, D., and C. Eisdorfer. 1986. *Loss of self: A family resource for the care of Alzheimer's disease and related disorders.* New York: W. W. Norton.

Cohen-Mansfield, J., and N. Billig. 1986. Agitated behaviors in the elderly. *Journal of the American Geriatric Society* 34 (10): 711–21.

Coons, D. H. 1983. The therapeutic milieu: Social-psychological aspects of treatment. In *Clinical aspects of aging,* 2d ed., ed. W. Reichel, 137–150. Baltimore: Williams & Wilkins.

Coons, D. H. 1987a. Overcoming problems in modifying the environment. In *Alzheimer's disease: Problems, prospects, and perspectives,* ed. H. Altman, 321–28. New York: Plenum.

Coons, D. H. 1987b. *Designing a residential care unit for persons with dementia.* Washington, DC: Congressional Office of Technology Assessment, Contract No. 633-1950.0.

Coons, D., A. Robinson, B. Spencer, and L. Green. 1987. *Designing the physical environment for persons with dementia.* A videotape unit distributed by Michigan Media Resources Center, Ann Arbor, MI.

Coons, D. H., and S. E. Weaverdyck. 1986. Wesley Hall: A residential unit for persons with Alzheimer's disease and related disorders. In *Therapeutic interventions for the person with dementia,* ed. E. D. Taira, 29–53. New York: Haworth Press.

Cummings, J. L., and D. F. Benson. 1983. *Dementia: A clinical approach.* Boston: Butterworth.

Eaton, M., I. L. Mitchell-Bonair, and E. Friedman. 1986. The effect of touch on nutritional intake of chronic organic brain syndrome patients. *Journal of Gerontology* 41 (5): 611–16.

Frengley, J. D., and L. C. Mion. 1986. Incidence of physical restraints on acute general medical wards. *Journal of the American Geriatric Society* 34 (8): 565–68.

George, L. K. 1984. *The dynamics of caregiver burden.* Washington, DC: American Association of Retired Persons. December.

Hiatt, L. G. 1985. Designing for mentally impaired persons: Integrating knowledge of people with programs, architecture, and interior design. Presented at the Annual Meeting of the American Association of Homes for the Aging. November.

Hodge, J. 1984. Toward a behavioral analysis of dementia. In *Psychological approaches to the care of the elderly,* ed. I. Hanley and J. Hodge, 61–87. London: Croom-Helm.

Kahana, E. 1982. A congruence model of person-environment interaction. In *Aging and the environment*, ed. M. P. Lawton, P. G. Windley, and T. O. Byerts, 97–121. New York: Springer.

Kahn, R. L., A. I. Goldfarb, M. Pollack, and A. Peck. 1960. Brief objective measures for the determination of mental status in the aged. *American Journal of Psychiatry* 117 (October): 326–28.

Kane, R. A., and R. L. Kane. 1981. *Assessing the elderly: A practical guide to management*. Lexington, MA: Lexington Books, D. D. Heath.

Koff, T. H. 1986. Nursing home management and Alzheimer's disease. *The American Journal of Alzheimer's Care and Related Disorders* 1 (Summer): 12–15.

Lawton, M. P. 1981. Sensory deprivation and the effect of the environment on management of the patient with senile dementia. In *Clinical aspects of Alzheimer's disease and senile dementia*, ed. M. Miller and A. Cohen, 227–49. New York: Raven Press.

Lawton, M. P. 1986. *Environment and aging*. Albany: Center for the Study of Aging.

Mace, N. L. 1987. Programs and services that specialize in the care of persons with dementing illnesses. In *Dementia prospects and policies*, Vol. 2. Washington, DC: Office of Technology Assessment.

Mace, N. L., and P. V. Rabins. 1981. *The 36-hour day*. Baltimore: Johns Hopkins University Press.

Metzelaar, L., and D. H. Coons. 1986. Visits: An opportunity for sharing. In *A better life*, ed. D. H. Coons, L. Metzelaar, A. Robinson, and B. Spencer, 47–91. Columbus, OH: Source for Nursing Home Literature.

Millard, P. H., and C. S. Smith. 1981. Personal belongings—a positive effect? *Gerontologist* 21 (1): 85–90.

Reichel, W. 1983a. Essentials in the care of the elderly. In *Clinical aspects of aging*, 2d ed., ed. W. Reichel, 1–10. Baltimore: Williams & Wilkins.

Reichel, W. 1983b. The evaluation and management of the confused, disoriented or demented elderly patient. In *Clinical aspects of aging*, ed. W. Reichel, 151–65. Baltimore: Williams & Wilkins.

Reisberg, B., S. Ferris, M. de Leon, and T. Cook. 1982. The Global Deterioration Scale for assessment of primary degenerative dementia. *American Journal of Psychiatry* 139:1136–39.

Robinson, A., B. Spencer, S. Weaverdyck, and S. Gardner. 1987. *Helping people with dementia in activities of daily living*. A videotape unit distributed by Terra Nova Films, Chicago, IL.

Wells, T. 1982. What does commitment to gerontological nursing really mean? *Journal of Gerontological Nursing* 8 (8): 434–37.

Wolanin, M. O., and L. R. F. Phillips. 1981. *Confusion: Prevention and care*. St. Louis: C. V. Mosby.

Woods, R. T., and P. G. Britton. 1985. *Clinical psychology with the elderly*. Rockville, MD: Aspen.

15

Changing Public Policy for Dementia Care

ROBERT MULLAN
COOK-DEEGAN, M.D.

Government pervasively influences how those who have dementia are treated, particularly after they enter the formal care system. This chapter reviews some of the ways that government affects care by describing the goals of governmental intervention, the ways that government acts, some of the specific programs that receive governmental support, and how such policies are enacted. A final section deals with how individuals can influence policy.

The real costs of dementia are family pain and loss of the mind of the afflicted person. It is these factors, more than economic cost, that will drive policy change, as policy makers realize the seriousness of the social destruction left in the wake of dementing illnesses. For policy purposes, however, it is useful to estimate economic costs, as they are indices for what government will be getting into should it choose to address long-term care for those with dementia.

The Hoover Institution at Stanford recently estimated the costs of Alzheimer's disease at $28 to $31 billion per year (Hay and Ernst 1987; Weiler 1987). An estimate prepared for the congressional Office of Technology Assessment estimated costs in 1985 at $24 to $48 billion in the United States (Battelle Memorial Institute 1984), and an estimate of 1983 costs done for the National Institute on Aging was set at $38 billion (Huang et al. 1986). The indirect costs borne by caregivers are estimated to add an additional $10 to $20 billion. These costs are caused by medical care, long-term care, and loss of income. The largest fraction of costs is due to dependency induced by brain failure that necessitates long-term care. An estimated 40 to 80 percent of residents in nursing homes suffer from dementia (U.S. Congress, Office of Technology Assessment 1987). The most likely figure is towards the upper, rather than the lower, end of this range, but data are so poor that the actual number cannot be known until further studies are done. The federal government paid an estimated $4.4 billion for nursing home care of people with dementia in 1986, and state governments paid another $4.1 billion (U.S. Congress 1987).

The cost of hospital, clinic, home, and day care is unknown. The majority of costs are borne by individuals and their families, but governmental programs set many of the rules for the practice of medicine and long-term care.

The direct costs are largely in the form of services for medical, nursing supervisory, and assistive services for those who cannot manage the vicissitudes of daily living due to dementia. These services are rendered by various providers. Those providing care can be divided into the informal network (family and friends who are not directly paid for their services) and formal care delivered by paid providers. Most public policy deals with formal care. Public policy dealing with dementia has begun to change rapidly in recent years. This is because the current care system only poorly addresses the formal care needs of those with dementia and does little to facilitate informal caregiving. Recent policy changes reflect a newly found awareness that there is a serious problem.

Adequate public policies will require that several factors all be readily apparent. There must be a consensus that there is a serious public problem, that the government could improve the situation, that the government should do so, that it has the resources to do so, and that there are well-defined solutions to the problem. Consensus does not imply unanimity, but merely enough political agreement to win the crucial votes in legislative bodies and to encourage executive actions at local, state, and federal levels. This, in turn, necessitates organization of people willing to work toward policy change by formulating plausible policy changes and to apply pressure to the crucial decision makers at the appropriate times.

There are already many policy makers committed to looking at and dealing with the various problems faced by those with dementia and their families. Their numbers are growing, but the Alzheimer's movement is only now developing a mechanism for prospectively formulating policies and is only beginning to be capable of applying pressure at the critical places and times. More effective efforts to improve public policy regarding Alzheimer's disease and dementia will require greater understanding of current government programs and learning about the political process involved in changing them.

The vast majority of people with dementia are covered under the federal Medicare program for their acute medical care because they are age sixty-five or older. The 5 to 15 percent of cases of dementia in people younger than sixty-five are directly affected by disability policies for federal and state income support programs, which in turn determine eligibility for Medicare. Failure to qualify for disability insurance also precludes Medicare coverage (unless the person suffers from kidney disease, which is a special eligibility category). The Medicare program determines payment rates for physicians, hospitals, and other providers of acute medical care and places constraints on how care is provided.

More than 70 percent of nursing home residents are covered under the Medicaid program, which is jointly funded by state and federal governments. The proportion of nursing home residents covered by Medicaid in a particular state varies widely, depending largely on how different states administer the Medicaid program. In general, those with the most restrictive criteria for eligibility (including many southern states) have the lowest fraction of residents covered by Medicaid. A few states have only a slight majority of nursing homes certified for Medicaid payment (e.g., Florida), but in most states the vast majority of nursing homes are thus certified. This requires that the facilities conform to guidelines determined by the federal and state governments. The certification criteria for Medicaid are, in fact, the major tools that the government has for ensuring quality of care in nursing homes. Facilities that do not meet minimal standards risk losing payments for their Medicaid patients. This is a strong incentive, but quality assurance policies have been notably ineffective. Recent focus on the problem of quality has brought about a new means of assessing patient status by focusing more directly on the services provided to individual patients (rather than the facilities and the paperwork) (Institute of Medicine 1986). At the same time, the federal government has encouraged states to use newly authorized and more flexible (and therefore perhaps more effective) enforcement procedures. New means of assessing quality of care and enforcing its delivery may improve care, but they have gone into effect so recently that their impact cannot yet be assessed.

State governments are also experimenting with mechanisms of payment to nursing homes for their services. Programs to test coverage of home care, respite care, day care, and other services have been mounted during the last three to four years, but results of the demonstrations have yet to be fully interpreted. These changes in long-term care are occurring when the acute system is in flux. There is some danger that the problem of dementia will be lost in the upheaval, but the process of change also brings many opportunities for the concerns of those dealing with dementia to "piggyback" on policy changes that are already occurring. The effectiveness with which American society deals with the problem of dementia for the next several decades depends in large part on the activities of individuals and organizations now and in the near future.

Goals of Public Policy

There are three primary goals for government programs in health and long-term care: improving access to care, assuring quality of care, and containing costs. Each of these goals is incorporated into the various programs that exist or have been proposed. Emphasis on the different goals has varied historically. The prime concern in the 1960s, for example, was to improve access to care. Both the Medicare and Medicaid programs were established in 1965 to broaden access to hospitals and clinics by the elderly and indigent, respectively. The dominant theme for the past decade has been cost containment. A renewed concern for quality of care in hospitals, nursing homes, and home services has surfaced in the last few years (Institute of Medicine 1986) and promises to continue. The issues of quality are likely to surface ever more frequently as long-term care becomes more central to health policy debates. These debates will encompass new attention to home care, respite care, and day care services in addition to hospital and nursing home care. The way to ensure quality service for day and respite care is not at all clear at present.

Overhaul of the long-term care system was discussed extensively in the 100th Congress, ending in October 1988, for the first time in American history. There was a tough fight in the House of Representatives about whether to vote on a long-term care bill proposed by the late Claude Pepper. The bill was not brought to the floor for debate, but the confrontation extracted promises from heads of all relevant committees seriously to entertain long-term care reform in the 101st Congress, beginning in 1989. There were three major bills in the House and two different ones in the Senate.

Governments have become active in providing, subsidizing, and regulating health care because the populations of developed countries have conferred special status on health care. This special status is addressed more explicitly in other developed countries (all of which have national health insurance or a government-administered health care system, although direct government involvement has waxed and waned in Australia's health care system). In most other countries, health care is regarded as a right or entitlement. In the United States, the mix of public and private health funding financing reflects ambivalence about whether heath care is an individual or a government responsibility.

Means of Public Policy

Governments have several ways to influence the care of those with dementia, including

- direct administration of health and long-term care services,
- payment to health and long-term care providers through public programs,
- licensing of facilities and services,
- inspection and enforcement of standards for services and facilities,
- financial incentives for delivery of services,
- training of caregivers and researchers,
- support of legal services,
- direct funding and indirect support of research, and
- dissemination of information.

The federal government pays directly for the medical care of veterans, those currently in military service (and their dependents), and Native Americans. It also pays for care rendered by other providers through Medicare and shares payment with states under Medicaid. (Eligibility and reimbursement under Medicare and Medicaid are described in Chapter 11.) Licensing of facilities is done by state and local governments. Licensing applies to nursing homes and home health care in all states and to day care facilities, home services and other health care, board and care facilities, and other services in some states. Physicians and nurses are licensed in all states; other health and social service personnel are licensed in most regions. Inspection and enforcement of care and facility standards are obligatory in all states for nursing homes, hospitals, and some other health facilities, although the rigor and frequency vary greatly. Federal guidelines on inspection frequency, flexibility of enforcement actions, and focus of attention are all changing in an attempt finally to address the chronic problems that have plagued long-term care for decades. Inspections and penalties for violation of state standards are far less common for board and care, adult day care, and home health care, but this may change as these settings and services are more widely used.

Financial incentives for the provision of services can be created by tax credits, tax deductions, direct funding of services for target groups, subsidy of insurance, mandating possession of private insurance, government-sponsored insurance programs, and many other mechanisms. Several states have recently enacted tax credits or deductions for those caring for someone with Alzheimer's disease, but the states doing this have not reported heavy use of the benefit. The limited impact of tax incentives may stem from the fact that they require knowledge by the taxpayer and benefit the fewer taxpayers in higher tax brackets more than many with lower incomes. For these and other reasons, health economists have argued that direct subsidy of insurance, reducing the risk of companies offering long-term care insurance, and encouraging employer-subsidized long-term care insurance as an employee benefit are more promising alternatives (U.S. Congress 1987; Davis and Neuman 1986). Many states have passed laws specifying the minimal requirements for long-term care insurance coverage and maximal profit margins. Two years ago, Maryland required that insurers offer coverage for dementia. Oregon has perhaps the most stringent law, which reduced the number of insurers offering long-term care insurance but limited available policies to the cream of the crop. Other states have followed guidelines set by the National Association of Insurance Commissioners. Those guidelines note the need to cover services needed by dementia patients, but stop short of requiring that policies explicitly include such language. This leaves some room for interpretation that thrusts the burden of anticipating which services will be needed onto families. Regulation of insurance is a state function, and there will doubtless be action in this arena during the next several years.

One of the most effective uses of public monies to benefit those with dementia has been the direct or indirect subsidy of services. In some states, administrators have creatively combined federal, state, and local resources to provide a wide array of services, such as respite care, home care (not only home *health* care), day care, and specialized nursing home care. In some areas, this is done by payment of those qualifying for existing programs, such as Medicaid. In others, targeting of services is less explicit. Some states and counties have announced "challenge" grants that match funding raised from private sources, and still others have created small pools of funds to support pilot projects of research on health service delivery. Some states pay for social workers or geriatric nurse practitioners to evaluate the needs of patients and their families, and then to coordinate services. Under these programs, recipients are limited to a maximal budget of governmental funding each month or year (which can be supplemented by private funds) or pay on a sliding scale based on income. States can also require that providers meet standards for reimbursement of services. Illinois has a law, for example, requiring that all persons admitted to nursing homes be evaluated for dementia.

Delivery of services to people suffering from dementia requires the availability of trained providers. Training programs are subsidized to a limited extent by the federal government, particularly medical education. States have a much larger role. States administer and fund a substantial proportion of undergraduate, graduate, and professional education through state and land grant colleges and universities. States also set standards for licensing of personnel. They can also require training for nurses' aides, nurses, physicians, and others delivering services in hospitals, nursing homes, and other settings reimbursed by the state. Maryland has recently required the training of nurses' aides for nursing homes receiving Medicaid funds, for example. Training provisions regarding nurses' aides were also included in the federal budget reconciliation act of 1987. These are currently being formulated at the federal level, to be passed down to the states for implementation.

Legal services for those with dementia deal primarily with two general functions: (1) understanding existing government programs and complying with their requirements and (2) arranging for someone to make decisions for the person who is becoming mentally incapacitated. These topics are covered in Chapter 11 and are not described here. Legal practices regarding guardianship and power of attorney are rapidly changing, and Medicaid and Medicare policies are also constantly changing. Legal issues are therefore in flux; early consultation with a competent attorney who is familiar with recent changes in the complex statutes and regulations is thus essential. This is of concern not only to family members, but also to providers who must comply with government regulations and must recognize when a designated person has the authority to make decisions on behalf of a patient. Some assistance on legal matters may be available through senior centers and legal service agencies. In general, however, care-givers and providers will need to have the services of their own counsel or have access to some other source of current legal information about federal, state, and local statutes, regulations, and administrative practices.

State and federal governments play a dominant role in the support of research. The private sector also has a stake in this and, in some selected areas such as drug research, private funding predominates. In general, however, research support derives from government. This is especially true for biomedical research. The federal government is expected to spend over $120 million in research on dementia in fiscal year 1989, up from $4 million in 1977. The vast majority of this will go for basic scientific and clinical research. Research on how to deliver services has, until recently, been largely uncoordinated and poorly funded. The federal government spent less than $2 million per year on health services research on dementia until 1987 (compared to its estimated $5 billion outlays for health and long term care). Recent legislation more than doubled this for 1987 and should more than double it again before 1991. The Robert Wood Johnson Foundation, in cooperation with the Alzheimer's Association and the Administration on Aging, is supporting a program of four-year funding of day and respite care at nineteen centers throughout the nation. Other private initiatives have focused on developing comprehensive care facilities that deliver both acute and long term care. Facilities developed in cooperation with the French Foundation in the Los Angeles area and the Hebrew Home of Riverdale in New York City are examples of these experiments.

Several states have supported a limited amount of biomedical or health services research. California, Illinois, Maryland, New Jersey, and Virginia have supported a small number of grants or contracts to fund research or to evaluate demonstration projects on respite or adult day care. Other states such as Massachusetts, New Jersey, Rhode Island, Hawaii, and Missouri have supported some form of evaluation of pilot projects of alternative care delivery systems. Until this year, however, there was no attempt by any group to support a program that could assess comparative advantages and costs of a complete array of services. The Philadelphia Geriatric Center recently studied a cost-limited program of day care, in-home care, institutional respite care, case management, and other services. Its main conclusion was that the services were judged useful and were appreciated, but that few were used. The Health Care Financing Administration is mounting a three-year, $40 million demonstration program of comprehensive services under the Medicare program at eight sites. The purpose is experimentally to test coverage of services not normally paid for by Medicare. The Medicare demonstration should yield data about which services are used, how much they cost, and who uses them. Future modifications of the long-term care system will doubtless build on this demonstration.

A final function of government is to disseminate information that is useful to the public. The mechanisms for informing citizens about health programs are generally poor. Most recipients do not understand the intricacies of the Medicare program, and Medicaid is even more obscure. It is not unusual for Medicaid eligibility determinations, for example, to differ from office to office within a state, and variations among states are even more marked. A more informed group of consumers would make such variations less acceptable and would encourage greater accountability among administrators and providers. Informed consumers would also give a competitive advantage to good providers. Demanding clearer public education programs would go a long way to ward making it possible to penetrate the system of care and to advocate for meaningful changes in the long-term care system.

Much of the technical information derived from research is disseminated through professional journals and meetings, but public education is generally left to the press. This is an efficient mechanism for conveying some information—scientific breakthroughs, for example—but fails to provide a stable source for those who wish to find out more. Reliance on the news media also breeds neglect of issues that do not tie directly to transient, highly conspicuous events. It also means that coverage is spotty and inconsistent for more mundane but highly relevant data about care delivery. Coverage of how poorly Medicaid functions, for example, is the subject of far fewer articles than are new drug therapies (that have often later proved to be errant scientific results affecting far fewer people).

The information void is filled by some lay books on Alzheimer's disease such as *The 36-Hour Day* (Mace and Rabins 1981), *The Loss of Self* (Cohen and Eisdorfer 1986), and *Understanding Alzheimer's Disease* (Aronson and ADRDA 1988). A caregiver journal—*The American Jour-

nal of Alzheimer's Care—started publication in 1985. What is often needed is an initial contact to direct those interested to these and other resources.

Several states have set up hot lines for callers, with variable success. The Alzheimer's Association has operated an 800 telephone number for several years to answer preliminary inquiries and to refer callers to its local chapters. The Alzheimer's Association, the French Foundation, and the National Institutes of Health also distribute leaflets and informative booklets. The National Institute on Aging will soon begin to manage a national information dissemination program that will likely include a national 800 number. This would greatly improve access to data about federally sponsored research and referral to local information sources. The challenge will be to also keep track of services. This cannot be done at the national level because the availability and quality of services vary dramatically from one city or town to the next, yet service-related information is among the most valuable to caregivers. Gathering and verifying information about local services is thus crucial to the success of a truly useful information clearinghouse. State, local, and private resources will thus be necessary to gather and forward information about services to any federally administered clearinghouse.

Description of Federal Programs

There are numerous programs that support, either directly or indirectly, the care of people with dementia. Many of the most useful services are available only through local or state governments or private providers. These are too variable and numerous to cover in this chapter. Instead, a few of the federal programs that most directly support care are listed and briefly described. For more detailed information, see other references (e.g., U.S. Congress 1987).

Medicare

Medicare is a federal program that funds acute medical care for those sixty-five and over, the disabled, and those with kidney disease. It is divided into two parts. One, covering primarily hospital services, is an insurance system supported in large part by a payroll tax on those currently working. The second part deals with physician charges and other services and is largely funded by premiums and from general revenues. Medicare is a government-sponsored health insurance program. For those sixty-five and over who develop dementia, it theoretically covers a fraction of the costs of diagnosis and medical treatment. It does not, in general, cover long-term care and does not cover most of the services needed on a continuing basis by those who develop a dementing illness.

Many proposals have been made in the past few years to modify Medicare by adding long-term care services to acute medical care. Several of these have been incorporated into bills before Congress, and there has been serious consideration of these proposals in federal agencies. To date, however, insufficient political might has gathered in support of any single proposal. As long-term care drifts further into the political limelight in coming years, however, this may well change. The goal in the meantime is to ensure that the services and financing mechanisms that are proposed meet the needs of dementia patients and their families.

Medicaid

Medicaid is a health and long-term care program for the indigent jointly funded by the state and federal governments. The federal government pays for over half of all Medicaid expenditures. The fraction paid by the federal government depends on the resources of the different states, with poorer states paying a lower proportion. The federal government mandates that a minimal set of services be covered. Beyond this minimum, states vary widely in the services covered. They also differ markedly in financial eligibility criteria, reimbursement practices, and levels of funding (see Chapter 11).

Medicaid can be roughly divided into two programs. The first, for which it was primarily created, is to provide acute medical care for those in poverty. The second, which has taken a progressively larger proportion of the funds over the last two decades, is a long-term care program for aged people. This second role has fallen to Medicaid because Medicare does not cover long-term care, and the expense of long-term care frequently exhausts the financial resources of those who develop illnesses that necessitate it. The elderly who pay for nursing home care thus become eligible because they become impoverished. This phenomenon of using up one's assets to become eligible for Medicaid coverage of long-term care (largely restricted to nursing home care) is called "spend-down" in the Medicaid argot. Spend-down will persist as long as the only alternative to paying for long-term care directly out-of-pocket is a welfare program like Medicaid. Progress could follow from a private long-term care insurance market or new public programs to assist in paying for long-term care.

Until 1988, the effects of spend-down were especially disastrous for older women who had never worked in jobs covered by Social Security. The spouse of someone needing health or long-term care could lose virtually all income and most assets by paying for it. "Spousal impoverishment" provisions of the new Catastrophic Health Care Act of 1988 limit the damage, principally by splitting assets and income (up to a fixed limit) so that the caregiving spouse's income and assets are not required as payment for the demented spouse's care.

Two features of Medicaid are especially important in understanding the political process. First, the two major programs—acute care for the poor and long-term care of aged people who become poor—are taken out of the same budget. This means that maternal and child care for inner city neighborhoods is funded out of the same pot as nursing home care for those with Alzheimer's disease. Second, the Medicaid programs has no one focus of responsibility. The history of Medicaid throughout its two decades is replete with the federal and state governments attempting to shift costs either to the other partner or to the users. Medicaid is thus a program that neither state nor federal governments can control.

Lack of focused responsibility has subverted political accountability. One symptom of this is the incredible complexity of Medicaid administration. There is no uniformity of any aspect of Medicaid—eligibility, organization, administration, reimbursement mechanism, extent of coverage, or type of service funded. State administrators are faced with directives emanating from federal and state legislatures and federal and state executive bureaucracies. Medicaid has been amended almost every year for the last decade at the federal level, and each legislative change spawns a regulatory response to implement it. State legislatures and health agencies add changes within their jurisdiction. Providers receive their guidance from local government administrators. They are faced with thick, impenetrable books of regulations that even the administrators rarely understand fully. Caregivers are presented with a befuddling array of mixed advice from caregiver organizations, state administrators, and providers. There has been little attempt to educate the public about Medicaid. This could perhaps cynically be attributed to a wish to keep the public ignorant but also stems in part from the hopelessness of the task.

(This is all the more reason to encourage public education, not only because of its direct public benefit, but also because it would force explanation of policies.) Yet Medicaid is the largest long-term care program in the United States, and reforms of long-term care typically focused on Medicaid until the last few years. The intractable problems of Medicaid are partly responsible for a shift in attention to Medicare for financing long-term care.

Medicare and Medicaid are the primary health programs in the United States. Five other federal programs are smaller and more focused. They provide fewer funds in total, but are often used to support services for those with dementia. These are Title XX, mental health services, Older Americans Act services, income support programs, and the Veterans Administration.

Title XX

Title XX is the federal block grant for social services. This is a way of transferring funds from the federal to state (and thereby local) governments. Discretion on how to spend these funds is left largely to state and county governments.

Mental Health Services

Mental health services are likewise funded through federal grants to states and are supplemented by state funds. Federal block grants are used to support counseling; psychiatric and psychological evaluation; treatment centers for those with psychiatric illness; drug abuse rehabilitation; programs on alcoholism; intervention in child abuse, rape, and family conflict; and other functions. Those with dementia are included as a group with psychiatric illness in some areas, particularly in community mental health centers that have some specialization in geriatrics.

The Older Americans Act

The Older Americans Act supports senior services of various sorts. The funds are typically distributed by the federal Administration on Aging to area or state Agencies on Aging, although there are some federally administered grants and contracts. In the past, the emphasis was on transportation, delivery of meals, senior recreation centers, and other programs of wide interest among the population sixty and older. In recent years, the Administration on Aging has increasingly concentrated on those elderly who suffer from disability. The problems faced by those with dementia have become a focus, particularly during the last three years. The services for those with dementia that have received more attention have included day care, coordination of care, provision of information about medical and social care, and support for research on care delivery to those with dementia.

Income Support Programs

Income support programs include Social Security and various government pension programs (through the civil services, the Veterans Administration, and military services). Although these do not directly cover services, the income made available to older citizens is often used to purchase health and social services. Some economists have argued that government programs should not be focused on a particular set of services, but rather should increase the funds available through government payments that transfer funds from younger to older individuals (or, alternatively, from less needy to more needy people), so that consumers could make their own choices about how to spend the money. In practice, income support and health care programs have grown dramatically over the last decade, whereas social programs other than health programs have been constricted. Income support programs have thus become the main governmental funding mechanism other than Medicaid for long-term care of aged people.

The Veterans Administration

The Veterans Administration (VA) has a wide variety of services for those who have served in military service. It has its own set of hospitals and clinics across the country and also supports some long-term care. Eligibility for VA services is first determined by being a veteran or, in some cases, a veteran's dependent. First priority for health care is given to those with a service-connected illness or disability. After that, services are made available when there is sufficient capacity at the local VA facility. Several VA centers have been at the forefront of innovation in the care of those with dementia. One of the first family support groups was established at a VA hospital in Washington state, for example, and evaluation centers and teaching nursing homes have been pioneered by the VA. Most VA hospitals will perform diagnostic and medical care for those with dementia. With some exceptions, depending usually on local administrators, the VA does not cover long-term care services for veterans who develop

Alzheimer's disease or another dementia (because dementia is not usually interpreted as a service-connected disability). Recent years have seen increasing fiscal pressure on the VA to reduce expenditures, on one hand, and increasing pressure from families and veterans to cover more long-term care services on the other. The most recent changes in veterans' health benefits are to require partial payments from veterans with higher incomes for services related to disabilities that are not service-connected.

One promising strategy at the state level is to pool the various streams of funding from the federal government and then more rationally reallocate funds to pay for needed services. Oregon has been a pioneer in this area. The same can be done at the county or local level. Food and Nutrition Services, Inc., of Santa Cruz County in California, for example, takes funds from more than thirty-five federal, state, and county sources and delivers a full spectrum of social services, including day and home care for dementia. This pooling permits efficiencies of scale and coordination of services and takes advantage of the flexibility of private sector management. On another tack, county governments in the suburbs of Minneapolis have managed to supply a full range of services for dementia by blending funds available from various government programs, and the services are coordinated by the county governments. It is clear that many approaches can improve the current system of long-term care, although it is not clear which way is best. The challenge is to combine existing federal, state, and local programs into a useful, coherent, and comprehensive (and comprehensible) system of care.

The Political Process

Changing government programs so that they are better adapted to the needs of those with dementia will require a substantial commitment of people, time, and money. In the prevailing austere fiscal environment, likely to persist well into the foreseeable future, those improvements that do not require direct government expenditure or restructuring will meet the least resistance. Changes that require restructuring without added expenditures are next most likely to succeed, but depend on minimizing the trauma of change. If money is to be taken from one group of people to be spent on another, then the political muscle must be there to contend with the inevitable conflict.

Options that require both restructuring and more government funding require the most political effort. Many argue that the problem of dementia, particularly the issues related to long-term care, will not be resolved without both increased funding and restructuring of government involvement in long-term care. The number of people with dementia will slowly rise over the next two decades and then rapidly grow for another two. Unless the course of Alzheimer's disease and other dementing illnesses is dramatically altered by prevention or treatment, political pressure to deal with long-term care will mount. More and more people will become caregivers or will know someone who has dementia, exposing the inadequacy of current policies. They will want policies to change.

The first step is to educate key decision makers about the consequences of dementia. Present coverage of dementia is unfair because it is less complete than that for other illnesses. Policies to correct this must address long-term care, bringing it into line with other health care programs.

State and federal legislatures are likely to be the places where policy changes originate. This is because legislators are, by design, more sensitive to public opinion than those in other branches of government. Legislators by and large respond to what they hear from constituents. As more of them learn about Alzheimer's disease and dementia, the political viability of legislation to deal with it increases. The dramatic growth of research funding is an indication that policy makers are increasingly aware of the problem. Research is one direct policy approach to a solution, and it has been vigorously supported.

The other major policy approach is to improve the delivery of long-term care, yet there is no consensus on how to do this. The problems of long-term care are more complex than simply increasing research funding. Gathering of data on long-term care has been relatively neglected, so that policy options are not clear, and there are strong philosophical disagreements about the role of government in paying for long-term care. Further, advocacy groups concentrated early on legislative support for research and are only now focusing on care delivery.

Future developments will doubtless involve continued increases in research funding, but a larger effort can be predicted for changing the care delivery system. The crucial element, missing to date, is a carefully elaborated proposal to deliver care that realistically appraises eligibility, costs, and side effects. Most proposals have been based on hopes that adding government funding will not increase costs or that adding eligible people will not increase the use of services.

Before such a proposal can be formulated, data must be gathered and analyzed about current care patterns, and there must be careful studies of alternative methods of delivering care. Much enthusiasm has been expressed in recent years for adding a Medicare long-term care entitlement, for funding special dementia units in nursing homes, for covering adult day care, and for reimbursing respite care. There is, however, a conspicuous void of solid information derived from the evaluation of real-world experiments and demonstrations. In many cases, there is not even agreement about definitions. Certainly, no program has been developed that could serve as a model for national policy. The experiments have finally begun during the past two or three years, and new data should combine with swelling demand for services to fuel progress toward a policy consensus. For the time being, efforts can concentrate on two primary objectives: to improve the policy formulation and advocacy skills of the various state and national organizations and to lay a base of health services research that can later yield a national policy agenda.

National voluntary organizations, providers, and caregivers must develop the political skills necessary to further their collective goals. Until recently, the Alzheimer's movement was dominated by a few groups. There were only limited attempts to form coalitions with other groups such as the American Association of Retired Persons (AARP) or disease-oriented organizations for Huntington's disease, Parkinson's disease, multiple sclerosis, stroke, spinal cord injury, and mental retardation.

The success of the Family Survival Project and the Alzheimer's Association in unifying many different constituencies to obtain services in the State of California shows that such coalitions can be powerful. Advocacy groups can better fight the inadequacies of the current long-term care system as part of a unified front. Even with the Alzheimer's movement, there has been marked divisiveness and failure to recognize common goals. Some of this can be explained by the rapidity of growth of the various organizations, which has made managing them quite difficult and rendered coalition building a lower priority. This is rapidly changing, however, and coalition building must become the norm. One promising development is the joint efforts of the Alzheimer's Association and the AARP (with the Villers Foundation and other sponsors) in promoting Long Term Care 88, a public interest group dedicated to focusing attention on long-term care issues.

What Can Providers and Caregivers Do to Influence Public Policy?

At the state and local level, access to legislators and executive agency administrators is relatively direct. At the federal level, the process is somewhat more complicated, but there are many open channels to influence policy. The key to success is clear and concise communication. If the intent of a meeting is merely to characterize a problem, then a policy maker may be interested, but will not be able to do much. If the goal is a change in policy, then the problem must be clearly stated, the solution presented, and the arguments both for and against the policy change explained. A personal meeting, supplemented by written material (including a one-page summary) is the most effective form of communication. Letters can be effective, but are often answered by an aide rather than the legislator or agency head. Quantitative information is strongly preferable when available, particularly when it is supported by a robust body of research. A legislator is unlikely to support an untested method for changing Medicaid reimbursement, for example, unless it has been thoroughly evaluated. If such evaluation is not available, then support for pilot projects to produce useful data is a viable objective. If there are specific problems with a current policy (e.g., a method of determining Medicaid eligibility that discriminates against those with dementia), then reference to practices in other states that have solved the problem are likely to be effective. Policy makers are pragmatic by reflex. They need a conceptual grasp of issues, but are helpless without concrete solutions to problems.

This places the burden of policy formulation, analysis, and communication on those who wish to advocate change. It is a heavy burden and requires homework, creativity, and tenacity. Often, even glaring social problems are left unsolved because there is no organization or individual who is able and willing to do all the work necessary. The problems related to dementia, particularly those dealing with long-term care, are in this category of unsolved social problems. To progress beyond this point will require substantial intellectual and practical effort by caregivers, providers, and policy makers.

References

Aronson, M. K., and Alzheimer's Disease and Related Disorders Association staff, eds. 1988. *Understanding Alzheimer's disease: What it is, how to treat it, how to cope with it.* New York: Scribners.

Battelle Memorial Institute. 1984. The economics of dementia. Contract report for the Office of Technology Assessment, U.S. Congress. Available from the National Technical Information Service (Springfield, VA) as *Losing a million minds, contractor documents, Part 2: Economics, social science, and health services research.* Accession Number PB-87-177-598/AS.

Cohen, D., and C. Eisdorfer. 1986. *The loss of self: A family resource for the care of Alzheimer's disease and related disorders.* New York: W. W. Norton.

Davis, K., and P. Neuman. 1986. Financing care for patients with Alzheimer's disease and related disorders. Contract report for the Senate Committee on Labor and Human Resources and the Congressional Office of Technology Assessment. Available from the National Technical Information Service (Springfield, VA) as *Losing a million minds, contractor documents, Part 2: Economics, social science, and health services research.* Accession Number PB-87-177-598/AS.

Hay, J. W., and R. L. Ernst. 1987. The economic costs of Alzheimer's disease. *American Journal of Public Health* 77:1169–75.

Huang, L.-F., T.-W. Hu, and W. S. Cartwright. 1986. The economic cost of senile dementia in the United States, 1983. Contract report prepared for the National Institute on Aging, No. 1-AG-3-2123.

Institute of Medicine. 1986. *Improving the quality of care in nursing homes.* Washington, DC: National Academy Press.

Mace, N., and P. Rabins. 1981. *The 36-hour day: A family guide to caring for persons with Alzheimer's disease, related dementing illnesses, and memory loss in later life.* Baltimore: Johns Hopkins University Press.

U.S. Congress. Office of Technology Assessment. 1987. *Losing a million minds: Confronting the tragedy of Alzheimer's disease and other dementias.* OTA-BA-323. Washington, DC: U.S. Government Printing Office. April. Also available as *Confronting Alzheimer's disease and other dementias.* Philadelphia: Lippincott.

Weiler, P. G. 1987. The public health impact of Alzheimer's disease. *American Journal of Public Health* 77:1157–58.

Index